ARKANA

Yoga

Mircea Eliade, a native of Romania, lectured in the École des Hautes-Études of the Sorbonne, and was subsequently chairman of the department of history of religions at the University of Chicago. His other works include *Shamanism: Archaic Techniques of Ecstasy* and *The Myth of the Eternal Return: or, Cosmos and History*, which are also published in the Arkana series.

MIRCEA ELIADE

YOGA

Immortality and freedom

Translated from the French by
Willard R. Trask

ARKANA

ARKANA

Published by the Penguin Group
27 Wrights Lane, London W8 5TZ, England
Viking Penguin Inc., 40 West 23rd Street, New York, New York 10010, USA
Penguin Books Australia Ltd, Ringwood, Victoria, Australia
Penguin Books Canada Ltd, 2801 John Street, Markham, Ontario, Canada L3R 1B4
Penguin Books (NZ) Ltd, 182–190 Wairau Road, Auckland 10, New Zealand

Penguin Books Ltd, Registered Offices: Harmondsworth, Middlesex, England

First published in the USA 1958
First published in Great Britain by Routledge 1988
Published by Arkana 1989
1 3 5 7 9 10 8 6 4 2

Filmset in Linotron Baskerville

Made and printed in Great Britain by
The Guernsey Press Co. Ltd,
Guernsey, Channel Islands.

To the memory of

my illustrious and venerable patron

Maharaja Sir Manindra Chandra Nandi of Kasimbazar, K.C.I.E.

my guru

Professor Surendranath Dasgupta

PRINCIPAL, SANSKRIT COLLEGE, CALCUTTA

and my teacher

Nae Ionescu

UNIVERSITY OF BUCHAREST

CONTENTS

*Shamanistic Magic and the Quest for Immortality, 311—Yoga
and Shamanism, 318—Ascent to Heaven. Mystical Flight,
326—"Magical Heat." "Inner Light," 330—Similarities and
Differences, 334—Coalescence and Degradation: Yoga and
Popular Religions, 341—The Dravidian Heritage, Mūṇḍā,
Proto-Mūṇḍā, 348—Harappā, Mohenjo-daro, 353*

NOTE TO THE SECOND EDITION (1969)

Throughout the text and the Additional Notes, an asterisk indicates that new reference material is supplied in the Addenda, pp. 531 ff. In the List of Works Cited, an asterisk indicates that a new translation has been substituted for citations (see p. 480). The author has made numerous minor corrections, of diacritical marks, etc.

FOREWORD

There is no more absorbing story than that of the discovery and interpretation of India by Western consciousness. I refer not only to its geographical, linguistic, and literary discovery, to expeditions and excavations—in short, to everything that constitutes the foundation for Western Indianism—but above all to the various cultural adventures inspired by the growing revelation of Indian languages, myths, and philosophies. Some of these cultural adventures have been described by Raymond Schwab in his fine book *La Renaissance orientale.* But the discovery of India is still in progress, and nothing entitles us to suppose that it is nearing its end. For the analysis of a foreign culture principally reveals what was sought in it or what the seeker was already prepared to discover. The discovery of India will not be accomplished until the day the creative forces of the West shall have run irremediably dry.

When spiritual values are in question, the contribution of philology, indispensable though it may be, does not exhaust the richness of the object. No doubt it would have been useless to attempt to understand Buddhism so long as the texts were not accurately edited, so long as the various Buddhistic philologies were not instituted. The fact remains that a comprehension of that vast and complex spiritual phenomenon was not infallibly guaranteed by the possession of such excellent tools as critical editions, polyglot dictionaries, historical monographs, and so on. When one approaches an exotic spirituality, one understands principally what one is predestined to understand by one's own vocation, by one's own cultural orientation and that of the historical moment to which one belongs. This truism is of general application. The image that our nineteenth century created of "inferior societies" was largely derived from the positivistic, antireligious, and ametaphysical attitude entertained by a number of worthy explorers and ethnologists who had approached the "savages" with the ideology of a contemporary of Comte, Darwin, or Spencer. Among the "primitives" they everywhere discovered "fetishism" and "religious infantilism"—simply because they could *see* nothing else. Only the resurgence of European metaphysical thought at the beginning of the present century, the religious renaissance, the many and various gains made by depth psychology, by poetry, by microphysics, have made it possible to understand the spiritual horizon of "primitives," the structure of their symbols, the function of their myths, the maturity of their mysticisms.

In the case of India the difficulties were even greater. On the one hand, the tools had to be forged, the philologies pursued; on the other, choice had to be made of the aspects of Indian spirituality that were most penetrable by the Western spirit. But, as was to be expected, what appeared to be most penetrable was precisely what answered to the most pressing needs of Western culture. It was chiefly interest in comparative Indo-Āryan philology that brought Sanskrit to the fore as a subject of study about the middle of the nineteenth century—just as, a generation or two earlier, minds had been stimulated to turn to India by idealistic philosophy or by the charm of the primordial images that German romanticism had just rediscovered. During the second half of the century, India was chiefly interpreted in terms of naturistic mythology and of the cultural fashion thereby launched in Europe and America. Finally, the resurgence of sociology and cultural anthropology in the first quarter of our own century inspired new perspectives.

All these experiments had their value, for they corresponded to problems natural to European culture. The various methods of approach practiced by Western scholars, though not always successful in revealing all the true values of Indian spirituality, were nevertheless of service. Little by little, India began to assert its presence in the consciousness of the West. For a considerable period, it is true, that presence was preponderantly manifested by comparative grammars. It was but rarely and timidly that India made its appearance in histories of philosophy—where, in accordance with the fashion prevailing at the moment, its place alternated between German idealism and "prelogical mentality." When interest in sociology became general, there was a great deal of solemn criticism of the caste system. But all these attitudes find their explanation in the horizons of modern Western culture. When a culture bestowed high priority among its problems upon the explanation of a linguistic law or of a social structure, India suffered no diminution by being invoked to solve one or another etymology or to illustrate one or another stage of social evolution—indeed, this was rather a mark of respect and admiration. In any case, the modes of approach were not bad in themselves; they were merely too specialized, and their chances of revealing the various contents of a great and complex spirituality were proportionately limited. Fortunately, methods are subject to improvement, and the failures of the past were not wasted—successive generations soon learned not to repeat the errors of their predecessors. We need only measure the progress in the study of Indo-European mythology from the time of Max Müller, and we shall realize the advantage that a Georges Dumézil has been able to gain, not only from comparative philology, but also from sociology, the history of religions, and ethnology, in presenting an infinitely more precise and infinitely more fertile image of the great categories of Indo-European mythical thought.

Everything leads to the belief that, at the present moment, a more accurate knowledge of Indian thought has become possible. India has entered the course of history; and, rightly or wrongly, Western consciousness tends to take a more serious view of the philosophies of peoples who hold a place in history. On the other hand, especially since the last generation of philosophers, Western consciousness is more and more inclined to define itself with reference to the problems of time and history. For over a century, the greater part of the scientific and philosophical effort of the West has been devoted to the factors that "condition" the human being. It has been shown how and to what degree man is conditioned by his physiology, his heredity, his social milieu, the cultural ideology in which he shares, his unconscious—and above all by history, by his historical moment and his own personal history. This last discovery of Western thought—that man is essentially a temporal and historical being, that he is, and can only be, what history has made him—still dominates Western philosophy. Certain philosophical trends even conclude from it that the only worthy and valid task proposed to man is to assume this temporality and this historicity frankly and fully, for any other choice would be equivalent to an escape into the abstract and nonauthentic and would be at the price of the sterility and death that inexorably punish any betrayal of history.

It does not fall to us to discuss these theses. We may, however, remark that the problems that today absorb the Western mind also prepare it for a better understanding of Indian spirituality; indeed, they incite it to employ, for its own philosophical effort, the millennial experience of India. Let us explain. It is the *human condition*, and above all the temporality of the human being, that constitutes the object of the most recent Western philosophy. It is this temporality that makes all the other "conditionings" possible and that, in the last analysis, makes man a "conditioned being," an indefinite and evanescent series of "conditions." Now, this problem of the "conditioning" of man (and its corollary, rather neglected in the West: his "deconditioning") constitutes the central problem of Indian thought. From the Upaniṣads onward, India has been seriously preoccupied with but one great problem—the structure of the human condition. (Hence it has been said, and not without reason, that all Indian philosophy has been, and still is, "existentialist.") The West, therefore, might well learn: (1) what India thinks of the multiple "conditionings" of the human being; (2) how it has approached the problem of the temporality and historicity of man; (3) what solution it has found for the anxiety and despair that inevitably follow upon consciousness of temporality, the matrix of all "conditionings."

With a rigor unknown elsewhere, India has applied itself to analyzing the various conditionings of the human being. We hasten to add that it has done so not in order to arrive at a precise and coherent explanation of man (as, for example, did nineteenth-century Europe when it believed that it explained man by his hereditary or social conditioning), but in order to learn how far the conditioned zones of the human being extend and *to see if anything else exists beyond these conditionings*. Hence it is that, long before depth psychology, the sages and ascetics of India were led to explore the obscure zones of the unconscious. They had found that man's physiological, social, cultural, and religious conditionings were comparatively easy to delimit and hence to master; the great obstacles to the ascetic and contemplative life arose from the activity of the unconscious, from the *saṃskāras* and the *vāsanās*—"impregnations," "residues," "latencies"—that constitute what depth psychology calls the contents and structures of the unconscious. It is not, however, this pragmatic anticipation of certain modern psychological techniques that is valuable; it is its employment for the "deconditioning" of man. Because, for India, knowledge of the systems of "conditioning" could not be an end in itself; it was not knowing them that mattered, but mastering them; if the contents of the unconscious were worked upon, it was in order to "burn" them. We shall see by what methods Yoga conceives that it arrives at these surprising results. And it is primarily these results which are of interest to Western psychologists and philosophers.

Let us not be misunderstood. We have no intention of inviting Western scholars to practice Yoga (which, by the way, is not so easy as some amateurs are wont to suggest) or of proposing that the various Western disciplines practice yogic methods or adopt the yogic ideology. Another point of view seems to us far more fertile—to study, as attentively as possible, the results obtained by such methods of exploring the psyche. A whole immemorial experience of human behavior in general here offers itself to Western investigators. It would be at least unwise in them not to take advantage of it.

As we said earlier, the problem of the human condition—that is, the temporality and historicity of the human being—is at the very center of Western thought, and the same problem has preoccupied Indian philosophy from its beginnings. It is true that we do not there find the terms "history" and "historicity" in the senses that they bear in the West today, and that we very seldom find the term "temporality." In fact, it was impossible that these concepts should be found under the particular designations of "history" and "historicity." But what matters is not identity in philosophical terminology; it is enough if the problems are homologizable. Now, it has long been known that Indian thought accords considerable importance to the concept of *māyā*, which has been translated—and with good reason—as "illusion," "cosmic illusion," "mirage," "magic," "becoming," "irreality," and the like. But, looking more closely, we see that *māyā* is illusion because it does not participate in Being, because it is "becoming," "temporality"—cosmic becoming, to be sure, but also historical becoming. It is possible, then, that India has been not unaware of the relation between illusion, temporality, and human suffering. Although its sages have generally explained human suffering in cosmic terms, we realize, if we read them with the attention they deserve, that they were thinking particularly of human suffering as a "becoming" conditioned by the structures of temporality. We have touched upon this problem elsewhere,[1] and we shall have occasion to return to it. What modern Western philosophy terms "being situated," "being constituted by temporality and historicity," has its counterpart, in Indian philosophy, in "existence in *māyā*." If we can homologize the two philosophical horizons—Indian and Western—everything that India has thought on the subject of *māyā* has a certain timeliness for us today. This becomes apparent if, for example, we read the *Bhagavad Gītā*. Its analysis of human existence is conducted in a language that is familiar to us; *māyā* is not only cosmic illusion but also, and above all, historicity; not only existence in the eternal cosmic becoming but above all existence in time and history. For

1 Cf. "Symbolisme religieux et angoisse" in the collective volume *L'Angoisse du temps présent et les devoirs de l'esprit.* [For full references, see the List of Works Cited.]

the *Bhagavad Gītā*, as in some measure for Christianity, the problem presented itself in these terms: how shall we resolve the paradoxical situation created by the twofold fact that man, on the one hand, finds himself *in* time, given over to history, and that, on the other hand, he knows that he will be "damned" if he allows himself to be exhausted by temporality and historicity; that, consequently, he must at all costs find *in this world* a road that issues upon a transhistorical and atemporal plane? The solutions proposed by the *Bhagavad Gītā* will be discussed later. What we wish to emphasize now is that all these solutions represent various applications of Yoga.

Here again, then, we encounter Yoga. For the fact is that, to the third question that is of concern to Western philosophy (the question, that is, what solution India proposes for the anxiety produced by our discovery of our temporality and historicity, the means by which one can remain in the world without letting oneself be exhausted by time and history), the answers offered by Indian thought all more or less directly imply some knowledge of Yoga. Hence it is apparent what familiarity with this problem can mean to Western investigators and philosophers. To repeat: it is not a matter of purely and simply accepting one of the solutions proposed by India. A spiritual value is not acquired after the fashion of a new make of automobile. Above all, it is not a matter of philosophical syncretism, or of "Indianization," still less of the detestable "spiritual" hybridism inaugurated by the Theosophical Society and continued, in aggravated forms, by the countless pseudomorphs of our time. The problem is more serious: it is essential that we know and understand a thought that has held a place of the first importance in the history of universal spirituality. And it is essential that we know it *now*. For, on the one hand, it is from *now* on that, any cultural provincialism having been outstripped by the very course of history, we are forced—Westerners and non-Westerners alike—to think in terms of universal history and to forge universal spiritual values. And, on the other hand, it is *now* that the problem of man's situation in the world dominates the philosophical consciousness of Europe—and, to repeat, this problem is at the very center of Indian thought.

Perhaps this philosophical dialogue will not be carried on, especially at first, without some disappointments. A number of Western investigators and philosophers may find the Indian analyses rather oversimplified and the proposed solutions ineffectual. Any technical language that is dependent upon a certain spiritual tradition always remains a jargon; Western philosophers may perhaps find the jargon of Indian philosophy outmoded, lacking in precision, unserviceable. But all these risks to which the dialogue is subject are of minor importance. The great discoveries of Indian thought will in the end be recognized, under and despite the philosophic jargon. It is impossible, for example, to disregard one of India's greatest discoveries: that of consciousness as witness, of consciousness freed from its psychophysiological structures and their temporal conditioning, the consciousness of the "liberated" man, of him, that is, who has succeeded in emancipating himself from temporality and thereafter knows the true, inexpressible freedom. The conquest of this absolute freedom, of perfect spontaneity, is the goal of all Indian philosophies and mystical techniques; but it is above all through Yoga, through one of the many forms of Yoga, that India has held that it can be assured. This is the chief reason we have thought it useful to write a comparatively full exposition of the theory and practices of Yoga, to recount the history of its forms, and to define its place in Indian spirituality as a whole.

It was after three years of study at the University of Calcutta (1928–31) under the direction of Professor Surendranath Dasgupta, and a residence of six months (1931) in the *āśram* of Rishikesh, Himālaya, that we entered upon the composition of this book. A first version, written in English, translated into Romanian by the author, and retranslated into French by some friends, was published in 1936, under the title *Yoga. Essai sur les origines de la mystique indienne*. Together with faults due to youth and inexperience, this version suffered from unfortunate misunderstandings resulting from the double translation; in addition, the text was disfigured by a large number of linguistic and typographical errors. Despite these serious imperfections, the work was well received by Indianists; the reviews by Louis de la Vallée Poussin, Jean Przyluski, Heinrich Zimmer, V. Papesso, to cite only those who have since died, long ago encouraged us to prepare a new edition. The corrections and the added material have resulted in a text that differs considerably from that of the 1936 publication. Except for a few paragraphs, the book has been entirely rewritten in order to adapt it as much as possible to our present views. (A portion of this new version was used in a little book published in 1948: *Techniques du Yoga.*) The bibliographies and the summaries of the present position of research in regard to the various questions, the details demanded by certain more special aspects of the problem, and, in general, all the technical discussions have been brought together at the end of the book in the form of short appendixes. We have sought to present a book that should be accessible to nonspecialists, without, however, departing from strict scientific practice; in the documentation collected at the end of the volume, Indianists will find supplementary material and bibliographical items. Need we add that none of the bibliographies is exhaustive?

We have used existing translations of Sanskrit and Pāli texts whenever good ones were available. If in translating the *Yoga-sūtras* and their commentaries we sometimes deviate from current interpretations, we do so in view of the oral teaching of our Hindu masters, especially of Professor Surendranath Dasgupta, with whom we translated and discussed all the important texts of the *yoga-darśana.*

In its present form, this book is addressed especially to historians of religions, psychologists, and philosophers. The greater part of it is devoted to an exposition of the various forms of yogic technique and of their history. Excellent books are available on the system of Patañjali—notably those by Dasgupta; hence we have not considered it necessary to discuss this subject at length. The same is true of the techniques of Buddhistic meditation, for which an abundant critical literature already exists. Instead, we have emphasized less known or inadequately studied aspects: the ideas, the symbolism, and the methods of Yoga, as they are expressed in tantrism, in alchemy, in folklore, in the aboriginal devotion of India.

We have dedicated this work to the memory of our protector, the Maharajah Sir Manindra Chandra Nandi of Kasimbazar, who made our residence in India possible by awarding us a scholarship, and to the memory of our most cherished masters: Nae Ionescu and Surendranath Dasgupta. To the teaching of the first we owe our philosophical initiation and orientation. As to Surendranath Dasgupta, not only did he lead us into the very center of Indian thought, but for three years he was our professor of Sanskrit, our master, and our *guru*. May all three rest in the peace of their faith!

We began the preparation of this present edition long ago, but we should not have been able to finish it except for a happy combination of circumstances. By according us a research grant, the Bollingen Foundation, of New York, allowed us to devote several years to the present work; may the Trustees of the Foundation accept our most sincere acknowledgments here. It is thanks to our dear friends Dr. René Laforgue and Délia Laforgue, who so tactfully put their house at our disposal, that, since 1951, we have been able to work in unhoped-for conditions; may they rest assured of our most sincere gratitude.

MIRCEA ELIADE

Paris, September 15, 1954

POSTSCRIPT

For the English edition, all quotations from the *Yoga-sūtras* and the commentaries on them and all texts of which reliable English translations do not exist have been translated directly from Sanskrit into English. We have also added a number of recent bibliographical references.

M. E.

Saint-Cloud, August, 1957

YOGA

Immortality and Freedom

CHAPTER ONE

The Doctrines of Yoga

Point of Departure

FOUR basic and interdependent concepts, four "kinetic ideas," bring us directly to the core of Indian spirituality. They are *karma*, *māyā*, *nirvāṇa*, and *yoga*. A coherent history of Indian thought could be written starting from any one of these basic concepts; the other three would inevitably have to be discussed. In terms of Western philosophy, we can say that, from the post-Vedic period on, India has above all sought to understand:

(1) The law of universal causality, which connects man with the cosmos and condemns him to transmigrate indefinitely. This is the law of *karma*.

(2) The mysterious process that engenders and maintains the cosmos and, in so doing, makes possible the "eternal return" of existences. This is *māyā*, cosmic illusion, endured (even worse—accorded validity) by man as long as he is blinded by ignorance (*avidyā*).

(3) Absolute reality, "situated" somewhere beyond the cosmic illusion woven by *māyā* and beyond human experience as conditioned by *karma*; pure Being, the Absolute, by whatever name it may be called—the Self (*ātman*), *brahman*, the unconditioned, the transcendent, the immortal, the indestructible, *nirvāṇa*, etc.

(4) The means of attaining to Being, the effectual techniques for gaining liberation. This corpus of means constitutes Yoga properly speaking.

With these four concepts in mind, we can understand how the fundamental problem of all philosophy, the search for truth, presents itself to Indian thought. For India, truth is not precious in itself; it becomes precious by virtue of its soteriological function, because knowledge of truth helps man to liberate himself. It is not the possession of truth that is the supreme end of the Indian sage; it is liberation, the conquest of absolute freedom. The sacrifices that the European philosopher is prepared to make to attain truth in and for itself: sacrifice of religious faith, of worldly ambitions, of wealth, personal freedom, and even life—to these the Indian sage consents only in order to conquer liberation. To "free oneself" is equivalent to forcing another plane of existence, to appropriating another *mode of being* transcending the human condition. This is as much as to say that, for India, not only is metaphysical knowledge translated into terms of *rupture* and *death* ("breaking" the human condition, one "dies" to all that was human); it also necessarily implies a consequence of a mystical nature: *rebirth to a nonconditioned mode of being*. And this is liberation, absolute freedom.

In studying the theories and practices of Yoga we shall have occasion to refer to all the other "kinetic ideas" of Indian thought. For the present, let us begin by defining the meaning of the term *yoga*. Etymologically, *yoga* derives from the root *yuj*, "to bind together," "hold fast," "yoke," which also governs Latin *jungere*, *jugum*, French *joug*, etc. The word *yoga* serves, in general, to designate any *ascetic technique* and any *method of meditation*. Naturally, these various asceticisms and meditations have been differently evaluated by the many Indian philosophical currents and mystical movements. As we shall soon see, there is a "classic" Yoga, a "system of philosophy" expounded by Patañjali in his celebrated *Yoga-sūtras;* and it is from the "system" that we must set out in order to understand the position of Yoga in the history of Indian thought. But, side by side with this "classic" Yoga, there are countless forms of "popular," nonsystematic yoga; there are also non-Brāhmanic yogas (Buddhist, Jainist); above all, there are yogas whose structures are "magical," "mystical," and so on.

1. *The Doctrines of Yoga*

Basically it is the term *yoga* itself that has permitted this great variety of meanings, for if, etymologically, *yuj* means "to bind," it is nevertheless clear that the "bond" in which this action of binding is to result presupposes, as its preliminary condition, breaking the "bonds" that unite the spirit to the world. In other words, liberation cannot occur if one is not first "detached" from the world, if one has not begun by withdrawing from the cosmic circuit. For without doing so, one could never succeed in finding or mastering oneself. Even in its "mystical" acceptation—that is, as signifying *union*—Yoga implies a preliminary detachment from matter, emancipation with respect to the world. The emphasis is laid on man's *effort* ("to yoke"), on his self-discipline, by virtue of which he can obtain concentration of spirit even before asking (as in the mystical varieties of Yoga) for the aid of the divinity. "To bind together," "to hold fast," "to yoke"—the purpose of all this is to *unify* the spirit, to do away with the dispersion and automatism that characterize profane consciousness. For the "devotional" (mystical) schools of Yoga this "unification," of course, only precedes the true union, that of the human soul with God.

What characterizes Yoga is not only its *practical* side, but also its *initiatory* structure. One does not learn Yoga by oneself; the guidance of a master (*guru*) is necessary. Strictly speaking, all the other "systems of philosophy"—as, in fact, all traditional disciplines or crafts—are, in India, taught by masters and are thus initiations; for millenniums they have been transmitted orally, "from mouth to ear." But Yoga is even more markedly initiatory in character. For, as in other religious initiations, the yogin begins by forsaking the profane world (family, society) and, guided by his *guru*, applies himself to passing successively beyond the behavior patterns and values proper to the human condition. When we shall have seen to what a degree the yogin attempts to dissociate himself from the profane condition,[1] we shall understand that he dreams of "dying to this life." We shall, in fact, witness a *death* followed by a *rebirth* to another mode of being—that repre-

1 Below, p. 95.

sented by liberation. The analogy between Yoga and initiation becomes even more marked if we think of the initiatory rites—primitive or other—that pursue the creation of a "new body," a "mystical body" (symbolically assimilated, among the primitives, to the body of the newborn infant). Now, the "mystical body," which will allow the yogin to enter the transcendent mode of being, plays a considerable part in all forms of Yoga, and especially in tantrism and alchemy. From this point of view Yoga takes over and, on another plane, continues the archaic and universal symbolism of initiation—a symbolism that, it may be noted, is already documented in the Brāhmanic tradition (where the initiate is called the "twice-born"). The initiatory rebirth is defined, by all forms of Yoga, as access to a nonprofane and hardly describable mode of being, to which the Indian schools give various names: *mokṣa*, *nirvāṇa*, *asaṃskṛta*, etc.

Of all the meanings that the word *yoga* assumes in Indian literature, the most explicit is that which refers to the Yoga "philosophy" (*yoga-darśana*), particularly as set forth in Patañjali's *Yoga-sūtras* and in the commentaries on them. Certainly, a *darśana* is not a system of philosophy in the Western sense (*darśana* = view, vision, comprehension, point of view, doctrine, etc., from the root *dṛś* = to see, to contemplate, to comprehend, etc.). But it is none the less a system of coherent affirmations, coextensive with human experience, which it attempts to interpret in its entirety, and having as its aim the "liberation of man from ignorance" (however various the meanings that the word "ignorance" is made to express). Yoga is one of the six orthodox Indian "systems of philosophy" ("orthodox" here meaning "tolerated by Brāhmanism," in distinction from the "heretical" systems, such as Buddhism or Jainism). And this "classic" Yoga, as formulated by Patañjali and interpreted by his commentators, is also the best known in the West.

So we shall begin our investigation with a review of Yoga theories and practices as formulated by Patañjali. We have several reasons for adopting this procedure: first, because Patañjali's exposition is a "system of philosophy"; second, because a great many practical indications concerning ascetic techniques and contemplative methods are summarized in it—indications that other (the nonsystematic) varieties of Yoga distort or, rather, color in accordance with their particular conceptions; finally, because Patañjali's *Yoga-sūtras* are the result of an enormous effort not only to bring together and classify a series of ascetic practices and contemplative formulas that India had known from time immemorial, but also to validate them from a theoretical point of view by establishing their bases, justifying them, and incorporating them into a philosophy.

But Patañjali is not the creator of the Yoga "philosophy," just as he is not—and could not be—the inventor of yogic techniques. He admits himself [2] that he is merely publishing and correcting (*atha yogānuśāsanam*) the doctrinal and technical traditions of Yoga. And in fact yogic practices were known in the esoteric circles of Indian ascetics and mystics long before Patañjali. Among the technical formulas preserved by tradition, he retained those which an experience of centuries had sufficiently tested. As to the theoretical framework and the metaphysical foundation that Patañjali provides for these practices, his personal contribution is of the smallest. He merely rehandles the Sāṃkhya philosophy in its broad outlines, adapting it to a rather superficial theism in which he exalts the practical value of meditation. The Yoga and Sāṃkhya systems are so much alike that most of the affirmations made by the one are valid for the other. The essential differences between them are few: (1) whereas Sāṃkhya is atheistic, Yoga is theistic, since it postulates the existence of a supreme God (Īśvara); (2) whereas, according to Sāṃkhya, the only path to salvation is that of metaphysical knowledge, Yoga accords marked importance to techniques of meditation. In short, Patañjali's effort, properly speaking, was especially directed to co-ordinating philosophical material—borrowed from Sāṃkhya—around technical formulas for concentration, meditation, and ecstasy. Thanks to Patañjali, Yoga,

2 *Yoga-sūtras*, I, 1.

which had been a "mystical" tradition, became a "system of philosophy."

Indian tradition regards Sāṃkhya as the oldest *darśana*. The meaning of the term *sāṃkhya* seems to have been "discrimination," the chief end of this philosophy being to dissociate the spirit (*puruṣa*) from matter (*prakṛti*). The earliest treatise is the *Sāṃkhya-kārikā* by Īśvarakṛṣṇa; its date is not definitely established, but it cannot be later than the fifth century of our era.[3] Among the commentaries on the *Sāṃkhya-kārikā*, the most useful is the *Sāṃkhya-tattva-kaumudī* by Vācaspatimiśra (ninth century). Another important text is the *Sāṃkhya-pravacana-sūtra* (probably fourteenth century), with the commentaries by Aniruddha (fifteenth century) and Vijñānabhikṣu (sixteenth century).

To be sure, the importance of the chronology of the Sāṃkhya texts must not be exaggerated. In general, any Indian philosophical treatise contains conceptions that antedate its composition and that are often extremely old. If we find a new interpretation in a philosophical text, this does not mean that it had not been entertained earlier. What seems to be "new" in the *Sāṃkhya-sūtras* may often be of unquestionable antiquity. Too much importance has been accorded to the allusions and polemics that can perhaps be discovered in these philosophical texts. Such references may very well be directed at opinions far more ancient than those to which they would seem to allude. If, in India, one can succeed in establishing the dates of different texts—and it is much more difficult there than elsewhere—it is still more difficult to establish the chronology of philosophical ideas themselves. Like Yoga, Sāṃkhya also has a prehistory. Very probably the origin of the system should be sought in an analysis of the constitutive elements of human experience, conducted from the point of view of distinguishing between the elements that forsake man at death and those that are "immortal," in the sense that they accompany the soul in its destiny beyond the grave. Such an analysis already occurs in the *Śatapatha Brāhmaṇa* (X, 1, 3, 4), which divides the human being into three "immortal" and three "mortal" parts. In other words, the "origins" of Sāṃkhya are bound up with a problem of a mystical nature: what subsists of man after death, what constitutes the veritable Self, the immortal element of the human being?

A long controversy, which still persists, concerns the historical per-

3 See Additional Note I, 1, at the end of this book.

sonality of Patañjali, the author of the *Yoga-sūtras.* Some Indian commentators (King Bhoja, Cakrapāṇidatta, the commentator on Caraka in the eleventh century, and two others, of the eighteenth century) have identified him with Patañjali the grammarian, who lived in the second century before our era. The identification has been accepted by Liebich, Garbe, and Dasgupta and contested by Woods, Jacobi, and A. B. Keith.[4] Whatever the fact may be, these controversies concerning the period of the *Yoga-sūtras* are of little relevance, for the techniques of *ascesis* and meditation set forth by Patañjali are certainly of considerable antiquity; they are not his discoveries, nor those of his time; they had been first tested many centuries before him. Indeed, Indian authors rarely present a personal system; in the great majority of instances, they are content to formulate traditional doctrines in the language of their own time. This is even more typically observable in the case of Patañjali, whose sole aim is to compile a practical manual of very ancient techniques.

Vyāsa (seventh–eighth century) composed a commentary, *Yoga-bhāṣya*, and Vācaspatimiśra (ninth century) a gloss, *Tattvavaiśāradī*, which are among the most important contributions to an understanding of the *Yoga-sūtras.* King Bhoja (beginning of the eleventh century) is the author of the commentary *Rājamārtaṇḍa*, and Rāmānanda Sarasvatī (sixteenth century) of the *Maṇiprabhā*. Finally, Vijñānabhikṣu annotated Vyāsa's *Yoga-bhāṣya* in his remarkable treatise, the *Yoga-vārttika.*[5]

For Sāṃkhya and Yoga, the world is *real* (not illusory—as it is, for example, for Vedānta). Nevertheless, if the world *exists* and *endures*, it is because of the "ignorance" of spirit; the innumerable forms of the cosmos, as well as their processes of manifestation and development, exist only in the measure to which the Self (*puruṣa*) is ignorant of itself and, by reason of this metaphysical ignorance, suffers and is enslaved. At the precise moment when the last Self shall have found its freedom, the creation in its totality will be reabsorbed into the primordial substance.

It is here, in this fundamental affirmation (more or less explicitly formulated) that the cosmos exists and endures because of man's lack of knowledge, that we can find the reason for the Indian

4 See Note I, 2.* [Concerning asterisk, see p. xi.]

5 For editions and translations of yogic texts, see Note I, 2.

depreciation of life and the cosmos—a depreciation that none of the great constructions of post-Vedic Indian thought attempted to hide. From the time of the Upaniṣads India rejects the world as it is and devaluates life as it reveals itself to the eyes of the sage—ephemeral, painful, illusory. Such a conception leads neither to nihilism nor to pessimism. *This* world is rejected, *this* life depreciated, because it is known that *something else* exists, beyond becoming, beyond temporality, beyond suffering. In religious terms, it could almost be said that India rejects the *profane* cosmos and *profane* life, because it thirsts for a *sacred* world and a *sacred* mode of being.

Again and again Indian texts repeat this thesis—that the cause of the soul's "enslavement" and, consequently, the source of its endless sufferings lie in *man's solidarity with the cosmos,* in his participation, active and passive, direct or indirect, in nature. Let us translate: solidarity with a *desacralized* world, participation in a *profane* nature. *Neti! neti!* cries the sage of the Upaniṣads: "No, no! thou art not *this;* nor art thou *that!*" In other words: you do not belong to the fallen cosmos, *as you see it now;* you are not necessarily engulfed in *this* creation; necessarily—that is to say, by virtue of the law of your own being. For *Being* can have no relation with *nonbeing*. Now, nature has no true ontological reality; it is, indeed, universal becoming. Every cosmic form, complex and majestic though it may be, ends by disintegrating; the universe itself is periodically reabsorbed by "great dissolutions" (*mahāpralaya*) into the primordial matrix (*prakṛti*). Now, whatever becomes, changes, dies, vanishes does not belong to the sphere of being—to translate once again, is not *sacred.* If solidarity with the cosmos is the consequence of a progressive desacralization of human existence, and hence a fall into ignorance and suffering, the road toward freedom necessarily leads to a desolidarization from the cosmos and profane life. (In some forms of tantric Yoga this desolidarization is followed by a desperate effort toward the resacralization of life.)

Yet the cosmos, life, have an ambivalent function. On the one hand, they fling man into suffering and, by virtue of *karma*, enmesh him in the infinite cycle of transmigrations; on the other hand, indirectly, they help him to seek and find "salvation" for his soul, autonomy, absolute freedom (*mokṣa, mukti*). For the more man suffers (that is, the greater is his solidarity with the cosmos), the more the desire for emancipation increases in him, the more intensely he thirsts for salvation. Thus the forms and illusions of the cosmos—and this by virtue of, not in spite of, their inherent magic, and by virtue of the suffering that their indefatigable becoming ceaselessly feeds—put themselves at the service of man, whose supreme end is emancipation, salvation. "From Brahman down to the blade of grass, the creation [*sṛṣti*] is for the benefit of the soul, until supreme knowledge is attained." [6] Supreme knowledge—that is to say, emancipation not only from ignorance, but also, and indeed first of all, from pain, from suffering.

The Equation Pain-Existence

"All is suffering for the sage" (*duḥkameva sarva vivekinaḥ*), writes Patañjali.[7] But Patañjali is neither the first nor the last to record this universal suffering. Long before him the Buddha had proclaimed: "All is pain, all is ephemeral" (*sarvam duḥkham, sarvam anityam*). It is a leitmotiv of all post-Upaniṣadic Indian speculation. Soteriological techniques, as well as metaphysical doctrines, find their justification in this universal suffering, for they have no value save in the measure to which they free man from "pain." Human experience of whatever kind engenders suffering. "The body is pain, because it is the place of pain; the senses, objects, perceptions are suffering, because they lead to suffering; pleasure itself is suffering, because it is followed by suffering." [8] And Īśvarakṛṣṇa, author of the earliest Sāṃkhya treatise, declares that the foundation stone of Sāṃkhya is man's desire to escape from the torture of the three sufferings—from celestial misery (provoked

6 *Sāṃkhya-sūtras*, III, 47. 7 *Yoga-sūtras*, II, 15.
8 Aniruddha, commenting on *Sāṃkhya-sūtras*, II, 1.

by the gods), from terrestrial misery (caused by nature), and from inner or organic misery.[9]

Yet this universal suffering does not lead to a "philosophy of pessimism." No Indian philosophy or gnosis falls into despair. On the contrary, the revelation of "pain" as the law of existence can be regarded as the *conditio sine qua non* for emancipation. Intrinsically, then, this universal suffering has a positive, stimulating value. It perpetually reminds the sage and the ascetic that but one way remains for him to attain to freedom and bliss—withdrawal from the world, detachment from possessions and ambitions, radical isolation. Man, moreover, is not alone in suffering; pain is a cosmic necessity, an ontological modality to which every "form" that manifests itself as such is condemned. Whether one be a god or a tiny insect, the mere fact of existing in time, of having duration, implies pain. Unlike the gods and other living beings, man possesses the capability of passing beyond his condition and thus abolishing suffering. The certainty that there is a way to end suffering—a certainty shared by all Indian philosophies and mysticisms—can lead neither to "despair" nor to "pessimism." To be sure, suffering is universal; but if man knows how to set about emancipating himself from it, it is not final. For, if the human condition is condemned to pain for all eternity—since, like every condition, it is determined by *karma* [10]—each individual who shares in it can pass beyond it, since each can annul the karmic forces by which it is governed.

To "emancipate" oneself from suffering—such is the goal of all Indian philosophies and all Indian mysticisms. Whether this deliverance is obtained directly through "knowledge" (according to the teaching of Vedānta and Sāṃkhya, for example) or by means of techniques (as Yoga and the majority of Buddhist schools hold), the fact remains that no knowledge has any value if it does not seek

9 *Sāṃkhya-kārikā*, 1.

10 Let us recall the meanings of the term: work, action; destiny (ineluctable consequence of acts performed in a previous existence); product, effect, etc.

the "salvation" of man. "Save for that, nothing is worth knowing," says the *Śvetāśvatara Upaniṣad* (I, 12). And Bhoja, commenting on a text of the *Yoga-sūtras* (IV, 22), declares that any knowledge whose object is not deliverance is valueless. Vācaspatimiśra begins his commentary on Īśvarakṛṣna's treatise: "In this world, the audience listens only to the preacher who sets forth facts whose knowledge is necessary and desired. To those who set forth doctrines that no one desires, no one attends, as comes to pass with fools or with men of the herd, who are good in their practical affairs but ignorant of the sciences and arts." [11] The same author, in his commentary on the *Vedānta-sūtra-bhāṣya*, specifies the necessary knowledge: "No lucid person desires to know what is devoid of all certainty or what is of no use . . . or of no importance." [12]

In India metaphysical knowledge always has a soteriological purpose. Thus only metaphysical knowledge (*vidyā*, *jñāna*, *prajñā*)—that is, the knowledge of ultimate realities—is valued and sought, for it alone procures liberation. For it is by "knowledge" that man, casting off the illusions of the world of phenomena, "awakens." By knowledge—and that means: by practicing withdrawal, the effect of which will be to make him find his own center, to make him coincide with his "true spirit" (*puruṣa*, *ātman*). Knowledge is transformed into a kind of meditation, and metaphysics becomes soteriology. In India not even "logic" is without a soteriological function in its beginnings. Manu uses the term *ānvīkṣaki* ("science of controversy," logic) as an equivalent to *ātmavidyā* ("knowledge of the soul," of the *ātman*)—that is, to metaphysics.[13] Correct argumentation, in conformity with the norms, frees the soul—this is the point of departure of the Nyāya school. Moreover, the earliest logical controversies, from which the Nyāya *darśana* will later develop, were concerned precisely with sacred texts, with the different interpretations that could be

11 *Tattva-kaumudī*, ed. Gangānātha Jhā, p. 1. [For full references, see the list of works cited.]

12 *Bhāmatī*, ed. Bāla Śāstri, pp. 1–2.

13 *Manu-Smṛti*, VII, 43.

put upon such and such an injunction in the Vedas; the purpose of all these controversies was to make possible the correct performance of a rite, in accordance with tradition. Now, this sacred tradition, of which the Vedas are the expression, is *revealed.* Under such conditions, to seek the meaning of words is to remain in permanent contact with the Logos, with the spiritual reality that is absolute, suprahuman, and suprahistorical. Just as the right pronunciation of the Vedic texts results in giving the ritual maximum efficacy, so *right comprehension* of a Vedic maxim results in purifying the intelligence and thus contributes to the spirit's liberation. All partial "ignorance," as it is abolished, carries man a step onward toward freedom and bliss.

The importance that all these Indian metaphysics, and even the ascetic technique and contemplative method that constitute Yoga, accord to "knowledge" is easily explained if we take into consideration the causes of human suffering. The wretchedness of human life is not owing to a divine punishment or to an original sin, but to *ignorance.* Not any and every kind of ignorance, but only ignorance of the true nature of *Spirit*, the ignorance that makes us confuse Spirit with our psychomental experience, that makes us attribute "qualities" and predicates to the eternal and autonomous principle that is Spirit—in short, a metaphysical ignorance. Hence it is natural that it should be a metaphysical knowledge that supervenes to end this ignorance. This metaphysical knowledge leads the disciple to the threshold of illumination—that is, to the true "Self." And it is this knowledge of one's Self—not in the profane sense of the term, but in its ascetic and spiritual sense—that is the end pursued by the majority of Indian speculative systems, though each of them indicates a different way of reaching it.

For Sāṃkhya and Yoga the problem is clearly defined. Since suffering has its origin in ignorance of "Spirit"—that is, in confusing "Spirit" with psychomental states—emancipation can be obtained only if the confusion is abolished. The differences between Sāṃkhya and Yoga on this point are insignificant. Only their methods differ: Sāṃkhya seeks to obtain liberation solely by *gnosis*, whereas for Yoga an *ascesis* and a *technique of meditation* are indispensable. In both *darśanas* human suffering is rooted in illusion, for man believes that his psychomental life—activity of the senses, feelings, thoughts, and volitions—is identical with Spirit, with the Self. He thus confuses two wholly autonomous and opposed realities, between which there is no real connection but only an illusory relation, for psychomental experience does not belong to Spirit, it belongs to nature (*prakṛti*); states of consciousness are the refined products of the same substance that is at the base of the physical world and the world of life. Between psychic states and inanimate objects or living beings, there are only differences of degree. But between psychic states and Spirit there is a difference of an ontological order; they belong to two different modes of being. "Liberation" occurs when one has understood this truth, and when the Spirit regains its original freedom. Thus, according to Sāṃkhya, he who would gain emancipation must begin by thoroughly knowing the essence and the forms of nature (*prakṛti*) and the laws that govern its evolution. For its part, Yoga also accepts this analysis of Substance, but finds value only in the practice of contemplation, which is alone capable of revealing the autonomy and omnipotence of Spirit experimentally. Hence, before expounding the methods and techniques of Yoga, we must see how the Sāṃkhya *darśana* conceives Substance and Spirit, together with the cause of their false solidarity; we must, in short, see in what the gnostic way advocated by this "philosophy" consists. We must also determine to what degree the Sāṃkhya and Yoga doctrines coincide, and distinguish, in the theoretical affirmations of the latter, those which are based on "mystical" experiences lacking in Sāṃkhya.

The "Self"

Spirit ("soul")—as a transcendent and autonomous principle—is accepted by all Indian philosophies, except by the Buddhists and the materialists (the Lokāyatas).[14] But it is by entirely different

14 See Note I, 3.

approaches that the various *darśanas* seek to prove its existence and explain its essence. For the Nyāya school, soul-spirit is an entity without qualities, absolute, unknowing. Vedānta, on the contrary, defines the *ātman* as being *saccidānanda* (*sat* = being; *cit* = consciousness; *ānanda* = bliss) and regards Spirit as a unique, universal, and eternal reality, dramatically enmeshed in the temporal illusion of creation (*māyā*). Sāṃkhya and Yoga deny Spirit (*puruṣa*) any attribute and any relation; according to these two "philosophies," all that can be affirmed of *puruṣa* is that it *is* and that it *knows* (its knowing is, of course, the metaphysical knowledge that results from its contemplation of its own mode of being).

Like the *ātman* of the Upaniṣads, *puruṣa* is inexpressible.[15] Its "attributes" are negative. "Spirit is that which sees [*sākṣin* = witness], it is isolated [*kaivalyam*], indifferent, mere inactive spectator," writes Īśvarakṛṣṇa,[16] and Gauḍapāda, in his commentary, insists on the eternal passivity of *puruṣa*. The autonomy and impassivity of Spirit are traditional epithets, as *Sāṃkhya-sūtras*, I, 147, attests; commenting on this text, Aniruddha cites the famous passage from the *Bṛhadāraṇyaka Upaniṣad* (IV, 3, 15), "This *puruṣa* is free" (*asaṇga*, "without attachments"), and Vijñānabhikṣu refers to *Śvetāśvatara Upaniṣad*, VI, 2, and *Vedāntasāra*, 158. Being irreducible, without qualities (*nirguṇatvat*), *puruṣa* has no "intelligence" (*ciddharma*),[17] for it is without desires. Desires are not eternal, hence they do not belong to Spirit. Spirit is eternally free,[18] for states of consciousness, the flux of psychomental life, are foreign to it. If *puruṣa* nevertheless appears to us to be an "agent" (*kartṛ*), this is owing both to human illusion and to the unique correlation termed *yogyatā*,[19] which designates a

15 The phrase *neti, neti*—"not thus! not thus!"—of *Bṛhadāraṇyaka Upaniṣad*, III, 9, 26, recurs in *Sāṃkhya-sūtras*, III, 75.

16 *Sāṃkhya-kārikā*, 19.

17 *Sāṃkhya-sūtras*, I, 146.

18 Ibid., I, 162.

19 Vyāsa (ad *Yoga-sūtras*, I, 4) and Vācaspatimiśra (ibid. and *Tattvakaumudī*, 31) state that "this unique correlation has no beginning," is not owing to a spatial or temporal correlation between the Self and intelligence;

kind of pre-established harmony between the two essentially distinct realities constituted by Self (*puruṣa*) and intelligence (*buddhi;* the latter, as we shall see further on, being only a "more refined product" of the primordial matter or substance).

Patañjali's position is the same. In *Yoga-sūtras*, II, 5, he repeats the statement that ignorance (*avidyā*) consists in regarding what is ephemeral (*anitya*), impure (*aśuci*), painful (*duḥkha*), and non-Spirit (*anātma*) as being eternal (*nitya*), pure (*śuci*), bliss (*sukha*), and Spirit (*ātman*). Vyāsa [20] reiterates that perception, memory, reasoning, etc., belong to the intelligence (*buddhi*) and that it is only by the effect of an illusion that these mental faculties are attributed to the *puruṣa*.[21]

Now, this conception of *puruṣa* at once raises difficulties. For if Spirit is eternally pure, impassive, autonomous, and irreducible, how can it acquiesce in being accompanied by psychomental experience? And how is such a relation possible? We may profitably postpone an examination of the solution that Sāṃkhya and Yoga propose for this problem until we shall have become better acquainted with the possible relationships between the Self and nature. We shall then see that the effort of the two *darśanas* is principally applied to the problem of the true nature of this strange "relation" that links *puruṣa* to *prakṛti*. However, neither the *origin* nor the *cause* of this paradoxical situation has been the object of a formal discussion in Sāṃkhya-Yoga. Why, finally, did the Self acquiesce in being drawn into a foreign orbit, more particularly that of life—and thus in engendering man as such, concrete, historical man, condemned to every catastrophe, assailed by every

---

it is a *yogyatā*—that is, a correspondence of a metaphysical order between Spirit (*puruṣa*) and the most subtle product of Substance, *buddhi*. This "correlation," which constitutes one of the greatest difficulties of Indian speculation in general, is explained by Sāṃkhya and Yoga through the teleological instinct of nature (*prakṛti*), which, without knowing it, "works" for the deliverance of Spirit. (See below, p. 30.) On the eight possible hypotheses to explain the relationships *puruṣa-prakṛti*, cf. Vyāsa, ad II, 23.

20 Ad *Yoga-sūtras*, II, 18.

21 See also Bhoja, ad *Yoga-sūtras*, II, 20, and Note I, 4.

suffering? *When*, and on what occasion, did this tragedy of the existence of man begin, if it is true that the ontological modality of Spirit is, as we have already seen, exactly opposite to the human condition, the Self being eternal, free, and passive?

The *cause* and the *origin* of this association between Spirit and experience—these are two aspects of a problem that Sāṃkhya and Yoga consider insoluble because it exceeds the present capacity of human comprehension. For man knows and comprehends by means of what Sāṃkhya-Yoga calls the "intellect," *buddhi*. But this intellect itself is only a product—an extremely refined product, to be sure—of matter, of the primordial substance (*prakṛti*). Being a product of nature, a "phenomenon," *buddhi* can enter into cognitional relations only with other phenomena (which, like it, belong to the infinite series of the creations of the primordial substance); under no circumstances could it know the Self, for it could by no possibility enter into any kind of relation with a transcendental reality. The cause and the origin of this paradoxical association between the Self and life (that is, "matter") could be understood only by an instrument of knowledge other than the *buddhi*, one in no way implying matter. Now, such knowledge is impossible in the present condition of humanity. It "reveals" itself only to him who, having broken his fetters, has passed beyond the human condition; "intellect" plays no part in this revelation, which is, rather, knowledge of one's Self, of the Self itself.

Sāṃkhya knows that the cause of "bondage"—that is, of the human condition, of suffering—is metaphysical ignorance, which, by force of the karmic law, is transmitted from generation to generation; but the historical moment at which this ignorance appeared cannot be established, just as it is impossible to determine the date of creation. The connection between the Self and life, and the resulting bondage (for the Self), have no history; they are beyond time, they are eternal. To insist upon finding a solution for these problems is vain, is childishness. They are problems wrongly posed; and in accordance with an old Brāhmanic practice,[22]

22 Śaṇkara, ad *Vedānta-sūtras*, III, 2, 17.

observed by Buddha himself on several occasions,[23] the sage responds to a wrongly posed problem by silence. The only certainty attainable on the subject is that man has been in this condition since the dawn of time, and that the goal of knowledge is not a fruitless search for the first cause and historical origins of this condition, but liberation.

Substance

It is only in passing that Patañjali refers to *prakṛti*[24] and its modalities, the *guṇas*,[25] and only to define their relationships with psychomental life and the techniques of liberation. He assumes a knowledge of the analysis of Substance, laboriously pursued by Sāṃkhya authors. It is primarily to these authors that we shall have recourse in order to understand the structure and the procession of Substance.

Prakṛti is as real and as eternal as *puruṣa;* but unlike Spirit, it is dynamic and creative. Though perfectly homogeneous and inert, this primordial substance possesses, so to speak, three "modes of being," which permit it to manifest itself in three different ways, which are termed *guṇas:* (1) *sattva* (modality of luminosity and intelligence); (2) *rajas* (modality of motor energy and mental activity); (3) *tamas* (modality of static inertia and psychic obscurity). However, these *guṇas* must not be regarded as different from *prakṛti,* for they are never given separately; in every physical, biological, or psychomental phenomenon all three *guṇas* exist simultaneously, though in unequal proportions (indeed, it is this inequality that permits the appearance of a "phenomenon," of whatever kind; otherwise, the primordial equilibrium and homogeneity by virtue of which the *guṇas* were in perfect equilibrium would persist forever). It is clear, then, that the *guṇas* have a two-

23 Cf., for example, Vasubandhu, *Abhidharmakośa,* V, 22; see also T. Stcherbatsky, *The Conception of Buddhist Nirvāṇa,* p. 22.

24 *Yoga-sūtras,* IV, 2, 3.

25 Ibid., I, 16; II, 15, 19; IV, 13, 34, 32.

fold character: objective on the one hand, since they constitute the phenomena of the external world, and, on the other hand, subjective, since they support, nourish, and condition psychomental life. (This is why *tamas* must be translated not only as "principle of the inertia of matter"—its objective meaning—but also as "darkness of consciousness," "obstacle created by the passions"—its psychophysiological meaning.)[26]

As soon as *prakṛti* departs from its original state of perfect equilibrium (*aliṅga, avyakta*) and assumes specific characteristics conditioned by its "teleological instinct" (to which we shall return), it appears in the form of an energetic mass called *mahat* ("the great").[27] Drawn on by the force of evolution (*pariṇāma*, "development," "procession"), *prakṛti* passes from the state of *mahat* to that of *ahaṃkāra*, which means: uniform apperceptive mass, as yet without "personal" experience, but with the obscure consciousness of being an ego (hence the term *ahaṃkāra; aham* = ego). From this apperceptive mass, the process of "evolution" bifurcates in opposite directions, one of which leads to the world of objective phenomena and the other to that of subjective phenomena (sensible and psychomental). The *ahamkāra* has the ability to transform itself qualitatively in accordance with which of the three *guṇas* predominates in it. When *sattva* (the modality of luminosity, of purity and comprehension) is predominant in the *ahaṃkāra*, the five cognoscitive senses (*jñānendriya*), and *manas*, "the inner sense," make their appearance; the latter serves as liaison center between perceptive and motor activity;[28] the base and receptacle of all impressions,[29] it co-ordinates biological and

26 On the *guṇas*, see also Note I, 5.

27 *Sāṃkhya-sūtras*, I, 61: "*Prakṛti* is the state of equilibrium of *sattva, rajas,* and *tamas*. From *prakṛti* issued *mahat; from mahat, ahaṃkāra;* from *ahaṃkāra*, the five *tanmātras* and the two series of sense organs; from *tanmātra* issued the *sthūlabhūtānis* [material elements, molecules]." This *sūtra* resumes all the processes of manifestation (or "cosmic procession") that we are engaged in analyzing. Further texts: *Sāṃkhya-sūtras*, I, 129; II, 10, 15; Īśvarakṛṣṇa, *Sāṃkhya-kārikā*, 3, 40, 56; Vyāsa, ad *Yoga-sūtras*, II, 19, etc.

28 Aniruddha, ad *Sāṃkhya-sūtras*, II, 40.

29 Ibid., II, 42.

psychic activities, particularly that of the subconscious. When, on the other hand, the equilibrium is dominated by *rajas* (the motor energy that makes all physical or cognoscitive experience possible), the five conative senses (*karmendriya*) appear. Finally, when *tamas* (inertia of matter, darkness of consciousness, the barrage of the passions) dominates, what appear are the five *tanmātras*, the five "subtle" (potential) elements, the genetic seeds of the physical world. By a process of condensation that tends to produce structures increasingly gross, these *tanmātras* give rise to atoms (*paramāṇu*) and molecules (*sthūlabhūtāni*; literally, "dense material particle"), which in turn give birth to vegetable organisms (*vrikṣa*) and animal organisms (*śarīra*). Thus man's body, as well as his "states of consciousness" and even his "intelligence," are all creations of one and the same substance.

It will be noted that, in accordance with Sāṃkhya and Yoga, the universe—objective or subjective—is only the evolution of an initial stage of nature (*ahaṃkāra*), that in which the homogeneous and energetic mass first gave birth to consciousness of individuality, to an apperception illuminated by the ego. By a twofold process of development and creation, the *ahaṃkāra* created a twofold universe—inner and outer—these two "worlds" having elective correspondences between them. Each sense corresponds to a specific atom, as each atom corresponds to a *tanmātra*.[30] But each of these products contains the three *guṇas*, though in unequal proportions; each product is characterized by the supremacy of a particular *guṇa* or, in the last stages of creation, by the predominance of a particular *tanmātra*.

It is important that we understand the notion of evolution in Sāṃkhya. *Pariṇāma* signifies development of what exists, *in posse*,

30 For example, "potential sound" (*śabdha-tanmātra*), by an agglutination with molecules, produces the "atom-space" (*ākāśa-aṇu*), to which—in the subjective order—sense of hearing corresponds; luminous and irradiating energy (*tejas-tanmātra*) produces the "irradiating atom" and the sense of sight, etc.

in the *mahat*. It is not a creation, nor a transcendence, nor the realization of new species of existence, but simply the realization of the potentialities that exist in *prakṛti* (under its living aspect, the *mahat*). To compare "evolution" in the Indian sense with Western evolutionism is to be guilty of great confusion. No new form, Sāṃkhya affirms, goes beyond the possibilities of existence that were already present in the universe. In fact, for Sāṃkhya, nothing is created, in the Western sense of the word. Creation exists from all eternity and can never be destroyed; but it will return to its original aspect of absolute equilibrium (in the great final resorption, *mahāpralaya*).

This conception of evolution is justified by a particular theory of causality. For if the effect exceeded the cause, there would be in the cause a nonexisting quantum, which would acquire existence in the effect. But, Sāṃkhya asks, how could this nonentity be the cause of an entity? How could *esse* come from *non esse?* Vācaspatimiśra says:[31] "If one affirms the production of an entity by a nonentity, then the latter, existing everywhere and at every moment, should give birth everywhere and at every moment to any effect and all effects." And, commenting on *Sāṃkhya-kārikā*, 9, he adds: "The effect is an entity, that is to say, it exists before the causal operation."[32] "If the effect were a nonentity before the causal operation, it could never be brought into existence."[33]

Between the cause and the effect there exists a real and definite relation. But if the effect did not exist in the cause, how should a *relation* be possible between *ens* and *non ens?* How should an intimate connection be possible between *absence* and *presence?* "Under these conditions," says Īśvarakṛṣṇa,[34] "all that can be brought about by the cause is the manifestation or the development of the pre-existing effect." To illustrate the theory of causality by an

31 *Tattva-kaumudī*, 62, and with more details in the *Nyāyavārtikatātparyaṭīkā*.

32 *Tattva-kaumudī*, 62.

33 Ibid., 64; cf. ibid., 68–69; *Sāṃkhya-sūtras*, I, 115 and 118, with the commentaries, especially Aniruddha, and I, 41. On Sāṃkhya logic, see Note I, 6.

34 *Sāṃkhya-kārikā*, 14.

example, Vijñānabhikṣu writes: "Just as the statue, already existing in the block of stone, is only revealed by the sculptor, so the causal activity only engenders the action by which an effect manifests itself, giving the illusion that it exists only in the present moment." [35]

Concerning the *ahaṃkāra,* Sāṃkhya texts give many details, but what is of interest to our brief exposition is that *ahaṃkāra* is defined as "self-knowledge." [36] We should bear in mind that this entity, though "material," does not manifest itself in sensory, physical forms, but is homogeneous, a pure and energetic mass without structure. According to Sāṃkhya, the *ahaṃkāra* acquires consciousness of itself, and, through this process, reflects itself (*sarva,* "emanation") in the series of the eleven psychic principles (*manas,* or the inner sense, which co-ordinates the faculties of the soul; the five cognitive and the five conative senses) and in the series of physical powers (*tanmātra*).

We should note the capital importance that Sāṃkhya, like almost all Indian systems, accords to the *principle of individuation through "consciousness of self."* We see that the genesis of the world is a psychic act, that it is from this self-knowledge (which, of course, is absolutely different from the "awakening" of the *puruṣa*) that the evolution of the physical world derives; and that objective and psychophysiological phenomena have a common matrix, the only difference between them being the *formula* of the *guṇas, sattva* predominating in psychic phenomena, *rajas* in psychophysiological phenomena (passion, activity of the senses, etc.), while the phenomena of "matter" are constituted by the increasingly inert and dense products of *tamas* (*tanmātra, aṇu, bhūtāni*).

Sāṃkhya-Yoga also provides a subjective interpretation of the three *guṇas* when it considers their psychic "aspects." When *sattva* predominates, consciousness is calm, clear, comprehensible, virtuous; dominated by *rajas,* it is agitated, uncertain, unstable; overwhelmed by *tamas,* it is dark, confused, passionate, bestial.[37]

35 *Sāṃkhya-pravacana-bhāṣya,* I, 120. 36 *Sāṃkhya-kārikā,* 24.

37 See *Yoga-sūtras,* II, 15, 19, with the commentaries.

But of course this subjective and human evaluation of the three cosmic modalities does not contradict their objective character—"outer" and "inner" being no more than verbal expressions.

With this physiological foundation, we can understand why Sāṃkhya-Yoga regarded all psychic experience as a simple "material" process. Ethics is affected—purity, goodness, is not a quality of spirit but a "purification" of the "subtle matter" represented by consciousness. The *guṇas* impregnate the whole universe and establish an organic sympathy between man and the cosmos, these two entities being pervaded by the same pain of existence and both serving the same absolute Self, which is foreign to the world and driven on by an unintelligible destiny. In fact, the difference between the cosmos and man is only a difference of degree, not of essence.

By virtue of *pariṇāma*, matter has produced an infinity of forms (*vikāra*), increasingly complex, increasingly varied. Sāṃkhya holds that such an immense creation, such a complicated edifice of forms and organisms, demands a justification and a signification outside of itself. A primordial, formless, and eternal *prakṛti* can have a meaning. But the world as we see it is not a homogeneous substance; on the contrary, it exhibits a number of distinct forms and structures. The complexity of the cosmos, the infinity of its "forms," are raised by Sāṃkhya to the rank of metaphysical arguments. The "creation" is, without any doubt, the product of our metaphysical ignorance; the existence of the universe and the polymorphism of life are owing to man's false opinion of himself, to the fact that he confuses the true Self with psychomental states. But, as we remarked above, it is impossible to know the origin and the cause of this false opinion. What we know, what we see, is that *prakṛti* has an extremely complicated evolution and that it is not simple but composite.

Now, common sense tells us that every compound exists in view of another. Thus, for example, a bed is a whole composed of various parts, but this provisional collaboration between the parts is not ordained for itself, it is in view of man.[38] Sāṃkhya thus brings out the teleological nature of creation; for if the mission of creation were not to serve Spirit, it would be absurd, meaningless. Everything in nature is composite; everything, then, must have a "superintendent" (*adhyakṣah*), someone who can make use of these compounds. This "superintendent" cannot be mental activity, nor states of consciousness (themselves extremely complex products of *prakṛti*). There must, then, be an entity that transcends the categories of Substance (*guṇa*) and that exists in view of itself. Yet more: there must be a subject to which mental activity is subordinated, toward which "pleasure and pain" are oriented. For, Vācaspatimiśra adds,[39] pleasure cannot be felt and distinguished by pleasure; and if it were felt by pain, it would no longer be an agreeable experience, but a painful one. Thus the two qualities (pain and pleasure) cannot exist, cannot be distinguished, save as oriented toward a single subject that transcends experience.

This represents the first proof found by Sāṃkhya for the existence of spirit: *saṃhataparārthatvāt puruṣasya*—that is, "knowledge of the existence of spirit by combination for the profit of another" —an axiom abundantly repeated in Indian literature[40] and adopted by Yoga.[41] Vācaspatimiśra adds: if anyone objects that the evolution and heterogeneity of Substance are intended to serve other "compounds" (as is the case, for example, with a chair, a "compound" created to serve another "compound," the human body), we can answer him that these "compounds" too must, in turn, exist for other "compounds" to use; the series of interdependences would inevitably lead us to a *regressus ad infinitum*. "And since we can avoid this *regressus*," Vācaspatimiśra continues, "by postulating

38 *Sāṃkhya-kārikā*, 17, with the commentaries, Vācaspatimiśra, 120; *Sāṃkhya-sūtras*, I, 140–44, with the commentaries of Aniruddha and Vijñānabhikṣu.

39 *Tattva-kaumudī*, 123.

40 *Sāṃkhya-sūtras*, I, 66; Vācaspatimiśra, ad *Sāṃkhya-kārikā*, 17; *Bṛhadāraṇyaka Upaniṣad*, II, 4, 5.

41 Cf. *Yoga-sūtras*, IV, 24.

the existence of a rational Principle, it is obviously stupid to go on needlessly multiplying the series of relations between compounds."[42] In accordance with this postulate, Spirit, the Self, is a simple and irreducible principle, autonomous, static, nonproductive, not implicated in mental or sensory activity, etc.

Although the Self (*puruṣa*) is veiled by the illusions and confusions of cosmic creation, *prakṛti* is dynamized by the "teleological instinct" that is wholly intent upon the "liberation" of *puruṣa*. Let us recall that "from Brahman down to the blade of grass, the creation is for the benefit of soul, until supreme knowledge is attained." [43]

The Relation Spirit-Nature

If the Sāṃkhya-Yoga philosophy explains neither the cause nor the origin of the strange association established between Spirit and experience, it nevertheless attempts to explain the nature of their association, to define the character of their mutual relations. They are not *real* relations, in the strict sense of the word—relations such as exist, for example, between external objects and perceptions. Real relations, of course, imply change and plurality; now, these are modalities essentially opposed to the nature of Spirit.

"States of consciousness" are only products of *prakṛti* and can have no kind of relation with Spirit—the latter, by its very essence, being above all experience. However—and for Sāṃkhya and Yoga this is the key to the paradoxical situation—the most subtle, most transparent part of mental life, that is, intelligence (*buddhi*) in its mode of pure luminosity (*sattva*), has a specific quality—that of reflecting Spirit. Comprehension of the external world is possible only by virtue of this reflection of *puruṣa* in intelligence. But the Self is not corrupted by this reflection and does not lose its ontological modalities (impassibility, eternity, etc.). The *Yoga-sūtras* (II, 20) say in substance: seeing (*draṣṭṛ*; i.e., *puruṣa*) is absolute consciousness ("sight par excellence") and, while remaining pure, it knows cognitions (it "looks at the ideas that are presented to

42 *Tattva-kaumudī*, 121. 43 *Sāṃkhya-sūtras*, III, 47.

it"). Vyāsa interprets: Spirit is reflected in intelligence (*buddhi*), but is neither like it nor different from it. It is not like intelligence because intelligence is modified by knowledge of objects, which knowledge is ever-changing—whereas *puruṣa* commands uninterrupted knowledge, in some sort it *is* knowledge. On the other hand, *puruṣa* is not completely different from *buddhi*, for, although it is pure, it knows knowledge. Patañjali employs a different image to define the relationship between Spirit and intelligence: just as a flower is reflected in a crystal, intelligence reflects *puruṣa*.[44] But only ignorance can attribute to the crystal the qualities of the flower (form, dimensions, colors). When the object (the flower) moves, its image moves in the crystal, though the latter remains motionless. It is an illusion to believe that Spirit is dynamic because mental experience is so. In reality, there is here only an illusory relation (*upādhi*) owing to a "sympathetic correspondence" (*yogyatā*) between the Self and intelligence.

From all eternity, Spirit has found itself drawn into this illusory relation with psychomental life (that is, with "matter"). This is owing to ignorance (*avidyā*),[45] and as long as *avidyā* persists, existence is present (by virtue of *karma*), and with it suffering. Let us dwell on this point a little. Illusion or ignorance consists in confusing the motionless and eternal *puruṣa* with the flux of psychomental life.[46] To say "I suffer," "I want," "I hate," "I know," and to think that this "I" refers to Spirit, is to live in illusion and prolong it; for all our acts and intentions, by the simple fact that they are dependent upon *prakṛti*, upon "matter," are conditioned and governed by *karma*. This means that every action whose point of departure is illusion (that is, which is based on *ignorance*, the confusion between Spirit and non-Spirit) is either the consummation of a virtuality created by a preceding act or the projection of another force that in turn demands its actualization, its consummation, in the present existence or in an existence to come. When one sets up the equation, "I want" = "Spirit wants," either a certain force is

44 Cf. *Yoga-sūtras*, I, 41.
45 *Yoga-sūtras*, II, 24.
46 *Sāṃkhya-sūtras*, III, 41.

set in motion or another force has been fertilized. For the confusion that this equation expresses is a "moment" in the eternal circuit of cosmic energies.

This is the law of existence; like every law, it is transsubjective, but its validity and universality are at the origin of the suffering by which existence is troubled. There is but one way to gain salvation—adequate knowledge of Spirit. Sāṃkhya only prolongs the tradition of the Upaniṣads: "He who knows the *ātman* crosses over [the ocean of suffering]." [47] "Through knowledge, liberation; through ignorance, bondage." [48] And the first stage of the conquest of this "knowledge" consists of one thing, in denying that Spirit has attributes—which is equivalent to denying suffering as something that concerns us, to regarding it as an objective fact, outside of Spirit, that is to say, *without value* and *without meaning* (since all "values" and all "meanings" are created by intelligence in so far as it reflects *puruṣa*). Pain exists only to the extent to which experience is referred to the human personality regarded as identical with *puruṣa*, with the Self. But since this relation is illusory, it can easily be abolished. When *puruṣa* is known, *values* are annulled; pain is no longer either pain or nonpain, but a simple *fact;* a fact that, while it preserves its sensory structure, loses its value, its meaning. This point should be thoroughly understood, for it is of capital importance in Sāṃkhya and Yoga and, in our opinion, has not been sufficiently emphasized. In order to deliver us from suffering, Sāṃkhya and Yoga *deny suffering as such*, thus doing away with all relation between suffering and the Self. From the moment we understand that the Self is free, eternal, and inactive, whatever happens to us—sufferings, feelings, volitions, thoughts, and so on—*no longer belongs to us*. All such things constitute a body of cosmic facts, which are conditioned by laws, and are certainly real, but whose reality has nothing in common with our *puruṣa*. Suffering is a cosmic fact, and man undergoes that fact, or contributes to its perpetuation, solely in so far as he allows himself to be seduced by an illusion.

47 *Chāndogya Upaniṣad*, VII, 1, 3.

48 *Sāṃkhya-sūtras*, III, 22, 23.

Knowledge is a simple "awakening" that unveils the essence of the Self, of Spirit. Knowledge does not "produce" anything; it reveals reality immediately. This true and absolute knowledge—which must not be confused with intellectual activity, which is psychological in essence—is not obtained by experience but by a revelation. Nothing divine plays a part here, for Sāṃkhya denies the existence of God; [49] Yoga accepts God, but we shall see that Patañjali does not accord him very much importance. The revelation is based on knowledge of the ultimate reality—that is, on an "awakening" in which object completely identifies itself with subject. (The "Self" "contemplates" itself; it does not "think" itself, for thought is itself an experience and, as such, belongs to *prakṛti.*)

For Sāṃkhya, there is no other way than this. Hope prolongs and even aggravates human misery; only he who has lost all hope is happy,[50] "for hope is the greatest torture that exists, and despair the greatest happiness." [51] Religious rites and practices have no value whatever,[52] because they are founded on desires and cruelties. Every ritual act, by the very fact that it implies an effort, engenders a new karmic force.[53] Morality itself leads to nothing decisive.[54] Indifference (*vairāgya* = renunciation), orthodoxy (*śruti*), and meditation are only indirect instruments of salvation. For Sāṃkhya the only perfect and definitive means is metaphysical knowledge.[55]

The cognitive process is naturally realized by the intellect; but

49 See Note I, 7. 50 *Sāṃkhya-sūtras*, IV, 11.

51 Text from the *Mahābhārata*, cited by the commentator Mahādeva Vedāntin, ad *Sāṃkhya-sūtras*, IV, 11.

52 *Sāṃkhya-sūtras*, III, 26. 53 Ibid., I, 84–85.

54 This was already an Upaniṣadic motif: the *Kauṣītaki Upaniṣad* (III, 1) affirms that sins are done away with by possession of true knowledge. The commentator Māṭhara asserts that one may eat flesh, drink wine, and make love, and that all these sins are abolished by knowledge of the doctrine of Kapila (that is, by Sāṃkhya). We shall later see the consequences of this spiritual position.

55 *Sāṃkhya-sūtras*, III, 23.

intellect itself is a highly evolved form of "matter." How, then, can deliverance (*mukti*) be accomplished through the collaboration of *prakṛti*? Sāṃkhya answers with the teleological argument: matter (*prakṛti*) instinctively acts in view of the enfranchisement of the soul (*puruṣa*). Intellect (*buddhi*), being the most perfect manifestation of *prakṛti*, is able, because of its dynamic possibilities, to aid the process of deliverance by serving as the preliminary stage of revelation. Yoga takes exactly the same position: *prakṛti* makes experience possible and, at the same time, pursues the liberation of the Self.[56] Commenting on this *sūtra*, Vyāsa adds an important detail; bondage, he says, is in fact only the situation of intelligence (*buddhi*) when the ultimate aim of the Self has not yet been attained, and liberation is only the state in which that end has been accomplished.

In the next chapter we shall see by what psychophysiological techniques one can, according to Yoga, attain this end. For Sāṃkhya, liberation is obtained almost automatically when intelligence (*buddhi*) leads man to the threshold of "awakening." As soon as this self-revelation is realized, intellect and all the other psychomental (hence material) elements that are wrongly attributed to *puruṣa* withdraw, detach themselves from Spirit, to be reabsorbed into *prakṛti*, like a "dancer who departs after having satisfied her master's desire." [57] "Nothing is more sensitive than *prakṛti*; as soon as it has said to itself, 'I am recognized,' it no longer shows itself before the eyes of the Spirit." [58] This is the state of the man who is "liberated in this life" (*jīvan-mukta*): the sage still lives, because his karmic residue remains to be consumed (just as the potter's wheel continues to turn from the velocity it has acquired, even though the pot is finished).[59] But when, at the moment of death, he abandons the body, the *puruṣa* is completely "liberated." [60]

56 *Yoga-sūtras*, II, 18, etc.

57 This comparison is frequent both in the *Mahābhārata* and in the Sāṃkhya treatises; cf. *Sāṃkhya-kārikā*, 59; *Sāṃkhya-sūtras*, III, 69.

58 *Sāṃkhya-kārikā*, 61.

59 Ibid., 67; *Sāṃkhya-sūtras*, III, 82.

60 *Sāṃkhya-kārikā*, 68.

How Is Liberation Possible?

Sāṃkhya-Yoga has, then, understood that "Spirit [*puruṣa*] can be neither born nor destroyed, is neither bound nor active [actively seeking deliverance], neither thirsts for freedom nor is liberated." [61] "Its mode is such that these two possibilities are excluded." [62] The Self is pure, eternal, free; it cannot be bound because it cannot enter into relations with anything but itself.[63] But man *believes* that *puruṣa* is bound and *thinks* that it can be liberated. These are illusions of our psychomental life. For, in fact, "bound" Spirit is free for all eternity. If its liberation seems to us a drama, it is because we place ourselves at a human point of view; Spirit is only spectator (*sākṣin*), just as liberation (*mukti*) is only a *becoming conscious* of its eternal freedom. *I* believe that I suffer, *I* believe that I am bound, *I* desire liberation. At the moment when—having "awakened"—I understand that this "I" (*asmitā*) is a product of matter (*prakṛti*), I at the same time understand that all existence has been only a chain of moments of suffering and that true Spirit "impassively contemplated" the drama of "personality." Thus, human personality does not exist as a final element; it is only a synthesis of psychomental experiences, and it is destroyed—in other words, ceases to act—as soon as revelation is an accomplished fact. Like all creations of the cosmic substance (*prakṛti*), the human personality (*asmitā*) also acted to bring about "awakening"; hence, once liberation is achieved, the personality is of no further use.

There is something of paradox in the way in which Sāṃkhya and Yoga conceive the situation of Spirit (*puruṣa*); though pure, eternal, and intangible, Spirit nevertheless consents to be associated, if

61 Gauḍapāda, *Māṇḍūkya-kārikā*, II, 32.

62 *Sāṃkhya-sūtras*, I, 160.

63 There is, however, a difference between liberated Spirit and that which is still in illusory bondage; this difference is *upādhi*. This "false relation" is the foundation of the mysterious association between *puruṣa* and psychomental states, precisely because man does not understand that it is an illusory relation.

only in an illusory manner, with matter; and, in order to acquire knowledge of its own mode of being and "liberate" itself, it is even obliged to make use of an instrument created by *prakṛti* (in this case, intelligence). Doubtless, if we view things in this way, human existence appears to be dramatic and even meaningless. If Spirit is free, why are men condemned to suffer in ignorance or to struggle for a freedom they already possess? If *puruṣa* is perfectly pure and static, why does it permit impurity, becoming, experience, pain, and history? Such questions could easily be multiplied. But Indian philosophy reminds us that we must not judge the Self from a logical or historical point of view—that is, by seeking the causes that have determined the present state of things. Reality must be accepted as it is.

It is nevertheless true that Sāṃkhya's position on this point is difficult to maintain. Hence, in order to avoid this paradox of a Self absolutely devoid of contact with nature and yet, in its own despite, the author of the human drama, Buddhism has entirely done away with the "soul-spirit," understood as an irreducible spiritual unity, and has replaced it by "states of consciousness." Vedānta, on the contrary, seeking to avoid the difficulty of the relations between the soul and the universe, denies the reality of the universe and regards it as *māyā*, illusion. Sāṃkhya and Yoga have been unwilling to deny ontological reality either to Spirit or to Substance. Hence Sāṃkhya has been attacked, principally because of this doctrine, by both Vedānta and Buddhism.[64]

Vedānta also criticizes the concept of the plurality of "selves" (*puruṣa*), as formulated by Sāṃkhya and Yoga. For these two *darśanas* affirm that there are as many *puruṣas* as there are human beings. And each of these *puruṣas* is a monad, is completely isolated; for the Self can have no contact either with the world around it (derived from *prakṛti*) or with other spirits. The cosmos, then, is peopled with these eternal, free, unmoving *puruṣas*—monads be-

64 See Śaṇkara's critique of Sāṃkhya metaphysics in his commentary on *Brahma-sūtras*, II, 2, 1–10. See Notes I, 8 and 9, on the relations between Sāṃkhya and Buddhism.

tween which no communication is possible. According to Vedānta, this conception is erroneous and the plurality of "selves" is an illusion. In any case, this is a tragic and paradoxical conception of Spirit, which is thus cut off not only from the world of phenomena but also from other liberated "selves." Nevertheless, Sāṃkhya and Yoga were obliged to postulate the multiplicity of *puruṣas;* for if there were but one Spirit, salvation would have been an infinitely simpler problem, the first man who should attain liberation would necessarily bring about that of the entire human race. If there had been but one universal Spirit, the concomitant existence of "liberated spirits" and "bound spirits" would have been impossible. Nor indeed, in such a case, could death, life, difference of sex, diversity in action, etc., have coexisted.[65] The paradox is obvious: this doctrine reduces the infinite variety of phenomena to a single principle, matter (*prakṛti*); it sees the physical universe, life, and consciousness as derived from a single matrix—and yet it postulates the plurality of spirits, although by their nature these are essentially identical. Thus it unites what would appear to be so different—the physical, the biotic, and the mental—and isolates what, especially in India, seems so unique and universal—Spirit.

Let us more closely examine the conception of liberation (*mokṣa*) in the doctrines of Sāṃkhya and Yoga. As it is for most Indian schools of philosophy—except, of course, those influenced by mystical devotion (*bhakti*)—so here, too, liberation is in fact a liberation from the *idea of evil and pain.* It is only a becoming conscious of a situation that was already in existence but over which ignorance had cast its veils. Suffering ceases of itself as soon as we understand that it is *exterior to Spirit,* that it concerns only the human "personality" (*asmitā*). For let us imagine the life of a "liberated" person. He will continue to act, because the potentialities of his earlier lives, and those of his own life before his "awakening," demand their actualization and consummation, in accordance with the karmic law.[66] But this activity is no longer *his;* it is objective, mechanical, disinterested—in short, it is not performed in view of

65 *Sāṃkhya-kārikā,* 18. 66 See above, p. 30.

its "fruit." When the "liberated" man acts, he is not conscious of an "I act" but of an "it acts"; in other words, he does not draw the Self into a psychophysical process. Since the force of ignorance no longer acts, new karmic nucleuses are no longer created. When all these "potentialities" are destroyed, liberation is absolute, final. It could even be said that the "liberated" man does not "experience" liberation. After his "awakening" he acts with indifference, and when the last psychic molecule detaches itself from him, he realizes a mode of being unknown to mortals, because absolute—a sort of Buddhist *nirvāṇa*.

Nevertheless, the "freedom" that the Indian gains through metaphysical knowledge or Yoga is real and concrete. It is not true that India has sought liberation only negatively, for it wishes to attain a positive realization of freedom. In fact, the man "liberated in this life" can extend the sphere of his action as far as he wishes; he has nothing to fear, for his acts no longer have any *consequences* for him and, hence, no *limits*. Since nothing can any longer bind him, the "liberated" man is free to do as he will, in any realm of activity; for he who acts is no longer *he*, as "Self," but a mere impersonal instrument. We shall see in later chapters how far the "situation of mere witness" in a transpersonal existence has been carried.

To us, Sāṃkhya's soteriological conception seems audacious. Starting from the original datum of every Indian philosophy, *suffering*, Sāṃkhya and Yoga, though promising to deliver *man* from suffering, are forced, at the end of their journey, to deny suffering as such, *human suffering*. Considered from the point of view of salvation, this road leads nowhere, since it starts from the axiom that Spirit is absolutely free—that is, not sullied by suffering—and arrives at the same axiom—that is, that the Self is only illusorily drawn into the drama of existence. The only term that matters in this equation—suffering—is left out of account. Sāṃkhya does not *do away* with human suffering; it *denies it as reality* by denying that it can have any real relationship with the Self. Suffering remains, because it is a cosmic fact, but it loses its significance. Suffering is done away with by *ignoring it as suffering*. Certainly, this suppression of suffering is not empirical (narcotics, suicide), for, from the Indian point of view, every empirical solution is illusory, since it is itself a karmic force. But Sāṃkhya's solution drives man outside of humanity, for it can be realized only through the destruction of the human personality. The Yoga practices proposed by Patañjali have the same goal.

These soteriological solutions may appear "pessimistic" to Westerners, for whom personality remains, in the last analysis, the foundation of all morality and all mysticism. But, for India, what matters most is not so much the salvation of the *personality* as obtaining *absolute freedom*. (We shall see later that the deep meaning of this freedom leaves the most extreme Western formulations far behind; what the Indian actually wants is, in a certain sense, to abolish creation by reincorporating all forms in the primordial Unity.) Once it is granted that this freedom cannot be gained in our present human condition and that personality is the vehicle of suffering and drama, it becomes clear that what must be sacrificed is the human condition and the "personality." And this sacrifice is lavishly compensated for by the conquest of absolute freedom, which it makes possible.

It could, obviously, be objected that the sacrifice demanded is too great for its fruits to be of any interest. For, after all, is not the human condition, whose suppression is demanded, man's sole patent of nobility? Sāṃkhya and Yoga answer this probable objection of the Westerner in advance when they affirm: as long as man has not risen above the level of psychomental life, he cannot but misjudge the transcendental "states" that will be the reward for the disappearance of normal consciousness; every value judgment in regard to these "states" is automatically invalidated by the mere fact that he who pronounces it is defined by his own condition, which is of an entirely different order from the condition upon which the value judgment is thought to bear.

Classic Yoga begins where Sāṃkhya leaves off. Patañjali takes over the Sāṃkhya dialectic almost in its entirety, but he does not believe that metaphysical knowledge can, by itself, lead man to final liberation. Gnosis, in his view, only prepares the ground for the acquisition of freedom (*mukti*). Emancipation must, so to speak, be conquered by sheer force, specifically by means of an ascetic technique and a method of contemplation, which, taken together, constitute nothing less than the *yoga-darśana*. The aim of Yoga, as of Sāṃkhya, is to do away with normal consciousness in favor of a qualitatively different consciousness, which can fully comprehend metaphysical truth. Now, for Yoga, this suppression of normal consciousness is not something easily attained. In addition to gnosis, the *darśana*, it also implies a practice (*abhyāsa*), an *ascesis* (*tapas*)—in short, a physiological technique, compared with which the strictly psychological technique is subsidiary.

Patañjali defines Yoga as "the suppression of states of consciousness" (*yogaḥ cittavṛtti-nirodhaḥ*).[67] Hence yogic technique presupposes an experimental knowledge of all the "states" that "agitate" a normal, secular, unilluminated "consciousness." These states of consciousness are limitless in number. But they fall into three categories, respectively corresponding to three possibilities of experience: (1) errors and illusions (dreams, hallucinations; errors in perception, confusions, etc.); (2) the sum total of normal psychological experiences (everything felt, perceived, or thought by the nonadept, by him who does not practice Yoga); (3) the parapsychological experiences brought on by the yogic technique and, of course, accessible only to adepts.

In Patañjali's view, for each of these "classes" (or categories) of experiences there is a corresponding science or group of sciences that furnishes a norm for the experience and, if it goes beyond designated limits, forces it to return within them. The theory of knowledge, for example, together with logic, has the duty of pre-

67 *Yoga-sūtras*, I, 2.

venting errors of the senses and conceptual confusions. "Psychology," law, ethics, have as their object the sum total of the normal man's states of consciousness, which, at the same time, they evaluate and classify. Since, for Yoga and Sāṃkhya, every psychological experience is produced by ignorance of the true nature of the Self (*puruṣa*), it follows that "normal" psychological events, although *real* from a strictly psychological point of view and validated from the point of view of logic (since they are not illusory, as are dreams and hallucinations), are nevertheless *false* from the metaphysical point of view. Thus metaphysics recognizes as valid only a third category of "states," principally those which precede enstasis (*samādhi*) and prepare deliverance.

The purpose of Patañjali's Yoga, then, is to abolish the first two categories of experiences (respectively produced by logical and metaphysical error) and to replace them by an "experience" that is enstatic, suprasensory, and extrarational. By virtue of *samādhi*, the yogin finally passes permanently beyond the human condition —which is dramatic, produced by suffering and consummated in suffering—and at last obtains the total freedom to which the Indian soul so ardently aspires.

Vyāsa [68] classifies the modalities of consciousness (or "mental planes," *citta bhūmi*) as follows: (1) unstable (*kṣipta*); (2) confused, obscure (*mūḍha*); (3) stable and unstable (*vikṣipta*); (4) fixed on a single point (*ekāgra*); (5) completely restrained (*niruddha*). Of these modalities, the first two are common to all men, for, from the Indian point of view, psychomental life is normally confused. The third modality of consciousness, *vikṣipta*, is obtained by fixing the mind "occasionally and provisionally," through the exercise of attention (for example, in an effort of memory or in connection with a mathematical problem, etc.); but it is transitory and is of no help toward liberation, since it was not obtained through Yoga. Only the last two of the modalities enumerated above are yogic "states"—i.e., brought on by *ascesis* and meditation.

68 Ad *Yoga-sūtras*, I, 1.

Vyāsa's analysis [69] continues with the doctrine that every normal consciousness can manifest itself in three different ways, according to which of the three *guṇas* is predominant in it. For man, his life, and his consciousness—together with the entire cosmos—are emanations of one and the same *prakṛti*, emanations that differ in designation only through the predominance in them of one of the three constituent modalities of substance—that is, the *guṇas*. Thus: (1) when *sattva* (purity, illumination through comprehension) predominates, consciousness manifests itself as *prakhyā* (vivacity, illumination; in general, state of mental clarity and serenity); (2) when *rajas* (energy) predominates, consciousness is *pravṛtti*, it is active and energetic, tense and willful; (3) when *tamas* (obscurity, heaviness) predominates, consciousness is *sthiti*, is inert, plunged in a state of repose and torpor. As we see, the immemorial Indian tradition according to which man (the microcosm) is homologous with the macrocosm is preserved intact by Patañjali's Yoga; it alters the tradition only by transposing the homology into the vocabulary of its own "physics," according to which the three *guṇas* are equally present in nature and life on the one hand and in states of consciousness on the other.

Clearly, this classification of the modalities and "dispositions" of consciousness is not made in view of mere knowledge. On the one hand, it sets Yoga "psychology" securely in the universal Indian tradition, in which classifications and homologies are the rule. On the other hand—and this is of greater importance to us—the gradation of states of consciousness in accordance with a hierarchical order is, in itself, a way of dominating them and getting rid of them at will. For, unlike Sāṃkhya, Yoga undertakes to destroy the different groups, species, and varieties of "states of consciousness" (*cittavṛtti*) one after the other. Now, this destruction cannot be accomplished unless one begins by having, as it were, "experimental knowledge" of the structure, origin, and intensity of that which is to be destroyed.

"Experimental knowledge" here means: method, technique,

69 *Yoga-sūtras*, I, 2.

practice. One can gain nothing without acting (*kriyā*) and without practicing asceticism (*tapas*)—this is a leitmotiv of yogic literature. Books II and III of the *Yoga-sūtras* are more particularly devoted to this yogic activity (purifications, bodily attitudes, breathing techniques, etc.).[70] This is why Yoga practice is indispensable. For it is only after having oneself experienced the first results of this technique that one can gain faith (*śraddhā*) in the efficacy of the method.[71] Indeed, Yoga practice demands a long series of exercises, which must be performed successively, without haste, without impatience, without any trace of "individual desire" to obtain "conjunction" (*samādhi*) quickly. Vyāsa[72] remarks in this connection that it is only after having conquered a certain "plane" (*bhūmi*)—that is, after having oneself experienced all the modalities of a certain yogic exercise (meditation, contemplation, etc.)—that one can pass to a higher "plane" (except, of course, for the rare cases in which the yogin, scorning certain lower exercises—reading the thoughts of strangers, etc.—concentrates his thought on God, Īśvara). "As for the nature of the next following [higher] plane," Vyāsa continues, "only Yoga practice can reveal it to us. Why? Because it is said [in the scriptures]: 'Yoga must be known by means of Yoga; Yoga manifests itself through Yoga,' etc."

Denial of the reality of the yogic experience, or criticism of certain of its aspects, is inadmissible from a man who has no direct knowledge of its practice, for yogic states go beyond the condition that circumscribes us when we criticize them. "It is always the mark of a weak, feminine nature to endeavor to establish one's superiority on the issue of a verbal quarrel, whereas it is the sign

70 Action, however, does not mean agitation, effort at any cost. Vācaspatimiśra (ad *Yoga-sūtras*, II, 1; cf. Vijñānabhikṣu, *Yogasāra-saṃgraha*, 42) particularly insists on the following two points: (*a*) that action (*kriyāyoga*) must not be exaggerated, so that physiological equilibrium shall not be disturbed; (*b*) that it must not be performed in view of its "fruits" (in other words, with "thirst," with "passion"); it must arise not from the "human" desire to satisfy appetites and ambitions, but from a *calm* desire to pass beyond the "human."

71 Vyāsa, ad *Yoga-sūtras*, I, 34.

72 Ibid., III, 6.

of a man to desire to conquer the world by the strength of one's own arms," says a text [73] that, though late, expresses a characteristic attitude of the yogic and tantric schools. The term *abhyāsa* ("practice," "exercise," "application") is very frequently employed in the Haṭha-yogic treatises. "Through practice [*abhyāsa*] success is obtained, through practice one gains liberation. Perfect consciousness is gained through practice. Yoga is attained through practice. . . . Death can be cheated of its prey through practice. . . . Through practice one gets the power of *vāc* [prophecy], and the power of going everywhere, through mere exertion of will." [74]

Texts to this purport could be cited indefinitely; all emphasize the necessity for direct experience, for realization, for practice. Patañjali, and after him countless yogic and tantric masters, know that the *cittavṛttis*, the "eddies of consciousness," cannot be controlled and, finally, done away with, unless they are first known "experimentally." In other words, one cannot free oneself from existence (*saṃsāra*) if one does not know life concretely. Herein lies the explanation of the paradoxical teleology of creation, which, according to Sāṃkhya and Yoga, fetters the human soul and at the same time urges it on to liberation. Thus, the human condition, although dramatic, is not desperate, since experiences themselves tend to deliver the spirit (especially by producing disgust with *saṃsāra* and longing for renunciation). Indeed, it is only through *experiences* that freedom is gained. Hence the gods (*videha*, "the disincarnate")—who have no experience because they have no body—are in a condition of existence inferior to the human condition and cannot attain to complete liberation.

The ambivalent function of experiences—which at once "enslave" man and stimulate him to "free" himself—is a concept peculiar to Indian thought. It will reveal more of its metaphysical implications when we come to deal with the "baroque" varieties

73 The *Tantratattva*, tr. in Arthur Avalon, *The Principles of Tantra*, I, 127.

74 *Śiva Saṃhitā*, IV, 9–11; tr. R. B. S. Chandra Vidyarṇava, cited in Theos Bernard, *Haṭha Yoga*, p. 47 n.

of Yoga (tantrism, mystical erotism, etc.). But at this point we can already recognize in Yoga a tendency that is specifically its own, and one that, therefore, we have not encountered in the Sāṃkhya *darśana.* It is a tendency toward the concrete, toward the act, toward experimental verification. Even Patañjali's "classic" Yoga (and still more the other kinds of Yogas) accords the greatest importance to experience—that is, to knowledge of the different states of consciousness. And there is nothing surprising in this, given the aim that Yoga in general pursues—which is to rarefy, to dislocate, and, finally, to do away with these states of consciousness. This tendency toward concrete, experimental knowledge, in view of finally mastering that of which one has, so to speak, taken possession through knowing it, will be carried to its extreme by tantrism.

The Subconscious

Analyzing the "psychic individuality," Patañjali discovers five classes or, rather, five "matrices" producing psychomental states (*cittavṛtti*): ignorance (*avidyā*), the feeling of individuality (*asmitā;* "persona"), passion (*rāga*), disgust (*dveśa*), and love of life, the "will to live" (*abhiniveśa*).[75] We must not think of these as five separate psychic functions; the psychic organism constitutes a whole, but its modes of behavior are many. All the classes of *vṛttis* are "painful" (*kleśa*); hence human experience in its entirety is painful. Only Yoga makes it possible to suspend the *vṛttis* and end suffering.

Thus the yogin must "work with" and "manipulate" these *vṛttis,* which constitute the psychomental stream. Their ontological cause is, of course, ignorance.[76] But, unlike Sāṃkhya, Yoga declares that abolition of metaphysical ignorance is not by itself enough to secure total destruction of the states of consciousness. The reason is that, even if the "eddies" existing at any given

75 *Yoga-sūtras,* II, 3, and Vyāsa's commentary. 76 Ibid., I, 8.

moment were done away with, others would immediately replace them, arising from the immense reserves of latencies in the subconscious. The concept of *vāsanā*, which designates these latencies, is of primary importance in Yoga psychology; in Patañjali's text, the term has the meaning "specific subconscious sensations." The obstacles that these subliminal forces raise on the path of liberation are of two kinds: on the one hand, the *vāsanās* constantly feed the psychomental stream, the infinite series of *cittavṛttis;* on the other hand, and this by reason of their specific (subliminal, "germinal") modality, the *vāsanās* constitute an immense obstacle—for they are in the highest degree elusive, difficult to control and master. By the very fact that their mode of being is that of "potentiality," their own dynamism forces the *vāsanās* to manifest, to "actualize," themselves under the form of acts of consciousness. Thus the yogin—even if he has long years of practice to his credit and has passed through several stages of his ascetic itinerary—is in danger of finding himself defeated by the invasion of a powerful stream of psychomental "eddies" precipitated by the *vāsanās.*

"The *vāsanās* have their origin in memory," Vyāsa writes,[77] thus emphasizing their subliminal nature. Life is a continual discharge of *vāsanās*, which manifest themselves through *vṛttis.* In psychological terms, human existence is a continuous actualization of the subconscious through experiences. The *vāsanās* condition the specific character of each individual; and this conditioning is in accordance both with his heredity and with his karmic situation. Indeed, everything that defines the intransmissible specificity of the individual, as well as the structure of human instincts, is produced by the *vāsanās*, by the subconscious. The subconscious is transmitted either "impersonally," from generation to generation (through language, mores, civilization—ethnic and historical transmission), or directly (through karmic transmigration; we remind the reader in this connection that the karmic potentials are transmitted through an "animic body," *liṅga*, literally "subtle body"). A considerable part of human experience is owing to this

77 Ad *Yoga-sūtras*, IV, 9.

racial and intellectual heritage, to these forms of action and thought which are created by the play of the *vāsanās*. These subconscious forces determine the lives of the majority of men. It is only through Yoga that they can be known, controlled, "burned."

All states of consciousness are "painful" (*kleśa*). This painful modality of the states of consciousness explains their frantic dynamism; one would say that states of consciousness attempt, by their sudden, dazzling, polymorphous, and vibrant appearance, to compensate for their "impurity" (*kliṣṭa* can also be translated "state of sin," "defilement"), their lack of ontological reality (for, as we have seen, they are only the provisional manifestation of cosmic matter). The rapidity with which these "eddies" succeed one another in the consciousness of the noninitiate is consoling. The destiny of matter is to be in continual transformation; and if this never-ceasing and never-resting transformation is "painful" (*kleśa*), it permits man (and even, by exacerbating pain, invites him) to escape from the cosmic circuit.

For what characterizes human consciousness—as well as the entire cosmos—is the continuous circuit established between the different biomental levels. Man's acts (*karma*), instigated by psychomental states (*cittavṛtti*), in their turn instigate other *cittavṛttis*. But these states of consciousness themselves result from the actualization of subliminal latencies, *vāsanās*. Hence the circuit latency-consciousness-acts-latencies, etc. (*vāsanā-vṛtti-karma-vāsanā*, etc.) offers no point at which there is a solution of continuity. And since they are manifestations of cosmic matter (*prakṛti*), all these modalities of "psychic substance" are real and, as such, cannot be destroyed through a simple act of cognition (as, in the example classic in Indian philosophy, the illusion that one is faced by a snake is "destroyed" when, looking more closely, one sees that the "snake" was really a stick). Thus the "burning" of these subliminal states, as it is termed in Yoga, means that the Self (*puruṣa*) detaches itself from the flux of psychic life. In this case, the mental energy—which, being determined by the karmic law and projected by ignorance, until then filled the horizon of consciousness, which it darkened—*also* emerges from the "individual" orbit within which it had operated (*asmitā*, "personality"), and, left to itself, ends by again finding its place in *prakṛti*, in the primordial matrix. The liberation of the man simultaneously "liberates" a fragment of matter, by allowing it to return to the primordial Unity from which it had proceeded. The "circuit of psychic matter" ends by virtue of the yogic technique. In this sense one can say that the yogin contributes, directly and personally, to the repose of matter, to abolishing at least a fragment of the cosmos. We shall later see the profoundly Indian meaning of this collaboration by the yogin in the repose of matter and the restoration of the primordial Unity.

We must add that, according to Patañjali, a consciousness filled with "painful" (*kliṣṭa*, "impure") states cannot also contain states that are "pure" (*akliṣṭa*). Indeed, even should they exist there, they could not manifest themselves, because they would be blocked by the *kliṣṭa* states. It is thus that the Yoga writers explain the solidarity of humanity in evil, in pain—and the resistance that the human condition itself opposes to the message of renunciation. Pain is a universal datum, but few are they who have the courage for renunciation and the strength to travel the road of deliverance to the end, for as long as life is dominated by *kliṣṭas*, every virtue that goes beyond them is immediately blocked, doomed to be abortive. From this longing for states that are isolated, pure (*akliṣṭa*, "pure" not in the moral but in the metaphysical sense), arises the desire for knowledge, and it is through knowledge that the nature of experience is revealed and that *kliṣṭas* can be cast aside as the result of a higher cognitive process (*viveka*, "metaphysical discrimination"). As we shall see further on, for yogic psychology and technique the role of the subconscious (*vāsanā*) is considerable, because it conditions not only a man's actual experience but also his native predispositions, as well as his future voluntary decisions. Hence it is useless to try to change states of consciousness (*cittavṛtti*) as long as the psychomental latencies (*vāsanā*) have not also been controlled and mastered. If the "destruction" of the *cittavṛttis* is to succeed, it is indispensable that the circuit "subconscious-consciousness" be broken. This is what Yoga attempts to attain by the application of a series of techniques, all of which, broadly speaking, aim at annihilating the psychomental flux, undertake to "arrest" it.

Before considering these various techniques, let us note in passing the profundity of the psychological analyses that we owe to Patañjali and his commentators. Long before psychoanalysis, Yoga showed the importance of the role played by the subconscious. Indeed, it is in the dynamism that characterizes the unconscious that Yoga sees the most serious obstacle that the yogin has to overcome. This is because the latencies—as if a strange impulse drove them to self-extinction—*want* to emerge into the light, *want*, by actualizing themselves, to become states of consciousness. The resistance that the subconscious opposes to every act of renunciation and asceticism, to every act that could result in the emancipation of the Self, is, as it were, the token of the fear that the subconscious feels at the mere idea that the mass of as yet unmanifested latencies could fail of their destiny, could be destroyed before having time to manifest and actualize themselves. This thirst for actualization on the part of the *vāsanās* is nevertheless interpenetrated by the thirst for extinction, for "repose," that occurs at all levels of the cosmos. Although the extinction of psychomental latencies that is bound up with their actualization represents only a change in the mode of being of nature, it is none the less true that every *vāsanā* manifested as a state of consciousness *perishes* as such; certainly, other *vāsanās* will replace it; but by actualizing itself *it* has simply ceased to be. The intensity of the biomental circuit arises precisely from the fact that "latencies" and "forms" always tend to cancel themselves. Yet every "appearance" and every "disappearance" within the horizon of life, as within the psychomental horizon, testifies to *refusal of self*, thirst to cease to be what one is. Viewed from this angle, every "form," every "appearance," and every "state"—of whatever kind—that inhabits the universe is driven by the same instinct for liberation by which man is driven. The whole cosmos has the same tendency as man to return to the primordial Unity. When certain forms of Mahāyāna Buddhism speak of the salvation of the entire cosmos, they are thinking of this final return and repose of "things," "beings," and "forms."

We referred above to the similarity between Yoga and psychoanalysis. And in fact the comparison can be made with certain reservations—all of them, by the way, in favor of Yoga. Unlike psychoanalysis, Yoga does not see in the unconscious merely the libido. For, in elucidating the circuit that connects consciousness and the subconscious, it is led to see the subconscious as at once the matrix and the receptacle of all egoistic acts, gestures, and intentions—that is, intentions dominated by the "thirst for fruit" (*phalatṛṣṇā*), by the desire for satisfaction of the self, for satiation, for multiplication. The source of everything that wants to manifest itself—that is, to have a "form," to show its "power," to define its "personality"—is the subconscious; thence they arise, and thither (because of karmic "sowings") they return. Even if this tendency to "form" is, basically, equivalent to the tendency to self-extinction possessed by the latencies (for, as we said above, the actualization of latencies is at the same time their "suicide"), it is none the less true that, from the point of view of pure spirit (*puruṣa*), this tendency to form is egoistic, its aim being "fruit"—that is, a gain.

Differing here, too, from psychoanalysis, Yoga believes that the subconscious can be dominated by asceticism and even conquered through employing the technique for unification of the states of consciousness, which we shall presently discuss. The psychological and parapsychological experience of the East in general, and of Yoga in particular, being incontestably more extensive and better organized than the experience upon which Western theories of the structure of the psyche have been built up, it is probable that, on this point too, Yoga is right and that—paradoxical as it may seem—the subconscious can be known, mastered, and conquered.

Techniques for Autonomy

Concentration "on a Single Point"

THE point of departure of Yoga meditation is concentration on a single object; whether this is a physical object (the space between the eyebrows, the tip of the nose, something luminous, etc.), or a thought (a metaphysical truth), or God (Īśvara) makes no difference. This determined and continuous concentration, called *ekāgratā* ("on a single point"), is obtained by integrating the psychomental flux (*sarvārthatā*, "variously directed, discontinuous, diffused attention").[1] This is precisely the definition of yogic technique: *yogaḥ cittavṛtti-nirodhaḥ*.[2]

The immediate result of *ekāgratā*, concentration on a single point, is prompt and lucid censorship of all the distractions and automatisms that dominate—or, properly speaking, *compose*—profane consciousness. Completely at the mercy of associations (themselves produced by sensations and the *vāsanās*), man passes his days allowing himself to be swept hither and thither by an infinity of disparate moments that are, as it were, external to himself. The senses or the subconscious continually introduce into consciousness objects that dominate and change it, according to their form and intensity. Associations disperse consciousness, passions do it violence, the "thirst for life" betrays it by projecting it

1 *Yoga-sūtras*, III, 11. 2 Ibid., I, 2.

outward. Even in his intellectual efforts, man is passive, for the fate of secular thoughts (controlled not by *ekāgratā* but only by fluctuating moments of concentration, *kṣiptavikṣipta*) is to *be thought* by objects. Under the appearance of thought, there is really an indefinite and disordered flickering, fed by sensations, words, and memory. The first duty of the yogin is to think—that is, not to *let himself* think. This is why Yoga practice begins with *ekāgratā,* which dams the mental stream and thus constitutes a "psychic mass," a solid and unified continuum.

The practice of *ekāgratā* tends to control the two generators of mental fluidity: sense activity (*indriya*) and the activity of the subconscious (*saṃskāra*). Control is the ability to intervene, at will and directly, in the functioning of these two sources of mental "whirlwinds" (*cittavṛtti*). A yogin can obtain discontinuity of consciousness at will; in other words, he can, at any time and any place, bring about concentration of his attention on a "single point" and become insensible to any other sensory or mnemonic stimulus. Through *ekāgratā* one gains a genuine will—that is, the power freely to regulate an important sector of biomental activity. It goes without saying that *ekāgratā* can be obtained only through the practice of numerous exercises and techniques, in which physiology plays a role of primary importance. One cannot obtain *ekāgratā* if, for example, the body is in a tiring or even uncomfortable posture, or if the respiration is disorganized, unrhythmical. This is why, according to Patañjali, yogic technique implies several categories of physiological practices and spiritual exercises (called *aṅgas,* "members"), which one must have learned if one seeks to obtain *ekāgratā* and, ultimately, the highest concentration, *samādhi.* These "members" of Yoga can be regarded both as forming a group of techniques and as being stages of the mental ascetic itinerary whose end is final liberation. They are: (1) restraints (*yama*); (2) disciplines (*niyama*); (3) bodily attitudes and postures (*āsana*); (4) rhythm of respiration (*prāṇāyāma*); (5) emancipation of sensory activity from the domination of exterior objects (*pratyā-*

hāra); (6) concentration (*dhāraṇā*); (7) yogic meditation (*dhyāna*); (8) *samādhi*.[3]

Each class (*aṅga*) of practices and disciplines has a definite purpose. Patañjali hierarchizes these "members of Yoga" in such a way that the yogin cannot omit any of them, except in certain cases. The first two groups, *yama* and *niyama*, obviously constitute the necessary preliminaries for any type of asceticism, hence there is nothing specifically yogic in them. The restraints (*yama*) purify from certain sins that all systems of morality disapprove but that social life tolerates. Now, the moral law can no longer be infringed here—as it is in secular life—without immediate danger to the seeker for deliverance. In Yoga, every sin produces its consequences immediately. Vyāsa [4] gives some interesting explanations on the subject of these five restraints (*ahiṃsā*, "not to kill"; *satya*, "not to lie"; *asteya*, "not to steal"; *brahmacarya*, "sexual abstinence"; *aparigraha*, "not to be avaricious"). "*Ahiṃsā* means not to cause pain to any creature, by any means or at any time. The restraints [*yama*] and the disciplines [*niyama*] that follow have their roots in *ahiṃsā* and tend to perfect *ahiṃsā*. . . . Veracity [*satya*] consists in according one's speech and thought with one's acts. Speech and thought correspond to what one has seen, heard, or deduced. One speaks in order to communicate knowledge. One cannot say that one has used speech for the good of another, and not for his harm, unless it has not been deceitful, confused, and sterile. If, however, it proves to have been harmful to creatures, even though spoken without deceit, confusion, or sterility, it is not the truth; it is only a sin. . . . Thus, everyone should reflect with great attention, and only then utter the truth, for the good of all creatures. . . . Stealing [*steya*] is illegally appropriating things that belong to another. Abstention from stealing [*asteya*] consists in destroying the desire to steal. *Brahmacarya* is restraining the

3 Ibid., II, 29. It is with this *sūtra* that Patañjali begins his exposition of Yoga technique, which he continues in Book III.

4 Ad *Yoga-sūtras*, II, 30.

secret forces [that is, the generative force: *brahmacaryam guptendriyasyopasthasya samyamaḥ*]. Absence of avarice [*aparigraha*] is the nonappropriation of things that do not belong to one and it is a consequence of one's comprehension of the sin that consists in being attached to possessions, and of the harm produced by the accumulation, preservation, or destruction of possessions."

These restraints can be recognized by all systems of ethics and realized by an apprentice yogin as well as by any pure and upright man. Their practice does not result in a specifically yogic state, but in a "purified" human state, higher than that of common humanity. This purity is necessary for the later stages. Through it, one suppresses one's egoistic tendencies; through it, one creates new centers of experience. Sexual abstinence is practiced to the end of conserving nervous energy. Yoga attaches the greatest importance to these "secret forces of the generative faculty," which, when they are expended, dissipate the most precious energy, debilitate mental capacity, and make concentration difficult; if, on the contrary, they are mastered and "restrained," they further contemplative ascent. It should, however, be added that sexual abstinence (*brahmacarya*) is not only refraining from sexual acts but "burning" carnal temptation itself. The instinct must not remain underground, diffused through the subconscious, or be "sublimated" as with the mystics, but simply destroyed, "rooted out" from consciousness and the senses.

Together with these restraints, the yogin must practice the *niyamas*—that is, a series of bodily and psychic "disciplines." "Cleanliness, serenity [*saṃtoṣa*], asceticism [*tapas*], the study of Yoga metaphysics, and the effort to make God [Īśvara] [5] the motive of all one's actions constitute the disciplines." [6] Cleanliness (*śauca*) means internal purification of the organs; thus alimentary residues and toxins are promptly eliminated. (This is obtained by

5 As Surendranath Dasgupta remarks (*Yoga as Philosophy and Religion*, pp. 87 ff.), only the late commentators—such as Vācaspatimiśra and Vijñānabhikṣu—believe that Īśvara removes the barriers created by *prakṛti*, barriers that are powerful obstacles on the yogin's path.

6 *Yoga-sūtras*, II, 32.

a series of artificial "purgations," which are especially emphasized by Haṭha Yoga—that is, the Yoga concerned almost exclusively with physiology and "subtle physiology.") Vyāsa adds that *śauca* also implies ridding oneself of mental impurities. "Absence of the desire to increase the necessities of life"—such is the definition of serenity (*saṃtoṣa*). "*Tapas* [asceticism] consists in bearing the 'pairs of opposites,' as, for example, the desire to eat and the desire to drink; heat and cold; the desire to remain standing and the desire to remain seated; the absence of words [*kāṣṭha mauna*] and the absence of gestures that could reveal one's feelings or thoughts [*ākāra mauna;* Vācaspatimiśra adds that "the absence of facial indications, by which the inner secrets of the mind are revealed, constitutes control over oneself, so that thought is not communicated by chance and to anyone at random"]. Study is knowledge of the sciences that relate to deliverance from existence [*mokṣa*], or repetition of the syllable *OṂ*,[7] etc." [8]

Obviously, even in the course of these exercises (which are, on the whole, ethical in nature and, in general, have no yogic structure), difficulties arise, most of them produced by the subconscious. The trouble arising from doubt is the most dangerous of the obstacles that bar the road of concentration. To overcome it, Patañjali recommends [9] implanting the contrary thought: "for (avoiding or dismissing) trouble from doubt, establishment of the opposites" (*vitarkabādhane pratipakṣabhāvanam:* some translators take *vitarka* to mean "guilty thoughts" and translate: "in order to avoid the trouble arising from guilty thoughts"; in fact, *vitarka* means "doubt, uncertainty," and Patañjali is evidently referring to the "temptation by doubt" that all ascetic treatises recognize and

7 The mystical syllable *OṂ* incarnates the mystical essence of the entire cosmos. It is nothing less than the theophany itself, reduced to the state of a phoneme (see below, p. 123). Speculations on the syllable *OṂ* are endless. It is nevertheless curious to note that Vyāsa homologizes *knowledge* of the sciences of salvation with a mystical *technique,* since the only requirement here is to repeat the syllable *OṂ*, without attempting any speculation concerning it.

8 Vyāsa, ad *Yoga-sūtras,* II, 32.

9 *Yoga-sūtras,* II, 33.

combat). In his commentary Vyāsa suggests certain thoughts to be actualized and produced at a moment of uncertainty. In the following *sūtra*,[10] Patañjali explains the nature of these "doubts" or "vices."[11] It is interesting to note, here and now, that the yogin's struggle against any of these "obstacles" is magical in character. Every temptation that he conquers is equivalent to a force that he appropriates. Such forces are obviously not moral; they are magical forces. To renounce a temptation is not only to "purify" oneself in the negative sense of the word; it is also to realize a true and positive gain; the yogin thereby extends his power over that which he had begun by renouncing. Even more: he reaches the point of *mastering* not only the objects that he had renounced, but also a magical force infinitely more precious than all objects as such. For example, he who realizes the restraint *asteya* (not to steal) "sees all jewels come to him."[12] We shall have occasion to return to this "magical power" (*siddhi*) that the yogin acquires through his discipline. To be sure, he is urged to renounce even this magical power, as he has renounced the human passions in exchange for which the particular power has been granted him. The concept of this almost physical equilibrium between renunciation and the magical fruits of renunciation is remarkable.

Physical purification, says Patañjali, produces a new and welcome feeling: disgust with one's own body, and cessation of contact with other bodies.[13] Through psychic purification one obtains *ekāgratā*—that is, authority over the senses and ability to know the soul.[14] Self-content, sobriety, give an "inexpressible happiness";[15] and asceticism *sensu stricto* (*tapas*, physical effort utilized as a means of purification) removes impurities and establishes a new power over the senses—that is, the possibility of passing beyond their limits (clairvoyance, clairaudience, mind reading, etc.) or of suppressing them at will.[16]

10 *Yoga-sūtras*, II, 34.
11 See Note II, 1, on the obstacles to yogic concentration.
12 *Yoga-sūtras*, II, 37. 13 Ibid., II, 40. 14 Ibid., II, 41.
15 Ibid., II, 42. 16 Vyāsa, ad II, 43.

Yogic Postures (āsana) *and Respiratory Discipline* (prāṇāyāma)

It is only with the third "member of Yoga" (*yogāṅga*) that yogic technique, properly speaking, begins. This third "member" is *āsana*, a word designating the well-known yogic posture that the *Yoga-sūtras* (II, 46) define as *sthirasukham*, "stable and agreeable." *Āsana* is described in numerous Haṭha Yoga treatises; Patañjali defines it only in outline, for *āsana* is learned from a *guru* and not from descriptions. The important thing is that *āsana* gives the body a stable rigidity, at the same time reducing physical effort to a minimum. Thus, one avoids the irritating feeling of fatigue, of enervation in certain parts of the body, one regulates the physical processes, and so allows the attention to devote itself solely to the fluid part of consciousness. At first an *āsana* is uncomfortable and even unbearable. But after some practice, the effort of maintaining the body in the same position becomes inconsiderable. Now (and this is of the highest importance), effort must disappear, the position of meditation must become natural; only then does it further concentration. "Posture becomes perfect when the effort to attain it disappears, so that there are no more movements in the body. In the same way, its perfection is achieved when the mind is transformed into infinity [*anantasamāpattibhyām*]—that is, when it makes the idea of its infinity its own content." [17] And Vācaspatimiśra, commenting on Vyāsa's interpretation, writes: "He who practices *āsana* must employ an effort that consists in suppressing the natural efforts of the body. Otherwise this kind of ascetic posture cannot be realized." As for "the mind transformed into infinity," this means a complete suspension of attention to the presence of one's own body.

Āsana is one of the characteristic techniques of Indian asceticism. It is found in the Upaniṣads and even in Vedic literature, but allusions to it are more numerous in the *Mahābhārata* and in the

17 Ibid., II, 47.

Purāṇas. Naturally, it is in the literature of Haṭha Yoga that the *āsanas* play an increasingly important part; the *Gheraṇḍa Saṃhitā* describes thirty-two varieties of them. Here, for example, is how one assumes one of the easiest and most common of the meditational positions, the *padmāsana*: "Place the right foot on the left thigh and similarly the left one on the right thigh, also cross the hands behind the back and firmly catch the great toes of the feet so crossed (the right hand on the right great toe and the left hand on the left). Place the chin on the chest and fix the gaze on the tip of the nose." [18] Lists and descriptions of *āsanas* are to be found in most of the tantric and Haṭha-yogic treatises.[19] The purpose of these meditational positions is always the same: "absolute cessation of trouble from the pairs of opposites" (*dvandvānabhighātaḥ*).[20] In this way one realizes a certain "neutrality" of the senses; consciousness is no longer troubled by the "presence of the body." One realizes the first stage toward isolation of consciousness; the bridges that permit communication with sensory activity begin to be raised.

Āsana is distinctly a sign of transcending the human condition. Whether this "arrest," this invulnerability in respect to the pairs of opposites, to the external world, represents a regression to the vegetable condition or a transcendence toward the divine archetype, iconographically formulated, is a question that we shall examine later. For the moment, we shall note only that *āsana* is the first concrete step taken for the purpose of abolishing the modalities of human existence. What is certain is that the motionless, hieratic position of the body imitates some other condition than the human; the yogin in the state of *āsana* can be homologized with a plant or a sacred statue; under no circumstances can he be homologized with man qua man, who, by definition, is mobile, agitated, unrhythmic. On the plane of the "body," *āsana* is an *ekāgratā*, a concentration on a single point; the body is "tensed," concentrated in a

18 *Gheraṇḍa Saṃhitā*, II, 8; tr. S. Chandra Vasu, cited in Bernard, *Haṭha Yoga*, p. 10, n. 12.

19 See Note II, 2.

20 *Yoga-sūtras*, II, 48.

single position. Just as *ekāgratā* puts an end to the fluctuation and dispersion of the states of consciousness, so *āsana* puts an end to the mobility and disposability of the body, by reducing the infinity of possible positions to a single archetypal, iconographic posture. We shall soon see that the tendency toward "unification" and "totalization" is a feature of all yogic techniques. The profound meaning of these "unifications" will become clear to us a little later. But their immediate purpose is even now obvious; it is to abolish (or to transcend) the human condition by a refusal to conform to the most elementary human inclinations. Refusal to move (*āsana*), to let oneself be carried along on the rushing stream of states of consciousness (*ekāgratā*), will be continued by a long series of refusals of every kind.

The most important—and, certainly, the most specifically yogic —of these various refusals is the disciplining of respiration (*prāṇāyāma*)—in other words, the "refusal" to breathe like the majority of mankind, that is, nonrhythmically. Patañjali defines this refusal as follows: "*Prāṇāyāma* is the arrest [*viccheda*] of the movements of inhalation and exhalation [*śvāsapraśvāsayoḥ*] and it is obtained after *āsana* has been realized." [21] Patañjali speaks of the "arrest," the suspension, of respiration; however, *prāṇāyāma* begins with making the respiratory rhythm as slow as possible; and this is its first objective. There are a number of texts that treat of this Indian ascetic technique, but most of them do no more than repeat the traditional formulas. Although *prāṇāyāma* is a specifically yogic exercise, and one of great importance, Patañjali devotes only three *sūtras* to it. He is primarily concerned with the theoretical bases of ascetic practices; technical details are found in the commentaries by Vyāsa, Bhoja, and Vācaspatimiśra, but especially in the Haṭha-yogic treatises.

A remark of Bhoja's [22] reveals the deeper meaning of *prāṇāyāma:* "All the functions of the organs being preceded by that of respiration—there being always a connection between respiration and consciousness in their respective functions—respiration, when all

21 Ibid., II, 49. 22 Ad *Yoga-sūtras*, I, 34.

the functions of the organs are suspended, realizes concentration of consciousness on a single object." The statement that a connection always exists between respiration and mental states seems to us highly important. It contains far more than mere observation of the bare fact that, for example, the respiration of a man in anger is agitated, while that of one who is concentrating (even if only provisionally and without any yogic purpose) becomes rhythmical and automatically slows down, etc. The relation connecting the rhythm of respiration with the states of consciousness mentioned by Bhoja, which has undoubtedly been observed and experienced by yogins from the earliest times—this relation has served them as an instrument for "unifying" consciousness. The "unification" here under consideration must be understood in the sense that, by making his respiration rhythmical and progressively slower, the yogin can "penetrate"—that is, he can experience, in perfect lucidity—certain states of consciousness that are inaccessible in a waking condition, particularly the states of consciousness that are peculiar to sleep.[23] For there is no doubt that the respiratory rhythm of a man asleep is slower than that of a man awake. By reaching this rhythm of sleep through the practice of *prāṇāyāma*, the yogin, without renouncing his lucidity, penetrates the states of consciousness that accompany sleep.

The Indian ascetics recognize four modalities of consciousness (besides the enstatic "state"): diurnal consciousness, consciousness in sleep with dreams, consciousness in sleep without dreams, and "cataleptic consciousness." By means of *prāṇāyāma*—that is, by increasingly prolonging inhalation and exhalation (the goal of this practice being to allow as long an interval as possible to pass between the two moments of respiration)—the yogin can, then, penetrate all the modalities of consciousness. For the noninitiate, there is discontinuity between these several modalities; thus he passes from the state of waking to the state of sleep unconsciously.

23 This is why the novice in *prāṇāyāma* almost always falls asleep as soon as he has succeeded in reducing his respiratory rhythm to that characteristic of the state of sleep.

The yogin must preserve continuity of consciousness—that is, he must penetrate each of these states with determination and lucidity.[24]

But experience of the four modalities of consciousness (to which a particular respiratory rhythm naturally corresponds), together with *unification* of consciousness (resulting from the yogin's getting rid of the discontinuity between these four modalities), can only be realized after long practice. The immediate goal of *prāṇāyāma* is more modest. Through it one first of all acquires a "continuous consciousness," which alone can make yogic meditation possible. The respiration of the ordinary man is generally arhythmic; it varies in accordance with external circumstances or with mental tension. This irregularity produces a dangerous psychic fluidity, with consequent instability and diffusion of attention. One can become attentive by making an effort to do so. But, for Yoga,

24 In the Himālayan *āśrams* of Hardwār, Rishikesh, and Svargashram, where we stayed from September, 1930, to March, 1931, numerous *sannyāsis* admitted to us that the goal of *prāṇāyāma* was to make the practitioner enter the state called *turīya*, the "cataleptic" state. We ourselves observed several *sannyāsis* who spent a great part of the day and night in a profound "meditation" in which their respiration was hardly perceptible. There is no doubt but that "cataleptic" states can be brought on at will by experienced yogins. Dr. Thérèse Brosse's mission to India (see Charles Laubry and Thérèse Brosse, "Documents recueillis aux Indes sur les 'yogins' par l'enregistrement simultané du pouls, de la respiration et de l'électrocardiogramme," *Presse médicale*, LXXXIII [Oct. 14, 1936]) showed that the reduction of respiration and of cardiac contraction to a degree that is usually observed only immediately before death is a genuine physiological phenomenon, which the yogins can realize by force of will and not as the result of autosuggestion. It goes without saying that such a yogin can be buried without any danger. "The restriction of respiration is sometimes so great that some [yogins] can allow themselves to be buried alive for a specified time, retaining a volume of air that would be completely inadequate to assure their survival. According to them, this small reserve of air is necessary in case an accident should bring them out of their yogic state during the experiment and put them in danger; it would allow them to make a few inhalations, by which they could return to their yogic state" (Jean Filliozat, *Magie et médecine*, pp. 115–16). Cf. id., review of *Daśopanishads*, ed. Kunhan Rāja, *Journal asiatique*, CCXXVIII (1937), 522.

effort is an exteriorization. Respiration must be made rhythmical, if not in such a way that it can be "forgotten" entirely, at least in such a way that it no longer troubles us by its discontinuity. Hence, through *prāṇāyāma*, one attempts to do away with the effort of respiration; rhythmic breathing must become something so automatic that the yogin can forget it.

Through *prāṇāyāma* the yogin seeks to attain direct knowledge of the pulsation of his own life, the organic energy discharged by inhalation and exhalation. *Prāṇāyāma*, we should say, is an attention directed upon one's organic life, a knowledge through action, a calm and lucid entrance into the very essence of life. Yoga counsels its disciples to live, but not to abandon themselves to life. The activities of the senses possess man, corrupt and disintegrate him. In the first days of practice, concentration on the vital function of respiration produces an inexpressible sensation of harmony, a rhythmic and melodic plenitude, a leveling of all physiological unevennesses. Later it brings an obscure feeling of presence in one's own body, a calm consciousness of one's own greatness. Obviously, these are simple data, accessible to everyone, experienced by all who attempt this preliminary discipline of respiration. Professor Stcherbatsky [25] writes that, according to O. Rosenberg, who tried certain yogic exercises in a Japanese monastery, this agreeable sensation could be compared "to music, especially when one plays it oneself."

Rhythmic respiration is obtained by harmonizing the three "moments": inhalation (*pūraka*), exhalation (*recaka*), and retention of the inhaled air (*kumbhaka*). These three moments must each fill an equal space of time. Through practice the yogin becomes able to prolong them considerably, for the goal of *prāṇāyāma* is, as Patañjali says, to suspend respiration as long as possible; one arrives at this by progressively retarding the rhythm.

The unit of measurement for the duration of respiration is a *mātrāprāmāṇa*. According to the *Skanda Purāṇa*, a *mātrā* is equal to the time necessary for one respiration (*ekaśvāsamapi mātrāprā-*

25 *Nirvāṇa*, p. 15, n. 2.

ṇāyāme nigadyate). The *Yogacintāmaṇi* adds that this respiration refers to that of sleep, which is equal to 2½ *palas* (a *pala* designating the time of a wink). In the practice of *prāṇāyāma* the *mātrā-pramāṇa* is used as the unit of measure—that is, one progressively retards each "moment" of respiration until, beginning with one *mātrā*, one reaches twenty-four. The yogin measures these *mātrās* either by mentally repeating the mystical syllable *OṂ* as often as necessary, or by moving the fingers of the left hand one after the other.[26]

Excursus: Prāṇāyāma *in Extra-Indian Asceticism*

Rhythmic breathing and holding the breath occur among the techniques of "mystical physiology" studied by Henri Maspéro in his essay "Les Procédés de 'Nourrir le principe vital' dans la religion taoïste ancienne";[27] it is there termed "embryonic respiration," *t'ai-chi*. The principal goal of this respiratory exercise is acquiring long life (*ch'ang shen*), which the Taoists conceive "as a material immortality of the body itself."[28] Unlike *prāṇāyāma*, then, "embryonic respiration" is neither an exercise preliminary to meditation nor an auxiliary exercise. It is self-sufficient. "Embryonic respiration" does not serve, as does *prāṇāyāma*, to prepare for spiritual concentration, for penetration into zones normally inaccessible to consciousness; instead, it accomplishes a process of "mystical physiology" in consequence of which the life of the body is indefinitely prolonged. In this, Taoism suggests Haṭha Yoga, which it resembles to a certain extent, just as some erotic practices employed in it (retention of semen) recall tantrism.[29] But the constant and primary preoccupation of China remains indefinite prolongation of the life of the material body, whereas India is obsessed by the idea of a spiritual freedom to be conquered through transfiguration, "deification," of the body.

We will cite some Taoist texts dealing with the technique of respiration. "One must withdraw to a retired chamber, shut the doors, seat oneself on a bed with a soft cover and a pillow two and a half inches high, lie

26 Cf. Rājendralāla Mitra, *Yoga Aphorisms*, pp. 42–43n. Cf. Dasgupta, *Yoga as Philosophy*, pp. 145–47; Richard Roesel, *Die psychologischen Grundlagen der Yogapraxis*, pp. 32–36, etc.

27 *Journal asiatique*, CCXXVIII (1937), 177–252, 353–430.

28 Maspéro, p. 178.

29 See below, p. 253.

down, with the body in the right position, close the eyes, and keep the breath shut in the diaphragm of the chest so that a hair laid on the nose and mouth will not move" (*Chen chong chi*).[30] A writer of the end of the sixth century, Li Ch'ien-ch'eng, gives the following directions: "Lie with the eyes shut and the hands closed, keep the breath shut up inside to 200, then expel it from inside the mouth." [31] This holding the breath is the essential thing. After long practice, one can reach the point of holding the breath during the time of 3, 5, 7, 9 respirations, then of 12, 120, etc. To become immortal, one must hold the breath for the time required for 1000 respirations.

The technique of "inner breathing"—that is, the form of respiration termed "embryonic"—is far more difficult. Since this breathing is purely internal, it is no longer a mere matter of checking respiration, as the early Taoists did. The following text is central: "Each time that, having absorbed the breath, one has leisure remaining, one must choose a quiet room where no one lives, loosen the hair, unfasten the clothes, and lie down, with the body in the right position, stretch out the feet and hands, not close (the hands), have a clean mat, the sides of which hang to the ground. . . . Then harmonize the breaths . . . when the breaths have (each) found their place (=the internal organ that respectively corresponds to each breath), swallow (the breath). Then shut in the breath until it becomes intolerable. Darken the heart [32] so that it does not think; let the breath go where it will and, when the breath is intolerable, open the mouth and let it out; when the breath has just escaped, respiration is rapid; harmonize the breaths; after seven or eight breaths, it rapidly becomes quieter. Then begin to melt the breath again in the same way. If one has time left over, stop after ten meltings. . . . Melting the breath cannot be done every day; every ten days, or every five days, if one has leisure, or if one feels that there is not communication everywhere, if the four limbs feel an intolerable heat, then do it." [33]

Some of the results to which this "embryonic breathing" leads resemble the yogic "powers" (*siddhi*). "One can then enter water (without drowning) or walk on fire (without being burned)," declares the celebrated treatise *Effective and Secret Oral Formula Concerning Several Methods of Absorbing the Breath*.[34]

30 After Maspéro, p. 203. 31 Ibid.

32 For the Chinese, the heart is the organ of thought.

33 After Maspéro, pp. 220–21. 34 Ibid., p. 229.

Holding the breath is practiced especially to cure certain maladies.[35] "One harmonizes the breath, then swallows it and holds it as long as possible; one meditates on the affected part, by thought one pours the breath upon it and by thought makes the breath fight the malady by attempting to force its way through the obstructed passage. When the breath is exhausted, one expels it, then begins again from twenty to fifty times; one stops when one sees sweat running over the affected part. One repeats the procedure daily at midnight or at the fifth watch, until a cure is effected." [36]

In neo-Taoistic practice the role of thought becomes more important. Ssŭ-ma Ch'eng-cheng writes in his "Discourse": "Those who absorb the breaths . . . must follow them by thought when they enter their viscera, so that the humors (of the viscera) shall be penetrated (by the breaths), each (breath) conformably with the (inner organ) over which it presides, and thus they can circulate through the whole body and cure all sicknesses." [37]

It is probable that, at least in its neo-Taoistic form, this discipline of the breaths was influenced by tantric Yoga; certain simultaneously respiratory and sexual practices reached China as early as the seventh century of our era.[38] Dr. Jean Filliozat definitely concludes in favor of a borrowing from India: "Taoism could not borrow a notion of the physiological role of the breath in this systematized form from ancient Chinese medicine, for ancient Chinese medicine includes no such notion." [39] On the other hand, there were in China certain archaic techniques, shamanic in structure, the purpose of which was to imitate the respiration of animals.[40] The "deep and silent" breathing of *ecstasy* resembled the respiration of animals during *hibernation*, and it is well known that the spontaneity and fullness of animal life was, for the Chinese, the pre-eminent example of an existence in perfect harmony with the cosmos. Marcel Granet [41] admirably synthesizes the simultaneously organic and spiritual function of this embryonic respiration, characteristic both of organic completeness and of ecstasy: "He who would avoid passion and vertigo must learn to breathe not from the throat alone, but with the whole body, from the heels up.

35 Ibid., p. 363 f.
36 Ibid., p. 364.
37 Ibid., p. 369.
38 See below, p. 415.
39 "Taoïsme et Yoga," *Dân Viêt-nam*, III (Aug., 1949), 120.
40 See M. Eliade, *Shamanism*, pp. 459 ff.
41 *La Pensée chinoise*, pp. 514–15.

Only this deep and silent breathing refines and enriches [man's] substance. It is, moreover, the respiration that establishes itself during both *hibernation* and *ecstasy*. By breathing with the neck . . . stretched, one succeeds, if I may so express it, in laminating the breath and quintessentializing its vivifying power. The supreme goal is to establish a kind of *inner circulation* of the vital principles, of such a nature that the individual can remain *perfectly impervious* and undergo the ordeal of immersion without harm. One becomes *impermeable*, autonomous, *invulnerable*, once one is in possession of the art of feeding and breathing in a closed circuit, as the *embryo* does." It is possible, then, that Indian influences reached the neo-Taoist groups who saw their ancestry not in Chinese scientific medicine but in the autochthonous "mystical" tradition; now, this tradition still preserved the immemorial nostalgia for the bliss and spontaneity of animals. In any case, Lao Tzŭ [42] and Chuang Tzŭ [43] were already familiar with "methodical respiration," and a Chou dynasty inscription attests the practice of a respiratory technique in the sixth century B.C.[44]

Respiratory technique is also employed by Islamic mysticism.[45] Whatever the case may be in regard to the *origin* [46] of this respiratory technique within the Islamic tradition, there is no doubt that certain Moslem mystics of India borrowed and practiced yogic exercises. (One of them, Prince Muḥammad Dārā Shikoh, even attempted a synthesis of Indian

42 *Tao Tê Ching*, VI. 43 *Chuang Tzŭ*, XV.

44 Hellmut Wilhelm, "Eine Chou-Inschrift über Atemtechnik," *Monumenta serica*, XIII (1948), 385–88. See also Arthur Waley, *The Way and Its Power*, pp. 44, 116 ff.; Chung-yuan Chang, "An Introduction to Taoist Yoga," *The Review of Religion*, XXI (1956), 131–48.

45 Cf. I. Goldziher, *Vorlesungen über den Islam*, p. 164; M. M. Moreno, "Mistica musulmana e mistica indiana," *Annali Lateranensi*, X (1946), 102–212, especially pp. 140 ff.; and particularly L. Gardet, "La Mention du nom divin (*dhikr*) dans la mystique musulmane," *Revue Thomiste*, LII (1952), 642–79; LIII (1953), 197–216, a study that we use below, pp. 217 ff.

46 Some writers—notably Max Horten, *Indische Strömungen in der islamischen Mystik*—have maintained that Ṣūfism received a strong Indian influence. Louis Massignon had already demonstrated the exaggeration of this thesis (*Essai sur les origines du lexique technique de la mystique musulmane*, pp. 63–80), and M. Moreno has recently arrived at negative results concerning the importance of the Indian contribution to the Islamic mystical tradition ("Mistica musulmana," pp. 210 ff.). But the more circumscribed problem of the origin of Moslem respiratory technique remains open.

and Islamic mysticism.)[47] The technique of *dhikr* sometimes bears striking formal resemblances to the Indian discipline of respiration. T. P. Hughes[48] mentions a monk living on the Afghan frontier of whom it was said that he had practiced *dhikr* so intensively that he was able to suspend his respiration for nearly three hours.[49]

An interesting problem is raised by Hesychasm. Some of the ascetic preliminaries and methods of prayer employed by the Hesychastic monks offer points of resemblance with yogic techniques, especially with *prāṇāyāma*. Father Irénée Hausherr thus summarizes the essentials of Hesychastic prayer: "It comprises a twofold exercise, omphaloskepsis and indefinite repetition of the Prayer of Jesus: 'Lord Jesus Christ, Son of God, have mercy on me!' By sitting in darkness, bowing the head, fixing the eyes on the center of the abdomen (in other words, the navel), trying to discover the place of the heart, by repeating this exercise indefatigably and always accompanying it with the same invocation, in harmony with the rhythm of respiration, which is retarded as much as possible, one will, if one perseveres day and night in this mental prayer, end by finding what one sought, the place of the heart, and, with it and in it, all kinds of wonders and knowledge."[50]

Here is a short passage, recently translated by Jean Gouillard,[51] from Nicephorus the Solitary[52] (second half of the thirteenth century): "As for you, as I have instructed you, sit down, compose your mind, introduce it —your mind, I say—into your nostrils; this is the road that the breath takes to reach the heart. Push it, force it to descend into your heart at the same time as the inhaled air. When it is there, you will see what joy will follow; you will have nothing to regret. As the man who returns home after an absence cannot contain his joy at again being with his wife and children, so the mind, when it is united with the soul, overflows with joy and ineffable delights. Therefore, my brother, accustom your mind not to hasten to depart from thence. At first, it has no zeal—that is the least that

47 Cf. M. Mahfuz-ul-Haq, ed., *Majma 'ul-Baḥrain; or, The Mingling of the Two Oceans.*

48 *Dictionary of Islam*, pp. 703 ff.

49 On *dhikr*, see below, p. 216.

50 *La Méthode d'oraison hésychaste*, p. 102.

51 *Petite Philocalie de la prière du cœur*, p. 204.

52 "The earliest datable witness for the Prayer of Jesus in combination with a respiratory technique" (Gouillard, p. 185).

can be said—for this enclosure and confinement within. But once it has contracted the habit, it will find no more pleasure in wanderings without. For 'the kingdom of God is within us,' and to him who turns his gaze upon it and pursues it with pure prayer, all the outer world becomes vile and contemptible."

In the eighteenth century the doctrines and techniques of Hesychasm were still familiar to the monks of Athos. The following extracts are from the *Encheiridion* of Nicodemus the Hagiorite. "Beginners must accustom themselves to performing this return of the mind as the divine Fasting Fathers have taught, bowing the head and pressing the beard against the upper part of the chest." [53] "*Why the breath must be held during prayer.* Since your mind or the act of your mind is from childhood accustomed to disperse and scatter itself among the sensible things of the outer world, therefore, when you say this prayer, breathe not constantly, after the habit of nature, but hold your breath a little until the inner word has once spoken the prayer, and then breathe, as the divine Fathers have taught. Because through this momentary holding of the breath, the heart becomes ill at ease and straitened and hence feels a pain, not receiving the air that its nature requires; and the mind, for its part, by this method, more easily collects itself and returns toward the heart. . . . Because through this momentary holding of the breath the hard and tough heart becomes thin, and the humidity of the heart, being properly compressed and warmed, becomes tender, sensitive, humble, and more disposed to compunction and to shedding tears freely. . . . Because during this short holding [of the breath] the heart feels uneasiness and pain, and through this uneasiness and this pain, it vomits the poisoned hook of pleasure and sin that it had swallowed." [54]

Finally, we must cite the fundamental treatise, the *Method of Holy Prayer and Attention*, long attributed to Simeon the New Theologian; "the little work may well be contemporary with that of Nicephorus, if it is not by Nicephorus himself, as I. Hausherr not improbably conjectures." [55] Father Hausherr had published an edition and translation of it in his "La Méthode d'oraison hésychaste." We cite it after the more recent translation by Gouillard: "Then seat yourself in a quiet cell, apart in a corner, and apply yourself to doing as I shall say: close the door, raise your mind above any vain or transitory object. Then, pressing your beard

53 After Hausherr, p. 107. 54 Ibid., p. 109. 55 Gouillard, p. 206.

against your chest, direct the eye of the body and with it all your mind upon the center of your belly—that is, upon your navel—compress the inspiration of air passing through the nose so that you do not breathe easily, and mentally examine the interior of your entrails in search of the place of the heart, where all the powers of the soul delight to linger. In the beginning, you will find darkness and a stubborn opacity, but if you persevere, if you practice this exercise day and night, you will find—O wonder!—a boundless felicity."[56] Finally, other Hesychastic texts could be cited—for example, Gregory of Sinai (1255–1346), some important passages from whose writings are given in Gouillard's *Petite Philocalie.*[57] The apology for Hesychasm by Gregory Palamas (*c.* 1296–1359), "the last great name in Byzantine theology," can be consulted with interest.[58]

But we must not be deceived by these external analogies with *prāṇāyāma*. Among the Hesychasts respiratory discipline and bodily posture are used to prepare mental prayer; in the *Yoga-sūtras* these exercises pursue unification of consciousness and preparation for meditation, and the role of God (Īśvara) is comparatively small. But it is none the less true that the two techniques are phenomenologically similar enough to raise the question of a possible influence of Indian mystical physiology on Hesychasm. We shall not enter upon this comparative study here.[59]

56 Ibid., p. 216.

57 On the ascetic "positions" during prayer, p. 248; on holding the breath, p. 249.

58 See some extracts in Gouillard, pp. 269–85.

59 On Hesychasm, see K. Holl, *Enthusiasmus und Bussgewalt beim griechischen Mönchtum*, pp. 214 ff.; M. Jugie, "Les Origines de la méthode d'oraison des hésychastes," *Echos d'Orient*, XXX (1931), 179–85; A. Bloom, "Contemplation et ascèse, contribution orthodoxe," *Études carmélitaines* (1948), pp. 49 ff.; id., "L'Hésychasme, yoga chrétien?" in Jacques Masui (ed.), *Yoga*, pp. 177–95; I. Hausherr, "L'Hésychasme: étude de spiritualité," *Orientalia Christiana Periodica*, XXII (1956), 5–40, 247–85; and the summaries of progress and the bibliographies compiled by Gouillard, pp. 22 ff., 37, and Gardet, pp. 645 ff.

Yogic Concentration and Meditation

Āsana, *prāṇāyāma*, and *ekāgratā* succeed—if only for the short time the respective exercise continues—in abolishing the human condition. Motionless, breathing rhythmically, eyes and attention fixed on a single point, the yogin experiences a passing beyond the secular modality of existence. He begins to become autonomous in respect to the cosmos; external tensions no longer trouble him (having passed beyond "the opposites," he is equally insensible to heat and cold, to light and darkness, etc.); sensory activity no longer carries him outward, toward the objects of the senses; the psychomental stream is no longer either invaded or directed by distractions, automatisms, and memory: it is "concentrated," "unified." This retreat outside the cosmos is accompanied by a sinking into the self, progress in which is directly proportional to progress in the retreat. The yogin returns to himself, takes, so to speak, possession of himself, surrounds himself with increasingly stronger "defenses" to protect him against invasion from without—in a word, he becomes invulnerable.

Needless to say, such a concentration, experienced on all levels (*āsana*, *prāṇāyāma*, *ekāgratā*), is accompanied by an increasing attention to the yogin's own organic life. While the exercise continues, the yogin's sensation of his body is wholly different from that of the noninitiate. Bodily stability, retardation of the respiratory rhythm, narrowing of the field of consciousness until it coincides with a point, together with the resultant vibration set up within him by the faintest pulsation of the inward life—all this apparently assimilates the yogin to a plant. This homology, by the way, would imply no pejorative judgment, even if it were adequate to the reality of the situation. For Indian consciousness, the vegetable modality is not an impoverishment but, quite the contrary, an enrichment of life. In Purāṇic mythology and in iconography, the rhizome and the lotus become the symbols of cosmic manifestations. The creation is symbolized by a lotus floating on the primordial waters. Vegetation always signifies superabundance, fertility, the sprouting of all seeds. As for Indian painting (the Ajaṇṭā frescoes, for example), the bliss of the personages is manifested in their soft, lithe gestures, like the stems of aquatic plants; one even has the impression that what flows in the veins of these mythical figures is not blood but vegetable sap.

A priori, then, this homology between a yogin in the state of concentration and a plant is not entirely improbable. The nostalgia that the Indian feels when he thinks of the closed and continuous circuit of organic life—a circuit without either inequalities or explosive moments (such, in a word, as is realized on the vegetative plane of life)—this nostalgia is a real fact. Yet we do not believe that this abolition of the human condition through immobility, this rhythm imposed on respiration, this concentration on a single point, have as their final aim the backward step that a return to the vegetable modality of life would signify. The goals pursued in Patañjali's *Yoga-sūtras*—and even more, the goals of other forms of Yoga—are definitely against such a hypothesis. The vegetable correspondences that can be found in yogic posture, respiration, and concentration seem to us to be fully explained by the archaic symbolism of "rebirth." Morphologically, one could homologize *āsana* and *prāṇāyāma* with the "embryonic respiration" employed by Taoism,[60] with the "embryonic" position in which so many peoples place their dead before burial (in the hope of a certain return to life), as well as with some ceremonies of initiation and regeneration performed in a closed place, the symbol of the womb. Space does not allow us to go into these ceremonies further here; we shall only say that they all presuppose the magical projection of the practitioner into an auroral time, into a mythical *illud tempus*. *Incipit vita nova* (and every regeneration is a "new birth")—but that is possible only if past time is abolished, and "history" with it,

60 The goal of this respiration is, according to Taoist sources, to imitate the respiration of the fetus in the maternal womb. "By returning to the base, by going back to the origin, one drives away old age, one returns to the state of the fetus," says the preface to the *T'ai-si K'ou Chüeh* ("Oral Formulas for Embryonic Respiration"), quoted after Maspéro, p. 198.

if the present moment coincides with the mythical moment of the beginnings of things—that is, with the creation of the worlds, with the cosmogony. In this sense, the yogin's bodily position and "embryonic respiration," although (at least in the *Yoga-sūtras*, but also in other forms of Yoga) they pursue a wholly different end, can be regarded as embryonic, vegetative ontological modalities.

Then again, *āsana* and *ekāgratā* imitate a divine archetype; the yogic position has a religious value in itself. It is true that the yogin does not imitate the "gestures" and "sufferings" of the divinity—and not without reason! For the God of the *Yoga-sūtras*, Īśvara, is a pure spirit who not only did not create the world but does not even intervene in history, either directly or indirectly. Hence—in default of his gestures—what the yogin imitates is at least the mode of being belonging to this pure spirit. Transcendence of the human condition, "deliverance," the perfect autonomy of the *puruṣa*—all this has its archetypal model in Īśvara. Renouncing the human condition—that is, Yoga practice—has a religious value in the sense that the yogin imitates Īśvara's mode of being: immobility, concentration on self. In other varieties of Yoga, *āsana* and *ekāgratā* can obviously acquire religious valences by the mere fact that, through them, the yogin becomes a living statue, thus imitating the iconographic model.

Making respiration rhythmical and, as far as possible, suspending it greatly promote concentration (*dhāraṇā*). For, Patañjali tells us,[61] through *prāṇāyāma* the veil of darkness is rent and the intellect becomes capable (*yogyata*) of concentration (*dhāraṇā*). The yogin can test the quality of his concentration by *pratyāhāra* (a term usually translated "withdrawal of the senses" or "abstraction," which we prefer to translate "ability to free sense activity from the domination of external objects"). According to the *Yoga-sūtras* (II, 54), *pratyāhāra* could be understood as the faculty through which the intellect (*citta*) possesses sensations *as if* the contact were real.

61 *Yoga-sūtras*, II, 52, 53.

Commenting on this *sūtra*, Bhoja says that the senses, instead of directing themselves toward an object, "abide within themselves" (*svarūpamātre svasthānam*). Although the senses are no longer directed toward external objects, and their activity ceases, the intellect (*citta*) does not thereby lose its property of having sensory representations. When the *citta* wishes to know an exterior object, it does not make use of a sensory activity; it is able to know the object by its own powers. Being obtained directly, by contemplation, this "knowledge" is, from the yogic point of view, more effective than normal knowledge. "Then," Vyāsa writes, "the wisdom [*prajñā*] of the yogin knows all things as they are." [62]

This withdrawal of sensory activity from the domination of exterior objects (*pratyāhāra*) is the final stage of psychophysiological *ascesis*. Thenceforth the yogin will no longer be "distracted" or "troubled" by the senses, by sensory activity, by memory, etc. All activity is suspended. The *citta*—being the psychic mass that orders and illuminates sensations coming from without—can serve as a mirror for objects, without the senses interposing between it and its object. The noninitiate is incapable of gaining this freedom, because his mind, instead of being stable, is constantly violated by the activity of the senses, by the subconscious, and by the "thirst for life." By realizing *cittavṛtti nirodhaḥ* (i.e., the suppression of psychomental states), the *citta* abides in itself (*svarūpamātre*). But this "autonomy" of the intellect does not result in the suppression of phenomena. Even though detached from phenomena, the yogin continues to contemplate them. Instead of knowing through forms (*rūpa*) and mental states (*cittavṛtti*), as formerly, the yogin now contemplates the essence (*tattva*) of all objects directly.

Autonomy with respect to stimuli from the outer world and to the dynamism of the subconscious—an autonomy that he realizes through *pratyāhāra*—allows the yogin to practice a threefold technique, which the texts call *saṃyama*. The term designates the last stages of yogic meditation, the last three "members of Yoga" (*yogaṇga*). These are: concentration (*dhāraṇā*), meditation prop-

62 *Yoga-bhāṣya*, II, 45.

erly speaking (*dhyāna*), and stasis (*samādhi*). These mental exercises become possible only after sufficient repetition of all the other physiological exercises, when the yogin has succeeded in attaining perfect mastery over his body, his subconscious, and his psychomental flux. The adjective "subtle" (*antarāṅga*) is applied to them to emphasize the fact that they imply no new physiological technique. They are so much alike that the yogin who attempts one of them (concentration, for example) cannot easily remain in it, and sometimes finds himself, quite against his will, slipping over into meditation or enstasis. It is for this reason that these last three yogic exercises have a common name—*saṃyama*.[63]

Concentration (*dhāraṇā*, from the root *dhṛ*, "to hold fast") is in fact an *ekāgratā*, a "fixing on a single point," but its content is strictly notional.[64] In other words, *dhāraṇā*—and this is what distinguishes it from *ekāgratā*, whose sole purpose is to arrest the psychomental flux and "fix it on a single point"—realizes such a "fixation" for the purpose of *comprehension*. Patañjali's definition of it is: "fixation of thought on a single point" (*deśabandhaścittasya dhāraṇā*).[65] Vyāsa adds that the concentration is usually on "the center [*cakra*] of the navel, on the lotus of the heart, on the light within the head, on the tip of the nose, on the tip of the tongue, or on any external place or object."[66] Vācaspatimiśra further adds that one cannot obtain *dhāraṇā* without the aid of an object on which to fix one's thought.

Commenting on *Yoga-sūtras*, I, 36, Vyāsa had referred to concentration on the "lotus of the heart" as leading to an experience of pure light. Let us note this detail—the "inner light" discovered through concentration on the lotus of the heart. The experience is already attested in the Upaniṣads, and always in connection with encountering one's true Self (*ātman*). The "light of the heart" will frequently recur in all the post-Upaniṣadic mystical methods of India. In connection with this text of Vyāsa, Vācaspatimiśra gives a long description of the lotus of the heart. It has eight petals,

63 Vācaspatimiśra, ad Vyāsa, III, 1.
64 See Note II, 3.
65 *Yoga-sūtras*, III, 1.
66 Ad *Yoga-sūtras*, III, 1.

and it is situated, head downward, between the abdomen and the thorax; the yogin must turn it head upward by stopping his breath (*recaka*) and concentrating his intellect (*citta*) on it. In the center of the lotus is the solar disk with the letter *A*, and here is the seat of the waking state. Above it is the lunar disk with the letter *U;* this is the seat of sleep. Higher again is the "circle of fire" with the letter *M*—the seat of deep sleep. Above all these is the "highest circle, whose essence is air"; this is the seat of the fourth state (*turīya*, "cataleptic state"). In this last lotus, or, more precisely, in its pericarp, is the "nerve [*nāḍī*] of Brahmā," oriented upward and reaching to the circle of the sun and the other circles. At this point begins the *nāḍī* named *suṣumṇā*, which also crosses the outer circles. This is the seat of the *citta;* by concentrating on it, the yogin acquires consciousness of the *citta* (in other words, *he becomes conscious of consciousness*).

At the risk of fatiguing the reader, we have followed Vācaspatimiśra's text as closely as possible. But it introduces us to a "mystical" or "subtle physiology," concerned with "organs" that reveal their existence only in the course of yogic exercises in concentration and meditation. This problem will occupy our attention again when we present the meditational techniques of tantrism; [67] it will then be necessary to demonstrate the relationships among the "subtle organs," the mystical letters, and the various states of consciousness. But it is important even now to point out that the tradition of classic Yoga, represented by Patañjali, knew and employed the schemata of "mystical physiology," which were later to play a considerable role in the history of Indian spirituality.

In his *Yogasāra-saṃgraha*,[68] Vijñānabhikṣu quotes a passage from the *Iśvara Gītā* according to which a *dhāraṇā* takes the time of twelve *prāṇāyāmas*. "The time necessary for concentration of the mind on an object [*dhāraṇā*] is equal to the time taken by twelve *prāṇāyāmas*" (i.e., by twelve controlled, equal, and retarded respirations). By prolonging this concentration on an object twelve times, one obtains "yogic meditation," *dhyāna*. Patañjali defines

67 See p. 241.

68 Ed. G. Jhā, pp. 43 ff.

dhyāna as "a current of unified thought," [69] and Vyāsa adds the following gloss to the definition: "Continuum of mental effort [*pratyayasyāikatānatā*] to assimilate the object of meditation, free from any other effort to assimilate other objects [*pratyayāntareṇa-parāmṛṣṭo*]." Vijñānabhikṣu [70] explains this process as follows: when, after achieving *dhāraṇā* on some point, one's mind has succeeded for a sufficient time in holding itself before itself under the form of the object of meditation, without any interruption caused by the intrusion of any other function, one attains *dhyāna*. As an example, he gives the contemplation of Viṣṇu or of some other god, whom one imagines to be in the lotus of the heart.

It is scarcely necessary to add that this yogic "meditation" is absolutely different from any secular meditation whatever. In the first place, in the framework of normal psychomental experience no "mental continuum" can reach the density and purity that yogic procedures permit attaining. Secondly, secular meditation stops either with the external form or with the value of the objects meditated upon, whereas *dhyāna* makes it possible to "penetrate" objects, to "assimilate" them magically. As an example, we cite the yogic meditation on the subject of "fire," as it is taught today (the meditation begins with concentration, *dhāraṇā*, on some glowing coals placed before the yogin). Not only does it reveal to the yogin the phenomenon of combustion and its deeper meaning; it allows him, in addition: (1) to identify the physiochemical process taking place in the coal with the process of combustion that occurs in the human body; (2) to identify the fire before him with the fire of the sun, etc.; (3) to unify the several contents of all these fires, in order to obtain a vision of existence as "fire"; (4) to penetrate within this cosmic process, now on the astral plane (the sun), now on the physiological plane (the human body), and finally even on the plane of infinitesimals ("the seed of fire"); (5) to reduce all these planes to a modality common to them all—that is, *prakṛti* as "fire"; (6) to "master" the inner fire, by virtue of *prāṇāyāma*, suspension of respiration (respiration = vital fire); (7) finally,

69 *Yoga-sūtras*, III, 2.

70 *Yogasāra-saṃgraha*, ed. Jhā, p. 45.

through a new "penetration," to extend this "mastery" to the glowing coals before him (for, if the process of combustion is exactly the same from one limit of the universe to the other, any partial mastery of the phenomenon infallibly leads to its "mastery" *in toto*), etc.

In giving this description (which, by the way, is no more than a rough approximation) of some of the exercises connected with the "meditation concerning fire," we have by no means undertaken to expose the mechanism of *dhyāna;* we have confined ourselves to suggesting a few examples of it. Its most specific exercises are, in any case, indescribable. There is nothing surprising in this. What is particularly difficult to explain is the act of "penetration" into the "essence of fire"; this act must be conceived neither under the species of the poetic imagination nor under that of an intuition of the Bergsonian type. What sharply distinguishes yogic meditation from these two irrational "flights" is its coherence, the state of lucidity that accompanies and continually orients it. For the "mental continuum" never escapes from the yogin's will. It is never enriched laterally, by uncontrolled associations, analogies, symbols, etc. At no moment does this meditation cease to be an *instrument* for penetrating into the essence of things—that is, finally, an instrument for taking possession of, for "assimilating," the real.[71]

The Role of Īśvara

Unlike Sāṃkhya, Yoga affirms the existence of a God, Īśvara. This God is, of course, no creator (the cosmos, life, and man having, as we have already noted, been "created" by *prakṛti,* for they all proceed from the primordial substance). But, in the case of *certain* men, Īśvara can hasten the process of deliverance; he helps them toward a more speedy arrival at *samādhi.* This God, to whom Patañjali refers, is more especially a god of yogins. He can come to the help only of a yogin—that is, a man who has already chosen

71 As we shall see further on, yogic meditation plays an extremely important part in Buddhist techniques.

Yoga. In any case, Īśvara's role is comparatively small. He can, for example, bring *samādhi* to the yogin who takes him as the object of his concentration. According to Patañjali,[72] this divine aid is not the effect of a "desire" or a "feeling"—for God can have neither desires nor emotions—but of a "metaphysical sympathy" between Īśvara and the *puruṣa*, a sympathy explained by their structural correspondence. Īśvara is a *puruṣa* that has been free since all eternity, never touched by the *kleśas*.[73] Commenting on this text, Vyāsa adds that the difference between Īśvara and a "liberated spirit" is as follows: between the latter and psychomental experience, there was once a relation (even though illusory); whereas Īśvara has always been free. God does not submit to being summoned by rituals, or devotion, or faith in his "mercy"; but his essence instinctively "collaborates," as it were, with the Self that seeks emancipation through Yoga.

What is involved, then, is rather a sympathy, metaphysical in nature, connecting two kindred entities. One would say that this sympathy shown by Īśvara toward certain yogins—that is, toward the few men who seek their deliverance by means of yogic techniques—has exhausted his capacity to interest himself in the lot of mankind. This is why neither Patañjali nor Vyāsa succeeds in giving any precise explanation of God's intervention in nature. It is clear that Īśvara has entered Sāṃkhya-Yoga dialectics, as it were, from outside. For Sāṃkhya affirms (and Yoga adopts the affirmation) that Substance (*prakṛti*), because of its "teleological instinct," collaborates in the deliverance of man. Thus the role of God in man's acquisition of freedom is of no importance; for the cosmic substance itself undertakes to deliver the many "selves" (*puruṣa*) entangled in the illusory meshes of existence.

Although it was Patañjali who introduced this new and (when all is said and done) perfectly useless element of Īśvara into the dialectics of the Sāṃkhya soteriological doctrine, he does not give Īśvara the significance that late commentators will accord to him. What is of first importance in the *Yoga-sūtras* is technique—in

72 *Yoga-sūtras*, II, 45.

73 Ibid., I, 24.

other words, the yogin's will and capacity for self-mastery and concentration. Why, then, did Patañjali nevertheless feel the need to introduce Īśvara? Because Īśvara corresponded to an experiential reality: Īśvara can, in fact, bring about *samādhi,* on condition that the yogin practice *Īśvarapraṇidhāna*—that is, devotion to Īśvara.[74] Having undertaken to collect and classify all the yogic techniques whose efficacy had been confirmed by the "classic tradition," Patañjali could not neglect a whole series of experiences that had been made possible by the single process of concentration on Īśvara. In other words: alongside the tradition of a purely magical Yoga—one that called upon nothing but the will and personal powers of the ascetic—there was another, a "mystical" tradition, in which the last stages of Yoga practice were at least made easier by devotion—even though an extremely rarefied, extremely "intellectual" devotion—to a God. In any case, at least as he appears in Patañjali and Vyāsa, Īśvara has none of the grandeur of the omnipotent Creator-God, none of the pathos that surrounds the dynamic and solemn God of various mystical schools. All in all, Īśvara is only an archetype of the yogin—a macroyogin; very probably a patron of certain yogic sects. At least Patañjali says that Īśvara was the *guru* of the sages of immemorial times, for, he adds, Īśvara is not bound by time.[75]

But let us now note a detail whose significance will not become clear until later. Into a dialectic of deliverance in which there was no need for a deity to figure, Patañjali introduces a "God," to whom, it is true, he accords but a minor role—for the yogin who takes him as the object of his concentration, Īśvara can facilitate the gaining of *samādhi.* But *samādhi*—as we shall see—can be gained without this "concentration on Īśvara." The Yoga practiced by the Buddha and his contemporaries can do without this "concentration on God." It is quite easy to imagine a Yoga that would accept the Sāṃkhya dialectic *in toto,* and we have no reason to believe that such a magical and atheistic Yoga did not exist. Patañjali nevertheless had to introduce Īśvara into Yoga, for Īśvara was, so to

74 Ibid., II, 45.

75 Ibid., I, 26.

speak, an experiential datum—the yogins did in fact appeal to him, although they could have obtained liberation by simply following the technique of Yoga.

Here we encounter the polarity "magic-mysticism," which we shall come to know better later on—in all its forms, which are innumerable. What is noteworthy is the increasingly active role that Īśvara comes to play in the late commentators. Vācaspatimiśra and Vijñānabhikṣu, for example, accord Īśvara great importance. It is true that these two commentators interpret Patañjali in the light of the spirituality that flourished in their own times. Now, they lived when all India was full of mystical and devotional currents. But it is precisely this almost universal victory of "mysticism" which is of extreme significance in the case of "classic" Yoga, which thereby moved away from what was typical of its beginnings—that is, "magic." Thus, under the combined influences of certain Vedāntic ideas and of *bhakti* (mystical devotion), Vijñānabhikṣu dwells on the "special mercy of God." [76] Another commentator, Nīlakaṇṭha, holds that God, though inactive, helps yogins "like a magnet." [77] The same author gives Īśvara a "will" capable of predetermining the lives of men, for "He makes him do good deeds whom He wants to raise, and He makes him commit bad deeds whom He wants to throw down." [78] How far we are here from the minor role that Patañjali gave Īśvara!

Enstasis and Hypnosis

It will be recalled that the last three "members of Yoga" (*yogaṅga*) represent "experiences" and "states" so closely connected that they are called by the same name—*saṃyama* (literally, "to go together," "vehicle"). Hence, to realize *saṃyama* on a certain "plane" (*bhūmi*) means simultaneous realization of "concentration" (*dhāraṇā*), "meditation" (*dhyāna*), and "stasis" (*samādhi*) on it; the "plane" or level can, for example, be that of inert matter

76 *Yogasāra-saṃgraha*, ed. Jhā, pp. 9, 18–19, 45–46.

77 Cf. Dasgupta, *Yoga as Philosophy*, p. 89.

78 Ibid., p. 88.

(earth, etc.) or that of incandescent matter (fire, etc.). The passage from "concentration" to "meditation" does not require the application of any new technique. Similarly, no supplementary yogic exercise is needed to realize *samādhi*, once the yogin has succeeded in "concentrating" and "meditating." *Samādhi,*[79] yogic "enstasis," is the final result and the crown of all the ascetic's spiritual efforts and exercises.

Innumerable difficulties must be overcome if we would understand precisely in what this yogic "stasis" consists. Even if we disregard the peripheral meanings that the concept *samādhi* acquires in Buddhist literature and in the "baroque" species of Yoga, and take into consideration only the meaning and value given it by Patañjali and his commentators, the difficulties remain. For one thing, *samādhi* expresses an experience that is completely indescribable. For another, this "enstatic experience" is not univalent—its modalities are very numerous. Let us see if, proceeding by stages, we can discover to what *samādhi* refers. The word is first employed in a gnosiological sense; *samādhi* is the state of contemplation in which thought grasps the form of the object directly, without the help of categories and the imagination (*kalpaṇā*); the state in which the object is revealed "in itself" (*svarūpa*), in its essentials, and as if "empty of itself" (*arthamātranirbhāsaṃ svarūpaśūnyamiva*).[80] Commenting on this text, Vācaspatimiśra cites a passage from the *Viṣṇu Purāṇa* (VI, 7, 90) where it is said that the yogin has ceased to employ "imagination," no longer regards the *act* and the *object* of meditation as distinct from each other. There is a real coincidence between *knowledge* of the object and the *object of knowledge;* the object no longer presents itself to consciousness in the relations that delimit and define it as a phenomenon, but "as if it were empty of itself." Illusion and imagination (*kalpaṇā*) are thus wholly done away with by *samādhi*. Or, as Vijñāna-

79 The meanings of the term *samādhi* are: union, totality; absorption in, complete concentration of mind; conjunction. The usual translation is "concentration," but this entails the risk of confusion with *dhāraṇā*. Hence we have preferred to translate it "enstasis," "stasis," "conjunction."

80 *Yoga-sūtras*, III, 3.

bhikṣu expresses it,[81] one arrives at *samādhi* "when *dhyāna* is freed from the separate notions of meditation, object of meditation, and meditating subject, and maintains itself only in the form of the object meditated on," that is, when nothing any longer exists besides the new ontological dimension represented by the transformation of the "object" (the world) into "knowledge-possession." Vijñānabhikṣu adds that there is a distinct difference between *dhyāna* and *samādhi;* meditation can be interrupted "if the senses enter into contact with alluring objects," whereas *samādhi* is an invulnerable state, completely closed to stimuli.

However, we must not regard this yogic state as a mere hypnotic trance. Indian "psychology" is familiar with hypnosis, and attributes it to a merely occasional and provisional state of concentration (*vikṣipta*). Some passages from the *Mahābhārata* show the popular Indian conception of the hypnotic trance; according to this conception, it is only an automatic damming of the "stream of consciousness" and not a yogic *ekāgratā.* The fact that the Indians did not confuse hypnosis with yogic trances is clear, for example, from a passage of the *Mahābhārata* (XIII, 40, 46, 50–51; 41, 13, 18). Devaśarman, obliged to go on a pilgrimage to perform a sacrifice, asks his disciple, Vipulā, to protect his wife, Ruci, from the charm of Indra. Vipulā looks into her eyes, and Ruci is unconscious of the magnetic influence of his look (*uvāsa rakṣaṇe yukto na ca sā tam abudhyata*).[82] Once the operator's eye is "fixed," his mind passes into Ruci's body and she is "petrified like a picture." When Indra enters the room, Ruci wants to rise and perform her duties as hostess, but, "having been immobilized and subjugated" by Vipulā, "she could not make a movement." Indra spoke: "Exhorted by Anaṇga, god of love, I am come for thy love, O thou of the gay smile!" But Ruci, who wanted to answer him, "felt unable to rise and speak" because Vipulā "had subjugated her senses by the bonds of yoga" (*babandha yogabandhāiś ca tasyāḥ sarvendriyāṇi saḥ*) and she had become unable to move (*nirvikāra,*

81 *Yogasāra-saṃgraha,* ed. Jhā, p. 44.
82 *Mahābhārata,* XIII, 40, 59.

"unalterable").[83] The hypnotic process is summarized as follows: "Uniting [*saṃyojya*] the rays of his own eyes with the rays of her eyes, he made his way into her body, as wind makes its way through the air." [84] Then again, Bhatta Kallata, in his *Spanda-kārikā*, describes the differences between hypnotic and somnambulistic trances and *samādhi*.[85] The state of *vikṣipta* is only a paralysis (emotional or volitional in origin) of the mental flux; this stoppage must not be confused with *samādhi*, which is obtained only through *ekāgratā*—that is, after the plurality of mental states (*sarvārtha*) has been suppressed.[86]

Samādhi "*with Support*"

Rather than "knowledge," however, *samādhi* is a "state," an enstatic modality peculiar to Yoga. We shall presently see that this state makes possible the self-revelation of the Self (*puruṣa*), by virtue of an act that does not constitute an "experience." But not any *samādhi* reveals the Self, not any "stasis" makes final liberation a reality. Patañjali and his commentators distinguish several kinds or stages of supreme concentration. When *samādhi* is obtained with the help of an object or idea (that is, by fixing one's thought on a point in space or on an idea), the stasis is called *samprajñāta samādhi* ("enstasis with support," or "differentiated enstasis"). When, on the other hand, *samādhi* is obtained apart from any "relation" (whether external or mental)—that is, when one obtains a "conjunction" into which no "otherness" enters, but which is

83 Ibid., XIII, 41, 3–12.

84 Ibid., XIII, 40, 56–57. To be sure, the hypnotic trance is brought on by yogic methods, but it is not in itself a yogic experience. The episode of Vipulā proves that, even in nontechnical literature, hypnosis was known and described with considerable accuracy. See below, p. 152.

85 Cf. Dasgupta, *Yoga Philosophy in Relation to Other Systems of Indian Thought*, pp. 352 ff. Sigurd Lindquist has devoted an entire book, *Die Methoden des Yoga*, to demonstrating the hypnotic nature of yogic experience. A minimum of living contact with Yoga would have saved him from such a foolhardy thesis.

86 *Yoga-sūtras*, III, 11.

simply a full comprehension of being—one has realized *asamprajñāta samādhi* ("undifferentiated stasis"). Vijñānabhikṣu [87] adds that *samprajñāta samādhi* is a means of liberation in so far as it makes possible the comprehension of truth and ends every kind of suffering. But *asamprajñāta samādhi* destroys the "impressions [*saṃskāra*] of all antecedent mental functions" and even succeeds in arresting the karmic forces already set in motion by the yogin's past activity. During "differentiated stasis," Vijñānabhikṣu continues, all the mental functions are "arrested" ("inhibited"), except that which "meditates on the object"; whereas in *asamprajñāta samādhi* all "consciousness" vanishes, the entire series of mental functions are blocked. "During this stasis, there is no other trace of the mind [*citta*] save the impressions [*saṃskāra*] left behind (by its past functioning). If these impressions were not present, there would be no possibility of returning to consciousness."

We are, then, confronted with two sharply differentiated classes of "states." The first class is acquired through the yogic technique of concentration (*dhāraṇā*) and meditation (*dhyāna*); the second class comprises only a single "state"—that is, unprovoked enstasis, "raptus." No doubt, even this *asamprajñāta samādhi* is always owing to prolonged efforts on the yogin's part. It is not a gift or a state of grace. One can hardly reach it before having sufficiently experienced the kinds of *samādhi* included in the first class. It is the crown of the innumerable "concentrations" and "meditations" that have preceded it. But it comes without being summoned, without being provoked, without special preparation for it. That is why it can be called a "raptus."

Obviously, "differentiated enstasis," *samprajñāta samādhi*, comprises several stages. This is because it is perfectible and does not realize an absolute and irreducible "state." Four stages or kinds are generally distinguished: "argumentative" (*savitarka*), "nonargumentative" (*nirvitarka*), "reflective" (*savicāra*), "superreflective" (*nirvicāra*).[88] Patañjali also employs another set

87 *Yogasāra-saṃgraha*, ed. Jhā, p. 4.
88 Cf. *Yoga-sūtras*, I, 42–44.

of terms: *vitarka, vićāra, ānanda, asmitā.*[89] But, as Vijñānabhikṣu, who reproduces this list, remarks, "the four terms are purely technical, they are applied conventionally to different forms of realization." These four forms or stages of *samprajñāta samādhi*, he continues, represent an ascent; in certain cases the grace of God (Īśvara) permits direct attainment of the higher states, and in such cases the yogin need not go back and realize the preliminary states. But when this divine grace does not intervene, he must realize the four stages gradually, always adhering to the same object of meditation (for example, Viṣṇu). These four grades or stages are also known as *samāpattis*, "coalescences." [90]

In the first stage, *savitarka* ("argumentative," [91] because it presupposes a preliminary analysis), thought identifies with the object of meditation in "its essential wholeness"; for an object is composed of a *thing*, a *notion*, and a *word*, and, during meditation, these three "aspects" of its reality are in perfect coincidence with the yogin's thought (*citta*). *Savitarka samādhi* is obtained through objects considered under their substantial (*sthūla*, "coarse") aspect; it is a "direct perception" of objects, but one that extends to both their past and their future. For example, Vijñānabhikṣu tells us, if one practices *savitarka samādhi* in relation to Viṣṇu, one visualizes the god under his substantial form and in the celestial region proper to him, but one also perceives him as he was in the past and as he will be in a more or less distant future. This is as much as to say that this species of *samādhi*, although produced by "coalescence" with the "coarse" aspect of a reality (in our example, direct perception of Viṣṇu's corporeality), is nevertheless not reduced to the immediacy of the object but also "pursues" and "assimilates" it in its temporal duration.

The following stage, *nirvitarka* ("nonargumentative"), is described by Vyāsa [92] as follows: "*Citta* becomes *nirvitarka* after the memory ceases to function, that is, after verbal or logical associa-

89 Ibid., I, 17. The parallelism between the four *samprajñāta samādhis* and the four Buddhist *dhyānas* was observed long ago. See Note II, 4.

90 *Yoga-sūtras*, I, 41, with the commentaries of Vyāsa and Vācaspatimiśra.

91 Ibid., I, 42.

92 Ad *Yoga-sūtras*, I, 43.

tions cease; at the moment when the object is empty of name and meaning; when thought reflects itself directly, by adopting the form of the object and shining solely with the object in itself [*svarūpa*]." In this meditation, thought is freed from the presence of the "I," for the cognitive act ("I know this object," or "This object is mine") is no longer produced; it is thought that *is* (becomes) the given object.[93] The object is no longer known through associations—that is to say, included in the series of previous representations, localized by extrinsic relations (name, dimensions, use, class), and, so to speak, impoverished by the habitual process of abstraction characteristic of secular thought—it is grasped directly, in its existential nakedness, as a concrete and irreducible datum.

Let us note that, in these stages, *samprajñāta samādhi* proves to be a "state" obtained by virtue of a certain "knowledge." Contemplation makes enstasis possible; enstasis, in turn, permits a deeper penetration into reality, by provoking (or facilitating) a new contemplation, a new yogic "state." This passing from "knowledge" to "state" must be constantly borne in mind, for, in our opinion, it is the characteristic feature of *samādhi* (as it is, indeed, of all Indian "meditation"). The "rupture of plane" that India seeks to realize, which is the paradoxical passage from *being* to *knowing*, takes place in *samādhi*. This suprarational experience, in which reality is dominated and assimilated by knowledge, finally leads to the fusion of all the modalities of being. That this is the deep meaning and the principal function of *samādhi*, we shall see somewhat later. What we would emphasize at the moment is that both *savitarka* and *nirvitarka samādhi* are "states-cognitions" obtained by concentration and meditation on the formal unity of "objects."

But one must go beyond these stages if one would penetrate into the very essence of things. And so it is that the yogin begins the meditation termed *savicāra* ("reflective"); thought no longer stops at the exterior aspect of material objects (objects that are

93 Ad *Yoga-sūtras*, I, 43.

formed by aggregates of atoms, of physical particles, etc.); on the contrary, it directly knows those infinitesimal nucleuses of energy which the Sāṃkhya and Yoga treatises call *tanmātras*. The yogin meditates on the "subtle" (*sūkṣma*) aspect of matter; he penetrates, Vijñānabhikṣu tells us, to *ahaṃkāra* and *prakṛti*, but this meditation is still accompanied by consciousness of time and space (not by an "experience" of a given space, a given duration, but by consciousness of the categories time-space). When thought "identifies" itself with the *tanmātras* without experiencing the "feelings" that, because of their energetic nature, these *tanmātras* produce (that is, when the yogin "assimilates them in an ideal fashion," without any resultant feeling of suffering, or pleasure, or violence, or inertia, etc., and without consciousness of time and space), the yogin obtains the state of *nirvicāra*. Thought then becomes one with these infinitesimal nucleuses of energy which constitute the true foundation of the physical universe. It is a real descent into the very essence of the physical world, and not only into qualified and individual phenomena.[94]

All these four stages of *samprajñāta samādhi* are called *bīja samādhi* ("*samādhi* with seed") or *sālambana samādhi* ("with support"); for, Vijñānabhikṣu tells us, they are in relation with a "substratum" (support) and produce tendencies that are like "seeds" for the future functions of consciousness.[95] *Asamprajñāta samādhi*, on the contrary, is *nirbīja*, "without seed," without support.[96] By realizing the four stages of *samprajñāta*, one obtains the "faculty of absolute knowledge" (*ṛtaṃbharāprajñā*).[97] This is already an opening toward *samādhi* "without seed," for absolute knowledge discovers the ontological completeness in which *being* and *knowing* are no longer separated. Fixed in *samādhi*, consciousness (*citta*) can now have direct revelation of the Self (*puruṣa*). Through the fact that this contemplation (which is actually a

94 Vyāsa and Vācaspatimiśra discuss these stages in their commentaries on *Yoga-sūtras*, I, 44, 45.

95 See also Bhoja, ad *Yoga-sūtras*, I, 17.

96 Vyāsa, ad I, 2.

97 *Yoga-sūtras*, I, 48.

"participation") is realized, the pain of existence is abolished.[98]

Still at this same point of enstasis—which is so difficult to define—we find two other varieties of contemplation: (1) *ānandānugata* (when, abandoning all perception, even that of "subtle" realities, one experiences the happiness of the eternal luminosity and consciousness of Self that belong to *sattva*) and (2) *āsmitānugata* (which one reaches at the moment that the intellect, *buddhi*, completely isolated from the external world, reflects only the Self). Vijñānabhikṣu [99] explains the name of this contemplation by the fact that the yogin reaches his true Self and understands, "I am [*asmi*] other than my body." It is also called *dharma-megha-samādhi*, the "cloud of *dharma*," [100] a technical term that is difficult to translate, for *dharma* can have many meanings (order, virtue, justice, foundation, etc.), but that seems to refer to an abundance ("rain") of virtues that suddenly fill the yogin. Simultaneously, he feels that he is saturated and that the world is breaking up; he has a feeling of "Enough!" in respect to all knowledge and all consciousness—and this complete renunciation leads him to *asamprajñāta samādhi*, to undifferentiated enstasis. For the mystical yogins, it is at this stage that the revelation of God (Īśvara) takes place; as Vijñānabhikṣu expresses it,[101] employing a traditional image (belonging to the *Smṛti*), when the twenty-fifth principle—that is, the *puruṣa*, the Self—becomes aware of its heterogeneity in respect to the other twenty-four principles (dependent upon *prakṛti*), one perceives the twenty-sixth principle, which is the Supreme Self, God. After contemplation of one's true Self—the goal of the Sāṃkhyayins—comes contemplation of God. But, as we have already remarked,[102] Vijñānabhikṣu interprets Yoga in the light of personal mysticism. We shall presently see what are the implications of this "reflection" of the Self, which is fully realized in *samādhi* "without support"; they are not exclusively enstatic in nature, for they raise the question of the ontological status of man in its entirety.

98 Vijñānabhikṣu, *Yogasāra-saṃgraha*, ed. Jhā, p. 5.

99 Ibid., p. 12.

100 *Yoga-sūtras*, IV, 29.

101 *Yogasāra-saṃgraha*, ed. Jhā, pp. 13 ff.

102 See above, p. 76.

The Siddhis *or "Miraculous Powers"*

Before attacking the problems raised by *asamprajñāta samādhi*, let us examine the results of the other species of *samādhi* more closely. The only results that can be of interest to the yogin are, obviously, those of a practical order—that is, penetration into regions inaccessible to normal experience, taking possession of zones of consciousness and sectors of reality that had previously been, so to speak, invulnerable. It is when he has reached this particular stage of his meditational discipline that the yogin acquires the "miraculous powers" (*siddhi*) to which Book III of the *Yoga-sūtras*, beginning with *sūtra* 16, is devoted. By "concentrating," "meditating," and realizing *samādhi* in respect to a certain object or an entire class of objects—in other words, by practicing *saṃyama* [103]—the yogin acquires certain occult powers in respect to the object or objects experienced.

Thus, for example, by practicing *saṃyama* on the distinction between "object" and "idea," the yogin knows the cries of all creatures.[104] By practicing *saṃyama* in regard to the subconscious residues (*saṃskāra*), he knows his previous existences.[105] Through *saṃyama* exercised in respect to "notions" (*pratyaya*), he knows the "mental states" of other men.[106] "But this knowledge of mental states does not imply knowledge of the objects that produced them, since these objects are not in direct connection with the yogin's thought. He knows the mental emotion of love, but he does not know the object of love." [107] *Saṃyama*, as we have just recalled, designates the last three "members of Yoga": *dhāraṇā*, *dhyāna*, and *samādhi*. The yogin begins by concentrating on an "object," on an "idea"; for example, on the subconscious residues (*saṃskāra*). When he has succeeded in obtaining *ekāgratā* concerning them, he begins to "meditate" them—that is, to assimilate

103 We remind the reader that *saṃyama* designates the last stages of yogic technique—i.e., concentration (*dhāraṇā*), meditation (*dhyāna*), and *samādhi*.

104 *Yoga-sūtras*, III, 17.

105 Ibid., III, 18.

106 Ibid., III, 19.

107 Vyāsa, ad III, 19.

them magically, to take possession of them. *Dhyāna*, "meditation," makes possible *samprajñāta samādhi*—in this case, *bīja samādhi*, *samādhi* with support (in the present instance the supports are, of course, the subconscious residues themselves). Through the yogic stasis realized on the basis of these residues, one becomes able not only to understand and assimilate them magically (this had already been made possible by *dhāraṇā* and *dhyāna*), but also to transform "knowledge" itself into "possession." *Samādhi* results in a constant identification between the meditator and the thing meditated. Needless to say, by understanding these residues to the point of becoming them, the yogin knows them not only as residues but at the same time by replacing them in the whole from which they were detached; in short, he can ideally (that is, without "experiencing" them) relive his previous existences. As we shall see, knowledge of former lives also plays an important part in Buddhism—a fact easy to understand if we bear in mind that "emerging from time" constitutes one of the major themes of Indian asceticism. One succeeds in emerging from time *by traveling back through it* ("against the fur," *pratiloman*)—that is, by reintegrating the primordial instant that had launched the first existence, the existence that is at the base of the entire cycle of transmigrations, the "seed-existence." The importance of this yogic technique will be discussed later.[108]

To go back to the other example: [109] by virtue of *saṃyama* concerning "notions," the yogin realizes the whole infinite series of other men's psychomental states; for as soon as a notion is "mastered from within," the yogin sees, as on a screen, all the states of consciousness that the notion is able to arouse in other men's souls. He sees an infinity of situations that the notion can engender, for not only has he assimilated the content of the "notion," he has also penetrated into its inner dynamism, he has made his own the human destiny that had the notion, etc. Some of these powers are even more miraculous. In his list of *siddhis*, Patañjali mentions all the legendary "powers" that obsess Indian mythol-

108 See below, p. 180.

109 *Yoga-sūtras*, III, 19.

ogy, folklore, and metaphysics with equal intensity. Unlike the folklore texts, Patañjali gives some very brief elucidations of them. Thus, wishing to explain why *saṃyama* concerning the form of the body can make him who practices it invisible, Patañjali says that *saṃyama* makes the body imperceptible to other men, and "a direct contact with the light of the eyes no longer existing, the body disappears." [110] This is the explanation he gives for the disappearances and appearances of yogins, a miracle mentioned by countless Indian religious, alchemical, and folklore texts. Vācaspatimisra comments: [111] "The body is formed from five essences [*tattva*]. It becomes an object perceptible to the eye by virtue of the fact that it possesses a form [*rūpa*, which also means color]. It is through this *rūpa* that the body and its form become objects of perception. When the yogin practices *saṃyama* on the form of the body, he destroys the perceptibility of the color [*rūpa*] that is the cause of perception of the body. Thus, when the possibility of perception is suspended, the yogin becomes invisible. The light engendered in the eye of another person no longer comes into contact with the body that has disappeared. In other words, the yogin's body is not an object of knowledge for any other man. The yogin disappears when he wishes not to be seen by anyone." This passage from Vācaspatimiśra attempts to explain a yogic phenomenon through the theory of perception, without recourse to miracle. Indeed, the general tendency of the more important yogic texts is to explain any parapsychological and occult phenomenon in terms of the "powers" acquired by the practitioner and to exclude any supernatural intervention.

Patañjali also mentions the other "powers" that can be obtained through *saṃyama*, such as the power of knowing the moment one is to die,[112] or extraordinary physical powers,[113] or knowledge of "subtle" things,[114] etc. *Saṃyama* practiced on the moon gives knowledge of the solar system; [115] on the umbilical

110 Ibid., III, 20.
111 Ad ibid.
112 Ibid., III, 21.
113 Ibid., III, 23.
114 Ibid., III, 24.
115 Ibid., III, 26.

plexus (*nābhicakra*), knowledge of the system of the body; [116] on the cavity of the throat (*kaṇṭhakūpe*), disappearance of hunger and thirst; [117] on the heart, knowledge of the mind.[118] "Whatever the yogin desires to know, he should perform *saṃyama* in respect to that object." [119] The "knowledge" obtained through the techniques of *saṃyama* is in fact a possession, an assimilation of the realities on which the yogin meditates. Whatever is meditated is—through the magical virtue of meditation—assimilated, possessed. It is easy to understand that the uninitiated have long confused these "powers" (*siddhi*) with the vocation of yoga. In India a yogin has always been considered a *mahāsiddha*, a possessor of occult powers, a "magician." [120] That this lay opinion is not wholly erroneous is shown by the entire spiritual history of India, in which the magician has always played, if not the principal role, at least an important one. India has never been able to forget that, under certain circumstances, man can become "man-god." It has never been able to accept the actual human condition, made up of suffering, impotence, and precariousness. It has always believed that there were men-gods, magicians, for it has always had the example of the yogins. That all these men-gods sought to exceed the human condition is obvious. But few of them succeeded in passing beyond the condition of the *siddha*, the condition of the "magician" or "god." In other words: very few indeed were those who succeeded in overcoming the second temptation, that of remaining permanently in a "divine condition."

As we know, in the Indian view, renunciation has a positive

116 *Yoga-sūtras*, III, 28. 117 Ibid., III, 29.

118 Ibid., III, 33. 119 Vācaspatimiśra, ad III, 30.

120 Bhoja (ad III, 44) gives the following list of the eight "great powers" (*mahāsiddhi*) of the yogin: (1) *aṇiman* (shrinking), that is, the power of becoming as small as an atom; (2) *laghiman* (lightness), the power of becoming as light as wool; (3) *gariman* (weight); (4) *mahiman* (illimitability), the power of touching any object at any distance (for example, the moon); (5) *prākāmya* (irresistible will); (6) *īśitva* (supremacy over the body and the *manas*); (7) *vaśitva* (dominion over the elements); (8) *kāmāvasāyitva* (fulfillment of desires). See also Note II, 5.

value. He who renounces feels not lessened thereby, but enriched —for the force that he gains by renouncing any pleasure far exceeds the pleasure that he has renounced. By virtue of renunciation, of asceticism (*tapas*), men, demons, or gods can become powerful to the point of threatening the economy of the entire universe. In the myths, legends, and tales of India, there are many episodes in which the principal character is an ascetic (man or demon) who, by virtue of the magical power he has gained through his renunciation, troubles even the repose of a Brahmā or a Viṣṇu. To prevent such an increase of sacred force, the gods tempt the ascetic. Patañjali himself refers to celestial temptations—that is, temptations proceeding from divine beings [121]—and Vyāsa [122] gives the following explanations: when the yogin approaches the last differentiated stasis, the gods come to him and tempt him, saying: "Come and rejoice here, in heaven. These pleasures are desirable, this maiden is adorable, this elixir conquers old age and death," etc. They continue to tempt him with celestial women, with supernatural sight and hearing, with the promise of turning his body into a "body of diamond"—in short, they offer him participation in the divine condition. But the divine condition is still far from absolute freedom. The yogin must reject these "magical hallucinations," these "false sensory objects that are of the nature of dreams," "desirable only for the ignorant," and persevere in his task of gaining final emancipation.

For as soon as the ascetic consents to make use of the magical forces gained by his disciplines, the possibility of his acquiring new forces vanishes. He who renounces secular life finally finds himself rich in magical forces, but he who succumbs to the desire to use them ultimately remains a mere "magician," without power to surpass himself. Only a new renunciation and a victorious struggle against the temptation of magic bring the ascetic a new spiritual enrichment. According to Patañjali and the whole tradition of classic Yoga—to say nothing of Vedāntist metaphysics, which contemns every kind of "power"—the yogin uses the innumerable

121 *Yoga-sūtras*, III, 51.

122 Ad ibid.

siddhis in order to regain supreme freedom, *asamprajñāta samādhi*, not in order to obtain a mastery over the elements, which, in any case, is only partial and provisional. For it is *samādhi*, not the "occult powers," which represents true "mastery." As Patañjali says,[123] these powers are "perfections" (this is the literal meaning of the term *siddhi*) in the waking state (*vyutthāna*), but represent obstacles in the state of *samādhi*—which is only natural, if we consider that, for Indian thought, all possession implies bondage to the thing possessed.

And yet, as we shall see later, nostalgia for the "divine condition" conquered by force, magically, has never ceased to obsess ascetics and yogins. The more so because, according to Vyāsa,[124] there is great similarity between certain gods inhabiting the celestial regions (in the Brahmāloka) and yogins at the stage of the *siddhis*—that is, possessing the "perfections" obtained through *samprajñāta samādhi*. For, Vyāsa says, the four classes of gods of the Brahmāloka are, by their very nature, in "states of mind" respectively corresponding to the four classes of differentiated *samādhi*. Because these gods stopped at the stage of *samādhi* with support ("with seed"), they are not liberated, they enjoy only an exceptional condition, the same condition that the yogins obtain when they become masters of the "perfections."

This gloss of Vyāsa's is important; it shows us that yogins are homologized with the gods; in other words, that, because of its "magical" and "religious" components, the way of Yoga leads to a mythological perfection, the very perfection enjoyed by the personages of the Indian pantheon. But, like the Vedāntin pursuing nothing save knowledge of the one absolute Being (Brahman), the true yogin does not let himself be tempted by the divine situation—which, glorious though it may be, is none the less "conditioned"—but strives to attain to knowledge and possession of the Self—that is, to the final liberation represented by *asamprajñāta samādhi*.

123 *Yoga-sūtras*, III, 37.

124 Ad III, 26.

Samādhi *"without Support" and Final Liberation*

Between the various degrees of *samprajñāta samādhi* there is a continual oscillation, owing not to the instability of thought but to the close organic connection existing between the types of *samādhi* with support. The yogin passes from one to another, his disciplined and purified consciousness practicing the several varieties of contemplation in turn. According to Vyāsa,[125] the yogin at this stage is still conscious of the difference between his own completely purified consciousness and the Self; that is, he is conscious of the difference between *citta* reduced to its luminous mode of being alone (*sattva*) and *puruṣa.* When this difference disappears, the subject attains *asamprajñāta samādhi;* now every *vṛitti* is eliminated, "burned"; nothing remains but the unconscious impressions (*saṃskāra*),[126] and at a certain moment even these imperceptible *saṃskāras* are consumed,[127] whereupon true stasis "without seed" (*nirbīja samādhi*) ensues.

Patañjali specifies [128] that there are two kinds of undifferentiated *samādhi,* or, more precisely, that there are two possible ways of attaining it: the way of technique (*upāya*) and the natural way (*bhava*). The first is that of the yogins, who conquer *samādhi* through Yoga; the second is that of the gods (*videha,* the "disincarnate") and of a class of superhuman beings (hence called *prakṛtilaya*) conceived as "absorbed in *prakṛti.*" Here again, as we have just noted in connection with the various stages of *samprajñāta samādhi,* we find the yogins homologized with gods and superhuman beings. Commenting on this *sūtra,* Vyāsa and Vācaspatimiśra emphasize the superiority of the enstasis obtained by yogins through technique (*upāya*), for the "natural" *samādhi* enjoyed by the gods is provisional, even if it may last for thousands

125 Ad I, 2.
126 *Yoga-sūtras,* I, 18, with Vyāsa's commentary.
127 Ibid., I, 51. 128 Ibid., I, 19.

of cosmic cycles. In passing, let us note the insistence with which human Yoga is proclaimed to be superior to the apparently privileged conditions of the gods.

Vijñānabhikṣu takes a somewhat different view.[129] For him, the *upāyapratyaya*, the "artificial" method (in the sense that it is not "natural," that it is a construction), consists in practicing *saṃyama* on Īśvara, or, if one has no mystical vocation, on one's own Self; this is the method commonly employed by yogins. As to the second way, the "natural" method (*bhavapratyaya*), some yogins can obtain undifferentiated enstasis (and hence final liberation) simply by desiring it; in other words, it is no longer a conquest achieved by technical means, it is a spontaneous operation; it is called *bhava*, "natural,"[130] Vijñānabhikṣu says, precisely because it results from the birth (*bhava*) of the beings who obtain it ("birth" meaning birth at a propitious hour, as a result of having practiced Yoga in a previous existence). This second way, *bhavapratyaya*, is characteristic of the *videhas* (bodiless beings), the *prakṛtilayas* (being absorbed in *prakṛti*), and other divinities. As an example of the *videhas*, Vijñānabhikṣu gives Hiraṇyagarbha and other gods who need no physical body because they are able to perform all their physiological functions in the "subtle" body. The *prakṛtilayas* are superhuman beings who, sunk in meditation on *prakṛti*, or on *prakṛti* animated by God, pierce the cosmic egg (mentally) and pass through all the envelopes (*āvaraṇa*, "case") —that is, all the levels of cosmic life down to the primordial *Grund*, *prakṛti* in its nonmanifested mode—and thereby obtain the situation of the Divinity.[131]

129 *Yogasāra-saṃgraha*, ed. Jhā, pp. 18 ff.

130 Vijñānabhikṣu here departs from the interpretation of Vyāsa and Vācaspatimiśra (ad *Yoga-sūtras*, I, 19), who take the term *bhava* to refer to the "world" and "worldly, secular life." In this case, the meaning of the *sūtra* would be: the gods enjoy a *samādhi* provoked by profane (*bhava*) means; not: the gods enjoy a *samādhi* provoked by natural means (that is, spontaneously), as Vijñānabhikṣu understands it.

131 Patañjali (*Yoga-sūtras*, I, 20) recapitulates the five means by which yogins obtain *asamprajñāta samādhi*: faith in the way of Yoga (*śraddhā*), energy (*vīrya*), memory (*smṛti*), *samādhi*, and wisdom (*prajñā*). Actually,

Vyāsa [132] summarizes the passage from *samprajñāta* to *asamprajñāta samādhi* as follows: through the illumination (*prajña*, "wisdom") spontaneously obtained when he reaches the stage of *dharma-megha-samādhi*, the yogin realizes "absolute isolation" (*kaivalya*)—that is, liberation of *purusa* from the dominance of *prakṛti*. For his part, Vācaspatimiśra [133] says that the "fruit" of *samprajñāta samādhi* is *asamprajñāta samādhi*, and the "fruit" of the latter is *kaivalya*, liberation. It would be wrong to regard this mode of being of the Spirit as a simple "trance" in which consciousness was emptied of all content. Nondifferentiated enstasis is not "absolute emptiness." The "state" and the "knowledge" simultaneously expressed by this term refer to a total absence of objects in consciousness, not to a consciousness absolutely empty. For, on the contrary, at such a moment consciousness is saturated with a direct and total intuition of being. As Mādhava says, "*nirodha* [final arrest of all psychomental experience] must not be imagined as a nonexistence, but rather as the support of a particular condition of the Spirit." It is the enstasis of total emptiness, without sensory content or intellectual structure, an unconditioned state that is no longer "experience" (for there is no further relation between consciousness and the world) but "revelation." Intellect (*buddhi*), having accomplished its mission, withdraws, detaching itself from the *puruṣa* and returning into *prakṛti*. The Self remains free, autonomous; it contemplates itself. "Human" consciousness is suppressed; that is, it no longer functions, its constituent elements being reabsorbed into the primordial substance. The yogin attains deliverance; like a dead man, he has no more relation with life; he

---

Patañjali returns in this *sūtra* to some of the "members of Yoga" (*yogaṅga*) that are the means of obtaining deliverance. Vijñānabhikṣu (*Yogasāra-saṃgraha*, ed. Jhā, p. 18) suggests that in case the yogin should hesitate to employ some of these means, he can gain *asamprajñāta samādhi* through devotion to God (cf. *Yoga-sūtras*, I, 23), for, he adds, devotion calls forth the grace of God. But, as we have noted before, Vijñānabhikṣu always emphasizes the theistic and mystical aspect of Yoga.

132 Ad III, 55. 133 Ad I, 21.

is "dead in life." He is the *jīvan-mukta*, the "liberated in life."[134] He no longer lives in time and under the domination of time, but in an eternal present, in the *nunc stans* by which Boethius defined eternity.[135]

Such would be the situation of the yogin in *asamprajñāta samādhi*, as long as it was viewed from outside and judged from the point of view of the dialectic of liberation and of the relations between the Self and Substance, as elaborated by Sāṃkhya. In reality, if we take into account the "experience" of the various *samādhis*, the yogin's situation is more paradoxical and infinitely more grandiose. Let us, then, more closely consider what is meant by the expression "reflection" of the *puruṣa*. In this act of supreme concentration, "knowledge" is equivalent to an "appropriation." For obtaining direct revelation of the *puruṣa* is at the same time to discover, to experience, an ontological modality inaccessible to the noninitiate. Such a moment can hardly be conceived otherwise than as a paradox; for, having once reached it, one could no longer in any way specify to what extent it would still be possible to speak of contemplation of the Self or of an ontological transformation of the human being. Simple "reflection" of the *puruṣa* is more than an act of mystical cognition, since it allows the *puruṣa* to gain "mastery" of itself. The yogin takes possession of himself through an "undifferentiated stasis" whose sole content is *being*. We should be false to the Indian paradox if we reduced this "taking possession" to a mere "knowing oneself," however profound and absolute. For "taking possession of oneself" radically modifies the human being's ontological condition. "Discovery of oneself," self-reflection of the *puruṣa*, causes a "rupture of plane" on the cosmic scale;

134 For an analysis of the "impersonal situation" of the *jīvan-mukta* who has only a "witnessing consciousness" without any reference to the ego, see Roger Godel, *Essais sur l'expérience libératrice.* The state of the *jīvan-mukta* can, of course, equally well be obtained by means other than those proposed by classic Yoga, but one cannot *prepare oneself* to obtain it except by employing the yogic disciplines of meditation and concentration.

135 See Eliade, "Indian Symbolisms of Time and Eternity," *Images and Symbols*, pp. 57–91.

when this occurs, the modalities of the real are abolished, being (*puruṣa*) coincides with nonbeing ("man," properly speaking), knowledge is transformed into magical "mastery," in virtue of the complete absorption of the known by the knower. And as, now, the object of knowledge is one's pure being, stripped of every form and every attribute, it is to assimilation with pure Being that *samādhi* leads. The self-revelation of the *puruṣa* is equivalent to a taking possession of being in all its completeness. In *asamprajñāta samādhi*, the yogin is actually all Being.

Clearly, his situation is paradoxical. For he is in life, and yet liberated; he has a body, and yet he knows himself and thereby *is puruṣa;* he lives in duration, yet at the same time shares in immortality; finally, he coincides with all Being, though he is but a fragment of it, etc. But it has been toward the realization of this paradoxical situation that Indian spirituality has tended from its beginnings. What else are the "men-gods" of whom we spoke earlier, if not the "geometric point" where the divine and the human coincide, as do being and nonbeing, eternity and death, the whole and the part? And, more perhaps than any other civilization, India has always lived under the sign of "men-gods."

Reintegration and Freedom

Let us recapitulate the stages of this long and difficult road recommended by Patañjali. From the first, its end is perfectly clear—to emancipate man from his human condition, to conquer absolute freedom, to realize the unconditioned. The method comprises a number of different techniques (physiological, mental, mystical), but they all have one characteristic in common—they are antisocial, or, indeed, antihuman. The worldly man lives in society, marries, establishes a family; Yoga prescribes absolute solitude and chastity. The worldly man is "possessed" by his own life; the yogin refuses to "let himself live"; to continual movement, he opposes his static posture, the immobility of *āsana;* to agitated, unrhythmical, changing respiration, he opposes *prāṇāyāma*, and even dreams of holding his breath indefinitely; to the chaotic flux of psychomental life, he replies by "fixing thought on a single point," the first step to that final withdrawal from the phenomenal world which he will obtain through *pratyāhāra.* All of the yogic techniques invite to one and the same gesture—to do exactly the opposite of what human nature forces one to do. From solitude and chastity to *saṃyama,* there is no solution of continuity. The orientation always remains the same—to react against the "normal," "secular," and finally "human" inclination.

This complete opposition to life is not new, either in India or elsewhere; the archaic and universal polarity between the sacred and the profane is clearly to be seen in it. From the beginning, the sacred has always been something totally different from the profane. And, judged by this criterion, Patañjali's Yoga, like all the other Yogas, preserves a religious value. The man who refuses his native condition and consciously reacts against it by attempting to abolish it is a man who thirsts for the unconditioned, for freedom, for "power"—in a word, for one of the countless modalities of the sacred. This "reversal of all human values" that the yogin pursues is, furthermore, validated by a long Indian tradition; for, in the Vedic perspective, the world of the gods is exactly the opposite of ours (the god's right hand corresponds to man's left hand, an object broken here below remains whole in the beyond, etc.). By the refusal that he opposes to profane life, the yogin imitates a transcendent model—Īśvara. And, even if the role that God plays in the struggle for emancipation proves to be small, this imitation of a transcendent model still has its religious value.

We should note that it is by stages that the yogin dissociates himself from life. He begins by suppressing the least essential habits of living—comforts, distractions, waste of time, dispersion of his mental forces, etc. He then attempts to *unify* the most important functions of life—respiration, consciousness. To discipline his breathing, make it rhythmical, reduce it to a single modality—that of deep sleep—is equivalent to a unification of all the varieties of respiration. On the plane of psychomental life, *ekāgratā* pursues the same end—to fix the flux of consciousness, to realize an unbroken psychic continuum, to "unify" thought. Even the most elementary of yogic techniques, *āsana*, has a similar goal; for if one is ever to become conscious of the "totality" of one's body, felt as a "unity," one can do it only by practicing one of these hieratic postures. The extreme simplification of life, the calm, the serenity, the static bodily position, the rhythmical breathing, the concentration on a single point, etc.—all these exercises pursue the same goal, which is to abolish multiplicity and fragmentation, to reintegrate, to unify, to make whole.

To say this is to say to what a degree, in withdrawing from profane human life, the yogin finds another that is deeper and truer (because "in rhythm")—the very life of the cosmos. Indeed, one can speak of the first yogic stages as an effort toward the "cosmicization" of man. To transform the chaos of biomental life into a cosmos—one divines this ambition in all the psychophysiological techniques of Yoga, from *āsana* to *ekāgratā*. We have elsewhere shown [136] that a number of yogic and tantric practices are explained by the intention to homologize the body and life of man with the celestial bodies and the cosmic rhythms, first of all with the sun and moon; and this important subject will claim our attention more than once during the course of this book.[137] Final liberation cannot be obtained without experience of a preliminary stage of "cosmicization"; one cannot pass directly from chaos to freedom. The intermediate phase is the "cosmos"—that is, realization of rhythm on all the planes of biomental life. Now, this rhythm is shown to us in the structure of the universe itself, by the "unifying" role played in it by the celestial bodies and especially the moon. (For it is the moon that measures time and makes an infinity of heterogeneous realities integral parts of the same complex.) A considerable proportion of Indian mystical physiology is based upon the identification of "suns" and "moons" in the human body.

To be sure, this "cosmicization" is only an intermediate phase,

136 "Cosmical Homology and Yoga," *Journal of the Indian Society of Oriental Art*, V (1937), 188–203. 137 See below, p. 269.

which Patañjali scarcely indicates; but it is exceptionally important in other Indian mystical schools. Obtained after "unification," "cosmicization" continues the same process—that of recasting man in new, gigantic dimensions, of guaranteeing him macranthropic experiences. But this macranthropos can himself have but a temporary existence. For the final goal will not be attained until the yogin has succeeded in "withdrawing" to his own center and completely dissociating himself from the cosmos, thus becoming impervious to experiences, unconditioned, and autonomous. This final "withdrawal" is equivalent to a rupture of plane, to an act of real transcendence. *Samādhi,* with all its tantric equivalents, is by its very nature a paradoxical state, for it is empty and at the same time fills being and thought to repletion.

Let us note that the most important yogic and tantric experiences realize a similar paradox. In *prāṇāyāma,* life coexists with holding the breath (a holding that is in fact in flagrant contradiction to life); in the fundamental tantric experience (the "return of semen"), "life" coincides with "death," the "act" becomes "virtuality."[138] It goes without saying that the paradox is implied in the very function of Indian ritual (as, of course, in every other ritual); for, by the power of ritual, some ordinary object incorporates the divinity, a "fragment" (in the case of the Vedic sacrifice, the brick of the altar) coincides with the "Whole" (the god Prajāpati), nonbeing with Being. Regarded from this point of view (that of the phenomenology of paradox), *samādhi* is seen to be situated on a line well known in the history of religions and mysticisms—that of the coincidence of opposites. It is true that, in this case, the coincidence is not merely symbolic, but concrete, experiential. Through *samādhi,* the yogin transcends opposites and, in a unique experience, unites emptiness and superabundance, life and death, Being and nonbeing. Nor is this all. Like all paradoxical states, *samādhi* is equivalent to a reintegration of the different modalities of the real in a single modality—the undifferentiated completeness of precreation, the primordial Unity. The yogin who attains to

138 See below, p. 270.

asamprajñāta samādhi also realizes a dream that has obsessed the human spirit from the beginnings of its history—to coincide with the All, to recover Unity, to re-establish the initial nonduality, to abolish time and creation (i.e., the multiplicity and heterogeneity of the cosmos); in particular, to abolish the twofold division of the real into object-subject.

It would be a gross error to regard this supreme reintegration as a mere regression to primordial nondistinction. It can never be repeated too often that Yoga, like many other mysticisms, issues on the plane of paradox and not on a commonplace and easy extinction of consciousness. As we shall see, from time immemorial India has known the many and various trances and ecstasies obtained from intoxicants, narcotics, and all the other elementary means of emptying consciousness; but any degree of methodological conscience will show us that we have no right to put *samādhi* among these countless varieties of spiritual escape. Liberation is not assimilable with the "deep sleep" of prenatal existence, even if the recovery of totality through undifferentiated enstasis seems to resemble the bliss of the human being's fetal preconsciousness. One essential fact must always be borne in mind: the yogin works on all levels of consciousness and of the subconscious, for the purpose of opening the way to transconsciousness (knowledge-possession of the Self, the *puruṣa*). He enters into "deep sleep" and into the "fourth state" (*turīya*, the cataleptic state) with the utmost lucidity; he does not sink into self-hypnosis. The importance that all authors ascribe to the yogic states of *super*consciousness shows us that the final reintegration takes place in *this* direction, and not in a trance, however profound. In other words: the recovery, through *samādhi*, of the initial nonduality introduces a new element in comparison with the primordial situation (that which existed before the twofold division of the real into object-subject). That element is *knowledge* of unity and bliss. There is a "return to the beginning," but with the difference that the man "liberated in this life" recovers the original situation enriched by the dimensions of *freedom* and *transconsciousness*. To express it differently, he does not return automatically to a "given" situation; he reintegrates the original completeness after having established a new and paradoxical mode of being—*consciousness of freedom,* which exists nowhere in the cosmos, neither on the levels of life nor on the levels of "mythological divinity" (the gods, *devas*)—which exists only in the Supreme Being, Īśvara. It is here that we become better aware of the initiatory character of Yoga. For in initiation, too, one "dies" to be "reborn"; but this new birth is not a repetition of natural birth; the candidate does not return to the profane world to which he has just died during his initiation; he finds a sacred world corresponding to a new mode of being that is *inaccessible to the "natural" (profane) level of existence.*

One would be tempted to see in this ideal—the conscious conquest of freedom—the justification offered by Indian thought for the fact, the apparently cruel and useless fact, that the world exists, that man exists, and that his existence in the world is an uninterrupted succession of suffering and despair. For, by liberating himself, man creates the spiritual dimension of freedom, and "introduces" it into the cosmos and life—that is, into blind and tragically conditioned modes of existence.

CHAPTER THREE

Yoga and Brāhmanism

Ascetics and Ecstatics in the Vedas

SO FAR, we have set forth the doctrines and techniques of Yoga as they are systematized and formulated in Patañjali's *Yoga-sūtras* and the commentaries on them. But, unlike the other *darśanas*, the *yoga-darśana* is not solely a "system of philosophy"; it sets its mark, so to speak, on a very considerable number of pan-Indian practices, beliefs, and aspirations. Yoga is present everywhere—no less in the oral tradition of India than in the Sanskrit and vernacular literatures. Naturally, this protean Yoga does not always resemble the "classic" system of Patañjali; rather, we find it in the form of traditional clichés, to which, during the course of the centuries, an increasing number of "popular" beliefs and practices has been added. To such a degree is this true that Yoga has ended by becoming a characteristic dimension of Indian spirituality. This prestige, this protean presence, raise a problem pregnant with consequences: may not Yoga be an autochthonous creation of the whole of India, the product not only of the Indo-Europeans but also, and especially, of the pre-Āryan populations?

Briefly, one could say that Yoga has succeeded in imposing itself as a universally valid technique by invoking two traditions: (1) that of the ascetics and ecstatics, documented from the time of the *Ṛg-Veda*, and (2) the symbolism of the Brāhmaṇas, especially the speculations justifying the "interiorization of sacrifice." This millennial process of integration, which issued in one of the greatest of Indian spiritual syntheses, is a striking illustration of what has been called the phenomenon of Hinduization; its mechanism will become increasingly clear as we approach the Middle Ages.

Only the rudiments of classic Yoga are to be found in the Vedas. On the other hand, those ancient texts refer to ascetic disciplines and "ecstatic" ideologies that, if they are not always directly related to Yoga properly speaking, finally found a place in the yogic tradition. It is for this reason that we refer to them here. But these two categories of spiritual facts must not be confused; ascetic methods and techniques of ecstasy are documented among the other Indo-European peoples, to say nothing of the other peoples of Asia, whereas Yoga is to be found only in India and in cultures influenced by Indian spirituality.

Thus, a hymn of the *Ṛg-Veda* (X, 136) tells of the *muni*, long-haired (*keśin*), clad in "soiled yellow," "girdled with wind," and into whom "the gods enter" (2). He proclaims: "In the intoxication of ecstasy we are mounted on the winds. You, mortals, can perceive only our body" (3). The *muni* flies through the air (4), he is the steed of the wind (*Vāta*), the friend of Vāyu, "impelled by the gods"; he inhabits the two seas, that of the rising and that of the setting sun (5); [1] "he travels by the road of the Apsarases, the Gandharvas, and wild beasts, he knows thoughts" (6) and "drinks with Rudra from the cup of poison" (7). Some have wished to see the prototype of the yogin in this long-haired *muni*. In reality, the figure is that of an ecstatic who only vaguely resembles the yogin, the chief similarity being his ability to fly through the air—but this *siddhi* is a magical power that is found everywhere.[2] The references to the horse of the wind, to the poison that he drinks with Rudra, to the gods whom he incarnates, point rather to a shamanizing technique. The description of his "ecstasy" is far more significant. The *muni* "disappears in spirit"; abandoning his body, he divines the thoughts of others; he inhabits the "two seas." All of these are experiences transcending the sphere of the profane, are states of

1 Cf. *Atharva Veda*, XI, 5, 5; XV, 7, 1.

2 See below, p. 276.

consciousness cosmic in structure, though they can be realized through other means than ecstasy.[3] The term is forced on us whenever we wish to designate an experience and a state of consciousness that are cosmic in scale, even if "ecstasy" in the strict sense of the word is not always involved.

The Vedas also refer to other supranormal experiences, in connection with mythical figures (Ekavrātya, Brahmacārin, Vena, etc.) who probably represent the divinized archetypes of certain ascetics and magicians. The divinization of man, the "man-god," remains a predominant motif of Indian spirituality. Ekavrātya, already documented in a celebrated and obscure hymn of the *Atharva Veda* (XV, 1), is regarded by the *Jaiminīya Upaniṣad Brāhmaṇa* (III, 21) as the divinity who originated the *vrātyas*, and in the *Praśna Upaniṣad* and the *Cūlikā Upaniṣad* he becomes a sort of cosmic principle.[4] Ekavrātya very probably represents the prototype of that mysterious group, the *vrātyas*, in whom various scholars have sought to see Śivaistic ascetics (Charpentier), mystics (Chaṭṭopādhyaya), precursors of the yogins (Hauer), or representatives of a non-Āryan population (Winternitz).[5] An entire book of the *Atharva Veda* (XV) is devoted to them, but the text is obscure; however, it is apparent that the *vrātyas* practice asceticism (they remain standing for a year, etc.), are familiar with a discipline of the breaths (which are assimilated to the various cosmic regions),[6] homologize their bodies with the macrocosm.[7] This mystical fellowship was in any case important, for a special sacrifice, the *vrātyastoma*, had been organized to restore its members to Brāhmanic society. The texts treating of the *vrātyastoma* and the *mahāvrata* (solstitial rite in which a number of archaic elements survive) give us a glimpse of these mysterious personages; they wore turbans, dressed in black, and had two ramskins, one white, one black, slung over their shoulders; as insignia, they

3 See above, p. 85.
4 Cf. J. W. Hauer, *Der Vrātya*, pp. 306 ff.
5 See Note III, 1.
6 *Atharva Veda*, XV, 14, 15 ff.
7 Ibid., XV, 18, 1 ff.

had a sharp-pointed stick, an ornament worn around the neck (*niṣka*), and an unstrung bow (*jyāhroḍa*). The stick-lance (prototype of the Śivaistic *śūla?*) and the bow, pre-eminently magical arms, recur in certain Asiatic shamanisms.[8] A cart drawn by a horse and a mule served them as a place of sacrifice. During the *vrātyastoma*, they were accompanied by other personages, the chief of whom were a *māgadha* and a *puṃścalī;* [9] the former seems to have filled the role of cantor, while the *puṃścali* was, literally, a prostitute; on the occasion of the *mahāvrata*, she engaged in ritual intercourse with the *māgadha* (or with a *brahmacārin*).[10] This latter ceremony contained a number of elements of archaic fertility magic: railing and obscene dialogues, ritual swaying, intercourse.

Sexual union is documented in the Vedic religion,[11] but it does not become a mystical technique until after the triumph of tantrism.[12] During the *mahāvrata* the *hotṛ* swung in a swing and also referred to the three breaths, *prāṇa*, *vyāna*, and *apāna;* [13] this probably represents a respiratory discipline implying the arrest of breathing, but it is very unlikely that the exercise was already a *prāṇāyāma*.[14] Later in the course of the *mahāvrata*, the *hotṛ* touched a hundred-stringed harp with a branch of *udumbara*, declaring: "I strike thee for the *prāṇa*, the *apāna*, and the *vyāna*." The swing is called "ship bound for heaven," the sacrificer "bird flying to

8 Cf. Eliade, *Shamanism*, p. 285 (the tree-lance among the Dyaks); Dominik Schröder, "Zur Religion der Tujen in Sininggebietes," *Anthropos*, XLVII (1952), 18 ff.; XLVIII (1953), 248 ff. ("lance of the spirits" among the Tu jen, etc.); on the bow in Asiatic shamanism, Eliade, pp. 174 f., etc.

9 *Atharva Veda*, XV, 2.

10 *Jaiminīya Brāhmaṇa*, II, 404 ff.; *Āpastamba Śrauta Sūtra*, XXI, 17, 18, etc.; Hauer, p. 264.

11 Cf. the erotic hymn, *Atharva Veda*, XX, 136; the *aśvamedha*, etc.

12 See below, p. 259.

13 *Śāṅkhāyana Śrauta Sūtra*, XVII; Hauer, pp. 258 ff.

14 From other references to the breaths in the *Atharva Veda* (V, 28; XV, 15 and 17) one could conclude that *recaka*, *pūraka*, and *kumbhaka* were also known; see Hauer, *Die Anfänge der Yogapraxis*, pp. 10 ff.; cf. id., *Der Vrātya*, pp. 291 ff. On the five breaths, see Note III, 2.

heaven"; [15] the girls who danced around the fire were likewise birds flying to heaven.[16] The images of the celestial ship and of the bird often recur in Brāhmanic literature; in any case, they do not belong only to the Indian tradition, since they are at the very heart of shamanistic symbolism, of the symbolism of the "center of the world," and of magical flight. As for the swing, it plays a part in fecundity rites, but it is also attested in shamanistic contexts.[17]

The entire complex is rather vague, and the traditions preserved in the texts are confused and sometimes contradictory. Besides Ekavrātya, the divinized archetype of the *vrātya*, we find the Brahmacārin, also conceived as a personage on a cosmic scale—initiated, clad in a black antelope skin, long-bearded, he journeys from the Eastern to the Northern Ocean and creates the worlds; he is praised as "an embryo in the womb of immortality"; clad in red, he practices *tapas*.[18] In the *mahāvrata*, as we have seen, a *brahmacārin* (= *māgadha*) entered into ritual union with the *puṃścalī*.

It is permissible to suppose that the *vrātyas* represented a mysterious brotherhood belonging to the advance guard of the Āryan invaders.[19] But they were not entirely distinct from the Keśins of the *Ṛg-Veda;* in some commentaries Rudra is called *vrātya-pati*,[20] and the *Mahābhārata* still uses the term *vrātya* to designate the Śivaistic bacchantes.[21] We must not let these orgiastic tendencies blind us to the cosmic structure of the *vrātyas'* "mystical" experiences. Now, experiences of this type also had a place of the first importance among the aboriginal, pre-Āryan populations—a fact that sometimes makes it difficult to separate the Indo-European contribution from the pre-Āryan substratum; at the time of their arrival in India, the Indo-Europeans also preserved a number of archaic cultural elements.

15 *Tāṇḍya-Mahā-Brāhmaṇa*, V, 1, 10.

16 Ibid., V, 6, 15.

17 Cf. J. G. Frazer, *The Dying God*, pp. 156 ff., 277 ff.; Eliade, *Shamanism*, pp. 129 ff.

18 *Atharva Veda*, XI, 5, 6–7.

19 Hauer, *Der Vrātya.*

20 Ibid., p. 191.

21 Ibid., p. 233 ff.

Tapas *and Yoga* *

The equivalence between this Indo-European religious archaism and that of the aborigines is very well illustrated by the theory and practice of *tapas*. This term (lit. "heat," "ardor") is used to designate ascetic effort in general. *Tapas* is clearly documented in the *Ṛg-Veda*,[22] and its powers are creative on both the cosmic and the spiritual planes; through *tapas* the ascetic becomes clairvoyant and even incarnates the gods. Prajāpati creates the world by "heating" himself to an extreme degree through asceticism [23]—that is, he creates it by a sort of magical sweating. For Brāhmanic speculation, Prajāpati was himself the product of *tapas*; in the beginning (*agre*) nonbeing (*asat*) became mind (*manas*) and heated itself (*atapyata*), giving birth to smoke, light, fire, and finally to Prajāpati.[24] Now, cosmogony and anthropogeny through sweating are mythical motifs also found elsewhere (for example, in North America). They are very probably connected with a shamanistic ideology; we know that the North American shamans make use of sweating cabinets to stimulate violent perspiration.[25] Moreover, the custom is only one aspect of a larger ideological complex that is earlier than shamanism, strictly speaking; we refer to "magical heat" and the "mastery of fire." [26] Magically increasing the heat of the body, and "mastering" fire to the point of not feeling the heat of burning coals, are two marvels universally attested among medicine men, shamans, and fakirs. Now, as we shall see later,[27] one of the most typical yogico-tantric techniques consists precisely in producing inner heat ("mystical heat"). The continuity between the oldest known magical technique and tantric Yoga is, in this particular, undeniable.

22 Cf., for example, VIII, 59, 6; X, 136, 2; 154, 2, 4; 167, 1; 109, 4, etc.

23 *Aitareya Brāhmaṇa*, V, 32, 1.

24 *Taittirīya Brāhmaṇa*, II, 2, 9, 1–10; in other texts, nonbeing is represented by the primordial waters; cf. *Śatapatha Brāhmaṇa*, XI, 1, 6, 1.

25 Eliade, *Shamanism*, p. 335.

26 Cf. ibid., pp. 363, 437 ff., 474 ff.

27 See below, p. 330.

"Creative sweating" and magical production of heat were also familiar to the Indo-Europeans. The human pair was born from the sweat of Ymir, and it was by causing the body of Gajōmard to sweat that Ahura-Mazda created man. The Irish hero Cuchulainn emerges from his first military exploit (equivalent to a military initiation) so "heated" that he bursts the staves and copper hoops of the tub in which he had been put; we find the same "heated fury" in Batradz, the hero of the Caucasian Narts.[28] As Georges Dumézil has shown, several terms in the Indo-European "heroic" vocabulary—*furor*, *ferg*, *wut*, *ménos*—express precisely this "extreme heat" and "rage" which, on other levels of sacrality, characterize the incarnation of power. Numerous episodes in the mythology or the religious folklore of India show us gods or mortals reduced to ashes by the power of a great ascetic's *tapas*. The Indo-Europeans were familiar with the technique and ideology of "magical heat" because, like a number of other ethnic groups in Asia, they were still under the influence of an archaic spiritual horizon. But it was especially in India that ascetic practices developed to a degree unknown elsewhere and that an extremely complex ideology grew up around the notion of *tapas*. In other words, it was on the soil of India that this incontrovertibly ancient and universally disseminated magical tradition reached a full flowering unparalleled anywhere else in the world.[29]

It is important to know how *tapas* was assimilated by yogic technique.[30] One preliminary observation is necessary: this ritual "heating" was not confined solely to ascetics and ecstatics. The *soma* sacrifice required the sacrificer and his wife to perform the *dīkṣā*, a rite of consecration comprising silent meditation, ascetic

28 Ymir, Gajōmard: A. Christensen, *Les Types du premier homme et du premier roi dans l'histoire légendaire des iraniens*, pp. 14 ff., 36 ff.; H. Güntert, *Der arische Weltkönig und Heiland*, pp. 346 ff.; Sven S. Hartman, *Gayōmart.* Cuchulainn, Batradz: G. Dumézil, *Horace et les Curiaces*, pp. 35 ff.; id., *Légendes sur les Nartes*, pp. 50 ff., 179 ff.

29 See Note III, 3.

30 The *Yoga-sūtras* contain four references to the spiritual value of *tapas:* II, 1, 32, 43; IV, 1.

vigil, fasting, and, in addition, "heat," *tapas;* and the rite could continue for from one day to as long as a year. Now, the *soma* was one of the most important sacrifices in Vedic and Brāhmanic India —which is as much as to say that *tapas* was part of the religious experience of the entire Indian people. It seems to follow that, as far as theory was concerned, there was no solution of continuity between ritual on the one hand and ascetic and contemplative techniques on the other—the difference between the sacrificer and the *tapasvin* was, in the beginning, a difference of degree. Continuity between ritual and asceticism can also be observed elsewhere; in the Christian world laymen and monks recite the same prayers and follow the same religious calendar, though the degree of their personal experiences differs. But it is important to emphasize that, from Vedic times on, there was a unity in fundamental conceptions; we shall thus understand the meaning of the later Hinduistic syntheses, brought about especially through assimilation and homologization of extra-Brāhmanic and even extra-Āryan religious values.

Now, *tapas,* which is obtained through fasting, through vigil kept in the presence of fire, etc., is also obtained by holding the breath. Holding the breath begins to play a ritual role from the period of the Brāhmaṇas: he who chants the Gāyatrīstotra should not breathe.[31] The reader will recall the reference to the breaths in the *Atharva Veda* (XV, 15–18). More precise information is given by the *Baudhāyana Dharma Sūtra* (IV, 1, 24), according to which "magical heat" is produced by holding the breath.[32] We see to what all these indications point: in order to consecrate himself to perform the *soma* sacrifice, the sacrificer must practice *tapas* and become "burning"—"magical heat" being pre-eminently the sign that one has passed beyond the human condition, has emerged from the "profane." But the heat can equally well be produced by disciplining or arresting respiration; this allows the assimilation of yogic techniques to orthodox Brāhmanic methods, just as it

31 *Jaiminīya Brāhmaṇa,* III, 3, 1; cf. *Kauṣītaki Brāhmaṇa,* XXIII, 5.

32 The *Majjhima-nikāya* (I, 244, etc.) transmits the same tradition.

allows the yogin to be assimilated to the *tapasvin;* in short, the bold homologization of the Vedic sacrifice with the techniques of ecstasy is already forecast here.

This homology was made possible especially by the Brāhmaṇas' speculations on sacrifice. We need hardly remind the reader of the importance of sacrifice, from Vedic times onward. It was all-powerful. The gods themselves subsist by virtue of ritual offerings: "It is sacrifice, O Indra, that has made thee so powerful. . . . It was worship that aided thy thunder when thou didst split the dragon." [33] Sacrifice is the principle of the life and soul of all the gods and all beings.[34] In the beginning, the gods were mortal; [35] they became divine and immortal through sacrifice; [36] they live by gifts from the earth, as men live by gifts from heaven.[37] But, above all, on the level of action, sacrifice expresses "works," the desire to *remake the world,* to reunite Prajāpati's scattered members.[38] The myth is well known: when Prajāpati created the world, his members fell from him, and the gods "recomposed" him.[39] Through sacrifice, Prajāpati is reconstructed,[40] but this can also be understood in the sense that Prajāpati is remade in order that he may repeat the cosmogony and that the world may endure and continue. As Sylvain Lévi remarks,[41] the sacrifice is not made, it is prolonged, it is continued; the sacrifice must be prevented from ceasing to be.

This paradoxical description of sacrifice—as a continuity that is nevertheless a *return to the primordial unity,* to the completeness of Prajāpati *before* the creation—does not affect its essential function:

33 *Ṛg-Veda,* III, 32, 12.
34 *Śatapatha Brāhmaṇa,* VIII, 6, 1, 10, etc.
35 *Taittirīya Saṃhitā,* VIII, 4, 2, 1, etc.
36 Ibid., VI, 3, 4, 7; VI, 3, 10, 2, etc.
37 Ibid., III, 2, 9, 7, etc.
38 The principal texts will be found in Sylvain Lévi, *La Doctrine du sacrifice dans les Brāhmaṇas;* cf. also A. K. Coomaraswamy, *Hinduism and Buddhism,* pp. 19 ff.
39 *Taittirīya Brāhmaṇa,* I, 2, 6, 1, etc.
40 *Taittirīya Saṃhitā,* V, 5, 2,1.
41 *La Doctrine,* pp. 79–80.

assuring the "second birth." In fact, the initiatory symbolism of sacrifice is emphasized by its sexual and gynecological symbolism. The texts are clear.[42] The *Aitareya Brāhmaṇa* (I, 3) expounds the homologization in detail: "Him whom they consecrate [with the *dīkṣā*] the priests make into an embryo again. With waters they sprinkle; the waters are seed. . . . They conduct him to the hut of the consecrated; the hut of the consecrated is the womb of the consecrated; verily thus they conduct him to his womb. . . . With a garment they cover him; the garment is the caul. . . . Above that is the black antelope skin; the placenta is above the caul. . . . He closes his hands; verily closing its hands the embryo lies within; with closed hands the child is born. . . . Having loosened the black antelope skin, he descends to the final bath; therefore embryos are born freed from the placenta; with the garment he descends; therefore a child is born with a caul." [43]

This symbolism is not a creation of the Brāhmaṇas. The initiate has everywhere been assimilated to a newborn infant, and in some cases the initiatory hut was regarded as the belly of a monster; [44] having entered it, the candidate was "swallowed," was ritually "dead" but also in the state of an embryo. Since the purpose of the sacrifice was to gain heaven (*svarga*), community of dwelling place with the gods, or the quality of a god (*devātma*) after death, here once again there is symmetry with the fundamental concept of archaic initiation, which was held to guarantee initiates the best possible condition in the beyond.

Still more: initiation is not reducible to the ritual of death and rebirth; it also comprises a secret gnosis. Now, the "science" of the Brāhmaṇas, although concentrated on the mysteries of sacrifice, also plays an important role.[45] "That world [the world of the gods]

42 Cf. Lévi, *La Doctrine*, pp. 104 ff.

43 Tr. A. B. Keith, *The Rigveda Brāhmaṇas*, pp. 108–09.

44 Frazer, *Spirits of the Corn and of the Wild*, I, 225 ff.

45 The gynecological and obstetric symbolism of initiation was continued in the imagery of philosophical apprenticeship. Socrates claims that his mission is that of a midwife; he delivers the "new man," he aids in the birth of "him who knows."

belongs only to those who know." [46] In the Brāhmaṇas the proposition "he who knows thus" (*ya evam veda*) is very frequently repeated. In the course of time, the "science" of sacrifice and of liturgical techniques loses some of its value, and a new science, *knowledge of brahman*, replaces it. Thus the way is opened to the Upaniṣadic *ṛṣis* and, later, to the masters of Sāṃkhya, for whom true "science" suffices for deliverance. For "unsafe boats . . . are these sacrificial forms," the *Muṇḍaka Upaniṣad* (I, 2, 7) will say.[47]

"Ritual Interiorization"

Sacrifice was early assimilated to *tapas*. The gods gained immortality not only through sacrifice,[48] but also through asceticism. The *Ṛg-Veda* (X, 167, 1) declares that Indra forced heaven through *tapas*, and this idea is carried very far in the Brāhmaṇas: "The gods gained their divine rank through austerity." [49] For *tapas*, too, is a "sacrifice." If, in Vedic sacrifice, the gods are offered *soma*, melted butter, and the sacred fire, in the practice of asceticism they are offered an "inner sacrifice," in which physiological functions take the place of libations and ritual objects. Respiration is often identified with an "unceasing libation." *Vaikhānasasmārtasūtra*, II, 18, refers to the *prāṇāgnihotra*—that is, the "daily sacrifice in respiration." [50] The concept of this "inner sacrifice" is a

46 *Śatapatha Brāhmaṇa*, X, 5, 4, 16.

47 Tr. R. E. Hume, *The Thirteen Principal Upanishads*, p. 368.

48 See above, pp. 106 ff.

49 *Taittirīya Brāhmaṇa*, III, 12, 3, 1, etc.

50 In the same text we find the physiological functions and the organs assimilated to the various ritual fires, to the objects employed in sacrifice, etc. "The self-luminous *ātman* is the sacrificer; the intellect is the bride; the lotus of the heart is the *vedi;* the body hair is the herb *dharba;* the *prāṇa* is the Gārhapatya; the *apāna* is the Ahavanīya; the *vyāna* is Dakṣiṇāgni; the *udāna* is the Sabhya fire; the *sāmana* is the Avasathya fire; these are the five fires [of the sacrifice]. The sense organs, the tongue, etc., are the sacrificial vessels; the objects of the senses, taste, etc., are the sacrificial substances." The *prāṇāgnihotra* also occurs in some Upaniṣads, but with a different meaning; cf. *Prāṇāgnihotra Upaniṣad*, 3–4.

fertile one, which will permit even the most autonomous ascetics and mystics to remain within the fold of Brāhmanism and later of Hinduism.

We shall quote a Brāhmanic text in which *prāṇāyāma* is homologized with one of the most famous of Vedic sacrifices, the *agnihotra* (oblation to fire, which the head of every household was required to perform twice daily, before sunrise and after sunset): "The 'Inner Agnihotra' . . . they call it.—As long, verily, as a person is speaking, he is not able to breathe. Then he is sacrificing breath in speech. As long, verily, as a person is breathing, he is not able to speak. Then he is sacrificing speech in breath. These two are unending, immortal oblations; whether waking or sleeping, one is sacrificing continuously, uninterruptedly. Now, whatever other oblations there are, they are limited, for they consist of works [*karma*]. Knowing this very thing, verily, indeed, the ancients did not sacrifice the Agnihotra sacrifice." [51]

The same conception, rather more discreetly expressed, is found in the *Chāndogya Upaniṣad* (V, 19–24): the true sacrifice consists in oblations to the breaths; "if one offers the Agnihotra sacrifice without knowing this [*sa ya idam avidvān*]—that would be just as if he were to . . . pour the offering on ashes." [52] This form of sacrifice is generally given the name "mental sacrifice." We should prefer to call it "ritual interiorization," for, besides mental prayer, it implies a profound assimilation of the physiological functions to the life of the cosmos. This homologizing the physiological organs and functions with the cosmic regions and rhythms is pan-Indian. Traces of it are to be found in the Vedas; strictly speaking, however, it is only in tantrism (and there largely because of the contribution of yogic techniques) that it will acquire the coherence of a "system."

The texts just cited doubtless refer to certain ascetics who practiced *prāṇāyāma*, which they homologized with the concrete sacrifice named the *agnihotra*. This is but one example of the way

51 *Kauṣītaki Brāhmaṇa Upaniṣad*, II, 5; tr. Hume, p. 310.
52 V, 24, 1; tr. Hume, p. 239.

in which the orthodox tradition often validated an exercise that, in itself, had no connections with orthodoxy. Now, the practical consequence of homologization is substitution (which it justifies). Thus asceticism becomes equivalent to ritual, to Vedic sacrifice. Hence it is easy to understand how other yogic practices made their way into the Brāhmanic tradition and were accepted by it.

However, we must not let ourselves suppose that these homologizations were always made in one direction. It was not always the fervent devotees of yogic practices who tried to obtain Brāhmanic approval of their attitude and method. Orthodoxy itself frequently took the first step. The very small number of "heresies" recorded during the three thousand years of Indian religious life is owing not only to the constant efforts of the innumerable sects and trends to gain formal admission to the traditional fold, but equally to the ceaseless assimilative and Hinduizing activity of orthodoxy. In India, orthodoxy means first of all the spiritual domination of a caste, that of the Brāhmans. Its theological and ritual "system" can be reduced to two fundamental points: (1) the Vedas are regarded as forming an unalterable scriptural corpus; (2) sacrifice outweighs everything else in importance. The two elements are pre-eminently "static." Yet the religious history of Indo-Āryan India proves to be essentially dynamic, in perpetual transformation. A double action—set in motion, and continued down to the present day, by Brāhmanic orthodoxy—explains this phenomenon: (1) by recourse to hermeneutics, the Vedas have been constantly reinterpreted; (2) by recourse to mythical, ritual, or religious homologizations, the complexities of extra-orthodox cults and mysticisms have been, so to speak, reduced to a common denominator and, finally, absorbed by orthodoxy. Assimilation of autochthonous "popular" divinities by Hinduism remains a current phenomenon.[53]

Naturally, orthodoxy performed this assimilation only at moments of crisis—that is, when its old ritual and doctrinal schemata no longer satisfied its own élites and when important ascetico-

53 See Note IV, 4.

mystical "experiences" or preaching had developed *extra muros.* All through the course of Indian history, we can detect a reaction against Brāhmanism's ritual schematization and also against its excessive "abstraction"—a reaction whose point of departure is to to be found in the very heart of Indian society. The reaction will increase in volume as India becomes increasingly Brāhmanized and Hinduized—that is, the absorption of extra-Brāhmanic and extra-Āryan elements will become more intense.

Symbolism and Gnosis in the Upaniṣads

The Upaniṣads, too, in their particular way, react against ritualism. They are the expression of experiences and meditations on the margin of Brāhmanic orthodoxy. They answered to a need for the absolute that the abstract schemata of ritualism were far from satisfying. In this respect, the Upaniṣadic *ṛṣis* took the same position as the yogins; both abandoned orthodoxy (sacrifice, civic life, the family) and, in all simplicity, set out in search of the absolute. It is true that the Upaniṣads remain in the line of metaphysics and contemplation, whereas Yoga employs asceticism and a technique of meditation. But this is not enough to halt the constant osmosis between the Upaniṣadic and yogic milieus. Some yogic methods are even accepted by the Upaniṣads as preliminary exercises in purification and contemplation. We shall not go into details here; out of the considerable body of Upaniṣadic meditations, we shall mention only the aspects that concern our subject directly.[54] The great discovery of the Upaniṣads was, of course, the systematic statement of the identity between the *ātman* and the *brahman*. Now, if we take into consideration what *brahman* had meant from Vedic times, the Upaniṣadic discovery entailed the following consequence: immortality and absolute power became accessible to every being who made the effort to reach gnosis and thus acquire knowledge of every mystery, for the *brahman* represented all that—it was the immortal, the imperishable, the powerful.

54 Texts and bibliographies in Note III, 5.

For if it is difficult to find a single formula that will include all the meanings given to *brahman* in Vedic and post-Vedic texts, there is no possible doubt that the term expressed the ultimate and inapprehensible reality, the *Grund* of every cosmic manifestation and of every experience, and, consequently, the *force* of every creation, whether cosmological (the universe) or simply ritual (sacrifice). There is no need to recall all of the nearly innumerable identifications and homologizations of the *brahman* (in the Brāhmaṇas, it is identified with fire, speech, sacrifice, the Vedas, etc.); the important fact is that, at all periods and on all cultural levels, the *brahman* was considered and expressly called the imperishable, the immutable, the foundation, the principle of all existence. It is significant that in the Vedas the mythical image of the *brahman* is the *skambha*, the cosmic pillar, the *axis mundi*, a symbol whose archaism no longer stands in need of proof, since it is found among the hunters and shepherds of central and northern Asia no less than in the "primitive" cultures of Oceania, Africa, and the two Americas.[55] In several hymns of the *Atharva Veda* (X, 7, 8, etc.) the *brahman* is identified with the *skambha* (lit., "stay," "support," "pillar")—in other words, the *brahman* is the *Grund* that supports the world, is at once cosmic axis and ontological foundation.

We can follow the process of dialectical elaboration to which the primordial symbol of the *axis mundi* was subjected: on the one hand, the axis is always placed at the "center of the world," it supports and connects the three cosmic regions (heaven, earth, underworld); this is as much as to say that it symbolizes both "cosmicization" (manifestation of forms) and the norm, the universal law; the *skambha* supports and divides heaven and earth; in other words, it assures and prolongs the world as a manifestation, prevents return to chaos, to confusion. On the other hand, "in the *skambha* is everything that is possessed by spirit [*ātmanvat*], everything that breathes." [56] Here we can already foresee the road that Upaniṣadic speculation will take; the Being identified in the

55 Cf. Eliade, *Shamanism*, pp. 259 ff.
56 *Atharva Veda*, X, 8, 2.

"axis" of the universe (in its "center," in its principle) is found again, on another level, in man's spiritual "center," in the *ātman*. "He who knows the *brahman* in man knows the Supreme Being [*parameṣṭhin*, the Lord] and he who knows the Supreme Being knows the *skambha*." [57] We see the endeavor to isolate the ultimate reality, the principle that cannot be formulated in words; *brahman* is recognized as the pillar of the universe, the support, the base, and the term *pratiṣṭhār*, which expresses all these notions, is already commonly employed in the Vedic texts; in the *Mahābhārata* and the Purāṇas *brahman* is called *dhruva*, "fixed," "motionless," "firm," "permanent." [58]

But to know the *skambha*, the *dhruva*, is to possess the key to the cosmic mystery and to find the "center of the world" in the inmost depths of one's being. Knowledge is a sacred force because it solves the enigma of the universe and the enigma of the Self. In ancient India, as in all other traditional societies, occult knowledge was the prerogative of a class, the specialists in the mysteries, the masters of rites—the Brāhmans. As might be expected, the universal principle, *brahman*, is identified with the man-Brāhman: *brahma hi brāhmaṇaḥ* is a leitmotiv of post-Vedic texts.[59] "The birth of the Brāhman is an eternal incarnation of the *dharma*"; [60] "it is those wise men who uphold all the worlds." [61]

The Brāhman is identified with *brahman* because he knows the structure and origin of the universe, because he knows the Word in which those things are expressed; for Vāc, the Logos, can transform anyone into a Brāhman.[62] As the *Bṛhadāraṇyaka Upaniṣad* will say (III, 8, 10), he who knows the imperishable (*akṣaram*—that is, *brahman*) is a Brāhman. In short, one becomes a Brāhman through knowledge of Being, of the ultimate reality, and the possession of this knowledge is revealed by the acquisition of the highest of powers, sacred power. By systematically formulating the

57 *Atharva Veda*, X, 7, 17.

58 See the texts collected by J. Gonda, *Notes on Brahman*, pp. 47–48.

59 Gonda, p. 51.

60 Manu, I, 98.

61 *Mahābhārata*, XIII, 151, 3; cf. other texts, Gonda, p. 52.

62 Already in *Ṛg-Veda*, X, 125, 5.

identity *ātman* (the Self) = *brahman* (= *skambha, dhruva, akṣara*), the classic Upaniṣads showed the way to emancipation from rituals and works. It is at this precise point that the Upaniṣadic *ṛṣis* meet with the ascetics and the yogins; setting out from other premises, and obeying vocations that are less speculative, more technical, more "mystical," the yogins also recognized that true knowledge of the cosmic mysteries found expression in the possession of an unbounded spiritual force; but they were more inclined to gain this knowledge of the Self by assault, through half-contemplative, half-physiological techniques. They will eventually identify the cosmos with their own body, by carrying to the extreme certain micro-macrocosmic homologies already attested in the *Ṛg-Veda;* the cosmic winds will be "mastered" as breaths; the cosmic *skambha*-pillar will be identified with the vertebral column; the "center of the world" will be found in a point (the "heart") or an axis (traversing the *cakras*) inside the body. In late texts, we begin to see a twofold osmotic movement: the yogins take advantage of the aura of sanctity that clings to the ancient Upaniṣads and adorn their treatises with the epithet "Upaniṣadic"; the Upaniṣadic *ṛṣis* turn to their profit the recent but already great fame of the yogins, of those who can simultaneously gain liberation and magical mastery of the world. It is for this reason that a rapid review of the yogic elements to be found in the Upaniṣads cannot but be instructive; it will help us to see the progress made in the acceptance of Yoga by Brāhmanism, as well as the prodigious polymorphism of the former. For henceforth—as we must not forget—it will be with the rich and sometimes strange morphology of "baroque" Yoga that we shall be concerned.

Immortality and Liberation

The term *yoga*, in its technical sense, first occurs in the *Taittirīya Upaniṣad* (II, 4: *yoga ātmā*) and the *Kaṭha Upaniṣad* (II, 12: *adhyātma yoga*).[63] But yogic practice is discernible in the earliest

63 Ibid., VI, 11 (the text closest to the classic meaning), etc.

Upaniṣads. Thus a passage from the *Chāndogya Upaniṣad* (VIII, 15: *ātmani sarvendrīyāṇi sampratiṣṭha*, "concentrating all one's senses upon one's self") allows us to infer the practice of *pratyāhāra;* similarly, *prāṇāyāma* is frequently to be found in the *Bṛhadāraṇyaka Upaniṣad.*[64]

In the Upaniṣads, *knowledge* brings deliverance from death: "Lead me from death to immortality!" [65] "They who know that become immortal." [66] Yoga practice, as the Upaniṣads apply it, pursues the same goal. It is significant that, in the *Kaṭha Upaniṣad*, it is Yama, king of the dead, who reveals supreme knowledge and Yoga together. The fable employed in this same Upaniṣad (its inspiration is an episode in the *Taittirīya Brāhmaṇa*) is original and mysterious: the young Brāhman Naciketas reaches the infernal regions, and, persuading Yama to grant him three wishes, asks him to tell him of man's lot after death. The descent into the infernal regions and the three days' sojourn there are well-known initiatory themes; obvious examples are the shamanic initiations and the Mysteries of antiquity. Yama tells Naciketas the secret of the "fire that leads to heaven," [67] a fire that can be referred either to a ritual fire or to a "mystical fire" produced by *tapas*. This fire is "the bridge to the supreme *brahman*"; [68] the image of the bridge, which is frequent even in the Brāhmaṇas, occurs again in the earliest Upaniṣads; [69] it is likewise attested in many traditions and generally signifies the initiatory passage from one mode of being to another.[70] But it is the teaching concerning the "great journey" that is particularly important. After vainly seeking to distract Naciketas from this problem by offering him a multitude of earthly goods, Yama reveals the great mystery to him—the *ātman*, who "is not to be obtained by instruction, nor by intellect, nor by much learning. He is to be obtained only by the one whom

64 E.g., I, 5, 23.

65 *Bṛhadāraṇyaka Upaniṣad*, I, 3, 28.

66 *Kaṭha Upaniṣad*, VI, 9; cf. ibid., VI, 18: *vimṛtyu*, "free from death."

67 Ibid., I, 14 ff.

68 Ibid., III, 2.

69 Cf. *Chāndogya Upaniṣad*, VIII, 4, 1–2.

70 Cf. Eliade, *Shamanism*, pp. 395 ff., 482 ff.

he chooses."[71] The last line has a mystical coloring, which is intensified by the reference to Viṣṇu in the following chapter.[72]

The man in perfect possession of himself is compared to a skillful driver, who is able to master his senses: it is such a man who gains liberation.

> Know thou the soul [*ātman*] as riding in a chariot,
> The body as the chariot.
> Know thou the intellect as the chariot-driver,
> And the mind as the reins.
>
> The senses, they say, are the horses;
> The objects of sense, what they range over.
>
> . . . He . . . who has understanding,
> Whose mind is constantly held firm—
> His senses are under control,
> Like the good horses of a chariot-driver.
>
> . . . He . . . who has understanding,
> Who is mindful and ever pure,
> Reaches the goal
> From which he is born no more.[73]

Although Yoga is not named, the image is specifically yogic; the harness, the reins, the driver, and the good horses are all related to the etymon *yuj*, "to hold fast," "to yoke."[74] And a strophe in another place is specific:

> This they consider as Yoga—
> This firm holding back of the senses.
> Then one becomes undistracted.[75]

Finally, we find a physiological detail that is yogic; resuming a

71 *Kaṭha Upaniṣad*, II, 23; tr. Hume, p. 350.

72 Ibid., III, 9.

73 Ibid., III, 3–4, 6, 8; tr. Hume, pp. 351–52.

74 Same image in the *Maitrāyaṇī Upaniṣad*, II, 6.

75 *Kaṭha Upaniṣad*, VI, 11. Cf. ibid., VI, 18: "Then Naciketas, having received this knowledge/Declared by Death, and the entire rule of Yoga,/Attained Brahma and became free from passion, free from death." Tr. Hume, pp. 360, 361.

śloka preserved in the *Chāndogya Upaniṣad,* our text tells us that

> There are a hundred and one arteries of the heart.
> Only one of these passes up to the crown of the head.
> Going up by it, one goes to immortality.[76]

This reference is of considerable importance; it reveals the existence of a system of mystical physiology concerning which later texts, especially the yogic Upaniṣads and the literature of tantrism, will give increasingly abundant details.

> He . . . who has the understanding of a chariot-driver,
> A man who reins in his mind—
> He reaches the end of his journey,
> That highest place of Vishṇu [*so'dhavanaḥ pāramāpnoti tadviṣṇoḥ paramaṃ padam*],

says the *Kaṭha Upaniṣad.*[77] This is not yet the Viṣṇu of the epic or of the Purāṇas, but his role in this first Upaniṣad in which Yoga is employed to obtain both knowledge of the *ātman* and immortality already shows us the direction of the great later syntheses; the three highest roads of liberation—Upaniṣadic *knowledge,* yoga *technique,* and *bhakti*—will be gradually homologized and integrated. The process is still further advanced in an Upaniṣad of the same period, the *Śvetāśvatara,* which, however, venerates Śiva instead of Viṣṇu. Nowhere else is the identity between mystical knowledge and immortality more frequently expressed.[78]

The predominance of the "motif of immortality" leads us to

76 VI, 16; tr. Hume, p. 361.

77 III, 9; tr. Hume, p. 352.

78 Immortality through God (I, 6); when Hara (=Śiva) is known, "birth and death cease" (I, 11); he who knows Rudra (Śiva) becomes immortal (III, 1); he who accepts the supreme *brahman* as Lord attains immortality (III, 7); "the man who truly knows him passes beyond death; there is no other way" (III, 8); immortality (III, 10; III, 13); Spirit is the "master of immortality" (III, 15); he who knows triumphs over death (IV, 15, 17, 20); the gods and the poets who have known the essence of *brahman*, concealed in the Vedas and the Upaniṣads, have become immortal (V, 6); immortality through Śiva alone (VI, 15, 17); the "supreme bridge to immortality" (*amṛtasya param setum;* VI, 19).

believe that the *Śvetāśvatara Upaniṣad* was composed in a "mystical" milieu, or rather that it was rewritten in such a milieu, for the text has been subjected to numerous additions in the course of the centuries. The term "liberation" appears in it less frequently (IV, 16). But a number of passages refer to the joy that is the fruit of the "eternal happiness" attained by those who know Śiva (VI, 12)—an expression that, with many others (IV, 11, 12, etc.), testifies to a concrete content of genuine mystical experience. The *brahman* is identified with Śiva, whose name is also Hara (I, 10), Rudra (III, 2), Bhagavat (III, 11). We need not here concern ourselves with the composite structure and Śivaistic coloring of this Upaniṣad.[79] But it was necessary to emphasize the element of experimental mysticism contained in it, in order better to explain the importance it gives to yogic practices (II, 8–13). That these are a matter of tradition and of the private "professional secrets" of certain anchoritic "experimenters," the author himself (or one of his "editors") gives us to understand. For he tells us:

By the efficacy of his austerity and by the grace of God (*devaprasāda*)
The wise Śvetāśvatara in proper manner declared Brahma
Unto the ascetics of the most advanced stage as the supreme means of purification—
This which is well pleasing to the company of seers.[80]

Thus yogic technique is made an integral part of the Upaniṣadic tradition, and it is a technique that bears considerable resemblance to that of the *Yoga-sūtras*. The essential passages are the following:

> Holding his body steady with the three [upper parts] [81] erect,
> And causing the senses with the mind to enter into the heart,
> A wise man with the Brahma-boat should cross over
> All the fear-bringing streams.

Having repressed his breathings here in the body, and having his movements checked,

79 See Note III, 5.

80 VI, 21; tr. Hume, p. 411.

81 I.e., chest, neck, head; cf. *Bhagavad Gītā*, VI, 13.

One should breathe through his nostrils with diminished breath.[82]
Like that chariot yoked with vicious horses,
His mind the wise man should restrain undistractedly.

In a clean, level spot,[83] free from pebbles, fire, and gravel,
By the sound of water and other propinquities
Favorable to thought, not offensive to the eye,
In a hidden retreat protected from the wind, one should practise Yoga.

Fog, smoke, sun, fire, wind,
Fire-flies, lightning, a crystal, a moon—
These are the preliminary appearances,
Which produce the manifestation of Brahma in Yoga.

When the fivefold quality of Yoga has been produced,
Arising from earth, water, fire, air, and space,
No sickness, no old age, no death has he
Who has obtained a body made out of the fire of Yoga.

Lightness, healthiness, steadiness [or, with another reading, "freedom from desires"],
Clearness of countenance and pleasantness of voice,
Sweetness of odor and scanty excretions—
These, they say, are the first stage in the progress of Yoga.[84]

The most important *aṅgas* of the *Yoga-sūtras* are here recognizable: *āsana*, *pratyāhāra*, *prāṇāyāma*. The acoustic and luminous phenomena that mark the stages of yogic meditation, which the later Upaniṣads will dwell upon, confirm the technical and experimental nature of the secret tradition transmitted by the *Śvetāśvatara*. Another Upaniṣad belonging to the same group, the *Māṇḍūkya*, adds decisive details concerning the four states of consciousness and their relations with the mystical syllable *OṂ*. The extreme brevity of this Upaniṣad (it has but twelve strophes) is more than compensated for by the importance of its revelations.

82 Cf. *Bhagavad Gītā*, V, 27.
83 Cf. ibid., VI, 11.
84 *Śvetāśvatara Upaniṣad*, II, 8–13; tr. Hume, p. 398.

For, although it repeats the Upaniṣadic speculations on dreams and the waking state,[85] the *Māṇḍūkya* for the first time offers a system of homologies among the states of consciousness, the mystical letters, and, as Zimmer so cogently saw, citing an allusion of Śaṇkara's, the four *yugas*. The tendency to homologize the different planes of reality is of the essence of every archaic and traditional spirituality; documented from Vedic times, it flourishes with the Brāhmaṇas and the Upaniṣads. But the *Māṇḍūkya* marks the triumph of a long labor of synthesis—that is, the integration of several levels of reference: Upaniṣadic, yogic, "mystical," cosmological.

Indeed, the first strophe of the *Māṇḍūkya* proclaims the mystery and grandeur of *OṂ*:[86] the syllable "is the Whole." Now, this Whole, which is the *brahman*, which is the *ātman*, has four quarters (*pāda*, "foot": "like the four feet of the cow," Śaṇkara annotates); four elements can likewise be distinguished in the mystical syllable: the letters *A*, *U*, *M*, and the final synthesis, the sound *OṂ*. This fourfold division opens the way to a daring homology; the four states of consciousness are related to the four "quarters" of the *ātman-brahman*, the four elements of *OṂ*, and, if Śaṇkara's commentary is included, with the four *yugas*. "What is in the waking state, cognitive outwardly . . . is the first quarter, called *vaiśvānara*" (the universal, what is common to all men); this *vaiśvānara* is the sound *A* (9). "What is in the dream state, cognitive inwardly . . . is the second quarter, called *taijasa*" (that which shines); this represents the sound *U* (10). "When one is asleep, and desires no desire, and sees no dream, that is deep sleep [*suṣupta*]: what is in the state of deep sleep . . . is the third quarter, called *prājña*" (he who knows); and *prājña* is the third sound, *M* (11). "The fourth state is held to be that which is cognitive neither outwardly nor inwardly, nor the two together,

85 E.g., *Bṛhadāraṇyaka Upaniṣad*, IV, 4, 7 ff.; *Chāndogya Upaniṣad*, VIII, 6, etc.

86 For the antiquity of meditation on the syllable *OṂ*, already traceable in the Vedas, see Paul Deussen, *Allgemeine Geschichte der Philosophie*, II, 349 ff.; Hauer, *Die Anfänge der Yogapraxis*, pp. 180–81.

nor is undifferentiated cognition, nor knowing, nor unknowing; which is invisible, ineffable, intangible, indefinable, inconceivable, not designable, whose essence is the experience of its own Self [*ekātmapratyayasāram*], which is beyond diversity, which is tranquil [*śāntam*], benign [*śivam*], without a second [*advaitam*]. This is the Self, which is to be known" (7). "And the fourth state . . . is the syllable *OṂ*" (12).[87]

A passage in the *Amṛtabindu Upaniṣad* (XI, 12) specifies that everything that is experienced in the state of waking, in dreams, and in dreamless sleep must be understood as the same unique *ātman*, but that liberation is gained only by him who has transcended these three dimensions of Spirit—that is, by him who has attained the state of *turīya*. In other words, the whole of experience belongs to the *ātman*, but freedom is conquered only when experience (in the sense of separate experience) has been transcended. The fourth state, *turīya*, corresponds to *samādhi;* it is the situation of total Spirit, without any specificity, a totality that, on the cosmic level, represents a complete cycle, comprising both the four *yugas* and the atemporal period of reabsorption in the primordial unity. *Turīya, samādhi*, represent Spirit in its undifferentiated unity. For India, as we know, unity can be realized only before or after creation, before or after time. Total reintegration—that is, return to unity—is, for Indian thought, the supreme goal of every responsible life. We shall soon meet this exemplary image again on all levels of spirituality and in all cultural contexts.

Yoga in the Maitri Upaniṣad

The *Maitrāyaṇī* (or *Maitri*) may be regarded as the point of departure for the whole group of middle-period Upaniṣads; it seems to have been composed at about the same time as the *Bhagavad Gītā*, or perhaps a little later (hence between the second century B.C. and the second century of our era), but in any case before the

87 Tr. Heinrich Zimmer (slightly modified), *Philosophies of India*, ed. Joseph Campbell, pp. 372–78.

didactic portions of the *Mahābhārata.*[88] As we shall see, Yoga technique and ideology are set forth more elaborately in the *Maitri* than in the earlier Upaniṣads. It is true that the sixth chapter, that in which the majority of the yogic elements occur and which is abnormally longer than the other chapters, would seem to have been composed later; but this detail, though of importance for the history of the text, is not decisive for an estimate of its content. (It cannot be too often repeated that the composition of Indian philosophic and religious texts never corresponds chronologically with the "invention" of their theoretic content.) All the verses of this sixth chapter begin with the formula "For it is said elsewhere"—which proves the dependence of the *Maitri Upaniṣad* on earlier yogic texts. In addition, although yogic technique is expounded in twelve strophes of Chapter VI, innumerable references or allusions to it occur almost throughout.[89] The *Maitri* knows only five of the eight *aṅgas* of classic Yoga; [90] *yama, niyama,* and *āsana* are absent, but we find *tarka,* "reflection," "strength of judgment" (a term quite rare in yogic texts, which the *Amṛtabindu Upaniṣad,* 16, explains as follows: "meditation that is not contrary to the *śāstra,*" i.e., the orthodox tradition). The physiological materialism of the explanation of *dhārāṇa* is interesting: "By pressing the tip of his tongue against the palate, by restraining voice, mind, and breath, one sees Brahma through contemplation [*tarka*]"; [91] the following paragraph (VI, 21) mentions the *suṣumṇā* artery, which "serves as channel for the *prāṇa*" and (through *prāṇāyāma* and meditation on the syllable *OṂ*) sustains the deep meditation by which *kevalatva* ("solitude," "isolation") is realized. These texts show what importance the *Maitri Upaniṣad* accords to auditory meditation. Several passages lay stress on the syllable *OṂ:* [92] meditation on it leads to deliverance (VI, 22), brings the vision

88 E. W. Hopkins, *The Great Epic of India,* pp. 33–46.

89 E.g., repugnance to the body, I, 3; all is perishable, I, 4; III, 4; the passions provoked by *tamas* and *rajas,* III, 5, etc.

90 Cf. *Yoga-sūtras,* II, 29.

91 *Maitri Upaniṣad,* VI, 20; tr. Hume, p. 436.

92 Cf. ibid., VI, 3–5, 21–26.

of the *brahman* and immortality (VI, 24); *OṂ* is identical with Viṣṇu (VI, 23), with all the gods, all the breaths, all sacrifices (VI, 5).

The explanation for this supremacy of meditation on the mystical syllable *OṂ* may perhaps lie not only in the spirit of synthesis and syncretism common to this class of Upaniṣads, but also in the practical success of a technique of auditory meditation that India had long known and still knows. Chapter VI, 22, offers a very obscure attempt to explain meditation on the "word" and the "nonword" (an attempt that may be regarded as a document in the prehistory of the theories of physical sound, *śabda*). The same chapter also describes another method for mystical auditory experience: "By closing the ears with the thumbs they hear the sound of the space within the heart. Of it there is this sevenfold comparison: like rivers, a bell, a brazen vessel, a wheel, the croaking of frogs, rain, as when one speaks in a sheltered place. Passing beyond this variously characterized [sound-Brahma], men disappear in the supreme, the non-sound, the unmanifest Brahma. There they are unqualified, indistinguishable, like the various juices which have reached the condition of honey." [93]

These details concerning "mystical sounds" testify to a highly elaborated technique of auditory meditation, to which we shall have occasion to return. Indeed, the interpretation of Yoga practice furnished by the *Maitri Upaniṣad* is based on these mystical auditions (VI, 25):

> Whereas one [the yogin] thus joins breath [*prāṇa*]
> and the syllable *OṂ*
> And all the manifold world . . .
> Therefore it has been declared to be Yoga.
>
> The oneness of the breath and mind,
> And likewise of the senses,
> And the relinquishment of all conditions of existence—
> This is designated as Yoga.[94]

93 Tr. Hume, pp. 437–38. 94 Ibid., p. 439.

He who practices correctly for six months realizes perfect union (VI, 28). But the "secret" must be communicated only to sons and disciples, and to them only if they are fit to receive it (VI, 29).

The Saṃnyāsa Upaniṣads

The *Cūlikā Upaniṣad* was probably written at the same period as the *Maitri*, and in it we find the simplest form of theistic Yoga.[95] Chronologically, these two are followed by two groups of short Upaniṣads in the nature of technical manuals for the use of ascetic disciples of either Vedānta or Yoga; the two groups are known as the Saṃnyāsa Upaniṣads and the Yoga Upaniṣads; the former are almost all in prose, the latter in verse.[96] As to their chronology, all that can be said is that they are contemporary with the didactic parts of the *Mahābhārata* and probably very little earlier than the *Vedānta-sūtras* and the *Yoga-sūtras*. As they have come down to us, they bear traces of the eclectic and devotional spirit of the period. They contain the same inexact, hazy, syncretistic, and poorly organized ideas as the epic, but crossed by the theistic and devotional experience that runs through the whole of Indian mystico-contemplative literature from the *Bhagavad Gītā* on.

In the group of Saṃnyāsa Upaniṣads, we must mention: the *Brahma Upaniṣad*, the *Saṃnyāsa* (both made up of sections written at various dates, some of them contemporary with the *Maitrāyaṇī Upaniṣad*, some later), the *Āruṇeya*, the *Kaṇṭhaśruti*, the *Jābāla*, and the *Paramahaṃsa Upaniṣad*. They glorify the ascetic (*sannyāsi*) who forsakes the world for the contemplative life. Concrete, experimental knowledge of the unity between the individual soul (*jīvātman*) and the supreme soul (*paramātman*) is regarded by the *Paramahaṃsa Upaniṣad* (I, 2) as a substitute for morning and evening prayer (*saṃdhyā*). This is yet another proof that all these

95 Cf. Paul Deussen, *Sechzig Upanishad's des Vedas*, p. 637; Hopkins, pp. 100, 110; Hauer, *Der Yoga als Heilweg*, p. 34.

96 Cf. Deussen, pp. 629–77, 678–715; J. N. Farquhar, *An Outline of the Religious Literature of India*, p. 95.

ascetic adventures in quest of the Absolute sought a warrant and a justification in Brāhmanism. The admonition to renounce the world is repeated *ad nauseam* by all these Upaniṣads, most of which are short and rather vapid. In the *Āruṇeya*, Brahmā advises Arjuna to renounce not only everything human (family, possessions, reputation, etc.) but also the seven higher spheres (Bhūr, Bhuvar, Svar, etc.) and the seven lower spheres (Atala, Pātāla, Vitala, etc.). In a few of these Saṃnyāsa Upaniṣads, we can discern allusions to some orders of heterodox ascetics representing the same "left-hand" tradition (*vāmacārī*) that has existed in India from Vedic times down to our day. (The *Paramahaṃsopaniṣad*, 3, mentions ascetics who are "slaves of the senses and without *jñāna*"; they will go to the "horrible hells known by the name of *Mahāraurava*." Does this indicate "left-hand" tantrism?) The *Brahmopaniṣad* (II, 9) expounds a curious theory of the "four places" inhabited by the *puruṣa:* the navel, heart, neck, and head. Each of these regions has a corresponding state of consciousness: the navel (or the eye), the state of diurnal waking; the neck, sleep; the heart, dreamless sleep (*suṣupta*); the head, the transcendental state (*turīya*). In the same way the four states of consciousness respectively correspond to Brahmā, Viṣṇu, Rudra, and Akṣara (the indestructible). This theory of "centers" and of the correspondence between different parts of the body and states of consciousness will later be elaborated by Haṭha Yoga and the tantras.

The Yogic Upaniṣads

In our brief exposition of yogic technique as found in the late Upaniṣads, we shall disregard the Saṃnyāsa group, for they add almost nothing new. Even among the group of yogic Upaniṣads a choice must be made. The principal texts of this group are the *Brahmabindu* (perhaps composed at the same period as the *Maitri Upaniṣad*), *Kṣurikā*, *Tejobindu*, *Brahmavidyā*, *Nādabindu*, *Yogaśikha*, *Yogatattva*, *Dhyānabindu*, *Amṛtabindu*, all composed at about the same timé as the chief Saṃnyāsa Upaniṣads and the didactic portions of the *Mahābhārata*.[97] Other collections include ten or eleven still later yogic Upaniṣads (*Yogakuṇḍalī*, *Varāha*, *Pāśupatabrahma*, etc.). The majority of these merely repeat the traditional clichés, and either adhere to or summarize the schemata of the most important yogic Upaniṣads—the *Yogatattva*, the *Dhyānabindu*, and the *Nādabindu*. Only these three are worth examining more thoroughly.

It is the *Yogatattva* that appears to be most minutely acquainted with yogic practices; it mentions the eight *aṅgas* (3) and distinguishes the four kinds of yoga: Mantra Yoga, Laya Yoga, Haṭha Yoga, and Rāja Yoga (19 ff.). To be sure, we are told near the beginning (14–15) that Yoga does not suffice for gaining *mokṣa* if one does not also possess *jñāna*, but the magical prowesses of the yogins are highly praised. For the first time, an Upaniṣad gives numerous and precise details concerning the extraordinary powers gained by practice and meditation. The four chief *āsanas* (*siddha*, *padma*, *sīṃha*, and *bhadra*) are mentioned (29), as are the obstacles encountered by beginners—sloth, talkativeness, etc. (30). A description of *prāṇāyāma* follows (36 ff.), together with a definition (40 ff.) of the *mātrā* (unit of measurement for the phases of respiration), and important details of mystical physiology (the purification of the *nāḍīs* is shown by external signs: lightness of body, brilliance of complexion, increase in digestive power, etc. [46]; *kevala kumbhaka*—i.e., complete suspension of respiration—is also manifested by physiological symptoms: at the beginning of practice, perspiration becomes abundant, etc. [52]). Through *kevala kumbhaka* one can gain mastery of anything in all the three worlds. The power of rising into the air, that of controlling and dominating any being (*bhūcāra siddhi*), are direct results of yoga practice. The yogin becomes as strong and beautiful as a god, and women desire him, but he must persevere in chastity; "on account

97 Cf. E. W. Hopkins, "Yoga-Technique in the Great Epic," *Journal of the American Oriental Society*, XXII (1901), 379.

of the retention of semen there will be generated an agreeable smell in the body of the yogin" (59 f.).[98] The definition of *pratyāhāra* is somewhat different from that given in the *Yoga-sūtras:* "completely withdrawing the sense organs from [sensory] objects during suspension of respiration" (68). A long list of *siddhis* (occult powers) shows that this Upaniṣad was composed in a magical milieu; among those mentioned are "clairaudience, clairvoyance, transportation across vast distances in a short time, yogic vocal powers, yogic power of transforming one's self into any form desired, yogic method of making oneself invisible and the power of transmuting iron and other baser metals into gold by smearing with the yogin's urine and excreta" (73 f.). This last *siddhi* clearly indicates the real connection between a certain form of Yoga and alchemy—a connection to which we shall have occasion to return.

The *Yogatattva Upaniṣad* sets forth a richer mystical physiology than the *Yoga-sūtras.* The "five parts" of the body correspond to the five cosmic elements (earth, water, fire, wind, ether), and each element corresponds to a particular mystical syllable and a particular *dhāraṇā,* governed by a god; by performing the appropriate meditation, the yogin becomes master of the corresponding element. The method is as follows (85 f.): "From the foot on to the knee is said to be the region of Pṛthivī [the earth]. Prthivī [99] is quadrilateral, is of yellow colour, and of the character of the syllable *laṃ.*[100] Having forced in the vital air in the region of Pṛthivī, along with the *lakāra* or the syllable *laṃ,* meditating on the four-faced Brahmā with the four arms and of the colour of gold, the yogin should hold the vital air for five *ghaṭikās.*[101] By doing so he will attain the conquest of Pṛthivī. From the Pṛthivī-yoga there will be no death for the yogin." The mystical syllable corresponding to the element *apas* (water) is *vaṃ,* and the *dhāraṇā*

98 This and the following translations from yogic Upaniṣads are taken from T. R. Śrīnivāsa Ayyaṇgār's version in *The Yoga Upaniṣads,* ed. G. Śrīnivāsa Murti. In some cases, the translations have been slightly modified.

99 I.e., its iconographic image.

100 I.e., its *mantra* is *laṃ.*

101 Two hours.

must be concentrated in the region extending from the knees to the rectum. If the yogin realizes this *dhāraṇā*, he need no longer fear death by water. (Some sources add that, after this meditation, the yogin is able to float on water.) For the element *agni* (fire) the corresponding syllable is *raṃ* and the corresponding region that which extends from the rectum to the heart; by realizing *dhāraṇā* here, the yogin becomes incombustible. The region between the heart and the middle of the eyebrows is that of *vāyu* (air), whose corresponding syllable is *yaṃ;* he who realizes this *dhāraṇā* need no longer fear the atmosphere. The region from the middle of the eyebrows to the top of the head is that of *ākāśa* (ether, cosmic space), whose corresponding syllable is *haṃ;* this *dhāraṇā* bestows the power of traveling through the air. All these *siddhis* are well known both to the mystico-ascetic traditions of India and to the folklore that has grown up about yogins.

Samādhi is described in this Upaniṣad as realizing the paradoxical situation in which the *jīvātma* (individual soul) and the *paramātma* (Universal Spirit) are placed from the moment when all distinction between them has ceased. The yogin can now do whatever he will; if he wishes, he can be absorbed into the *parabrahman;* if, on the contrary, he prefers to keep his body, he can remain on earth and possess all the *siddhis*. He can also become a god, live surrounded by honors, in the heavens, take whatever form pleases him. Having become a god, he can live as long as he chooses. Toward the end, the *Yogatattva Upaniṣad* also gives a list of *āsanas* and *mudrās* (112 ff.), some of which, as we shall find, recur in the *Haṭhayogapradīpikā*. Among them is the singular meditative position that consists in balancing on the crown of the head, feet up, which has therapeutic effects; wrinkles and gray hairs disappear three months after this exercise (126). Other *mudrās* result in the acquisition of well-known *siddhis:* the power of flying through the air, knowledge of the future, even immortality (through the *vajrolīmudrā*). Immortality, we may note, is frequently mentioned.

The *Yogatattva Upaniṣad*, then, presents a yogic technique revalorized in the light of the Vedāntic dialectic; the *puruṣa* and

Īśvara, "Self" and "God," are replaced by *jīvātma* and *paramātma*. But even more significant than this Vedāntic coloring is the experimental tone that characterizes the entire Upaniṣad. The text retains the character of a technical manual, with precise directions for the use of ascetics. The end pursued by all this discipline is clearly expressed: it is to gain the condition of "man-god," of unlimited longevity, and of absolute freedom. This is the leitmotiv of all the baroque varieties of Yoga, which tantrism will develop to the utmost.[102]

The *Nādabindu Upaniṣad* presents a mythical personification of the mystical syllable *OṂ*, imagined as a bird whose right wing is the letter *A*, etc., and describes its cosmic value—the different worlds that correspond to it, etc. (1–5). Next comes a series of twelve *dhāraṇās*, with details as to what becomes of yogins who die at one or another degree of meditation (to what worlds they will pass, with what gods they will associate, etc.). The famous Vedāntic motif of the serpent and the rope, which serves to illustrate the discussion of the theory of illusion, is also mentioned. But the most interesting part of this Upaniṣad is its description of the auditory phenomena that accompany certain yogic exercises. By virtue of the sound he hears in the *siddhāsana* posture, which makes him deaf to every noise from the outer world, the yogin obtains the *turīya* state in two weeks (31–32). At first, the sounds perceived are violent (like those of the ocean, thunder, waterfalls), then they acquire a musical structure (of *mardala*, of bell and horn), and finally the hearing becomes extremely refined (sounds of the *vīṇā*, the flute, the bee; 33–35). The yogin must exert himself to obtain sounds as subtle as possible, for this is the only way in which he can progress in his meditation. Finally, the yogin will experience union with the *parabrahman*, which has no sound (*aśabda*). This state of meditation probably resembles a state of catalepsy, for the text says that "the yogin will remain like a dead

102 Tantric elements, however, are not lacking; there is mention of the *kuṇḍalinī* (82 ff.) and of the two *mudrās* with sexual valences, *vajrolī* and *khecarī* (126).

man. He is liberated [*mukta*]." In this *unmanī* state (realized at the moment that the yogin has passed beyond even mystical hearing), his body is "as a piece of wood, he has cognizance of neither cold nor heat, nor pain nor pleasure" (53–54). He no longer hears any sound.

This Upaniṣad, too, evinces its "experimental" origin; it was certainly composed in a yogic circle that specialized in "mystical auditions"—that is, in obtaining "ecstasy" through concentration on sounds. But we must not forget that such concentration is acquired only by the application of a yogic technique (*āsana*, *prāṇāyāma*, etc.) and that its final objective is to transform the whole cosmos into a vast sonorous theophany.[103]

Of all the late Upaniṣads, the richest in technical details and "mystical" revelations is undoubtedly the *Dhyānabindu*. Its magical and antidevotional character is apparent from the first line, where we are told that, however grave a man's sins, they are destroyed by *dhyānayoga*. This is precisely the point of view of extremist tantrism: the adept is totally emancipated from all moral and social laws. Like the *Nādabindu*, the *Dhyānabindu* begins with an iconographic description of the syllable *OṂ*, which is to be "contemplated" as identical with Brahman. Each of its letters ($a + u + m$) has a "mystical" color and is homologized with a god. Nor is assimilation to the gods (here devoid of all religious value, since they are mere iconographic symbols) connected only with the syllable *OṂ*. *Prāṇāyāma* is similarly identified with the three chief gods of the Vedic pantheon: "Brahmā is said to be inhalation, Viṣṇu suspension [of breath], Rudra exhalation." However, the yogin is advised to obtain *prāṇāyāma* through concentration on the syllable *OṂ* (19 f.).

"Subtle" physiology is particularly well developed in this Upaniṣad. The "lotus of the heart" has eight petals and thirty-two filaments (25). Special value is accorded to *prāṇāyāma;* inhalation should be through the three "mystical veins," *suṣumṇā*, *iḍā*, and *piṅgalā*, and should be absorbed "at the middle of the eyebrows,"

103 On "mystical sounds," see Note III, 6.

which is at once "the root of the nostrils and the seat of immortality" (40). The text mentions four *āsanas*, seven *cakras* ("centers"), and gives two names of *nāḍīs* (the "veins" of Indian mystical physiology).[104] It also mentions (66 f.) the "awakening" of Parameśvarī—that is, of Kuṇḍalinī—a specifically tantric process, to which we shall have occasion to return. In addition, there is an element of erotic magic, a technique in some ways similar to the "orgiastic" gestures of the *vāmacārīs* ("left-hand" tantrism) and of the Sahajīyā sect. Of course, these are only suggestions, not precise and detailed instructions. Thus, for example, it is said of him who accomplishes the *khecarīmudrā*[105] that his "semen never wastes away, when he is in the embrace of a beautiful woman" (84). (The reference, then, is to an arrest of semen in the tantric fashion.) And later: "As long as the *khecarīmudrā* is firmly adhered to, so long the semen does not flow out. Even if it should flow and reach the region of the genitals, it goes upwards, being forcibly held up by the power of the *yonimudrā* sanctified by the *vajrolī*. The selfsame *bindu* is of two varieties: the white and the reddish. The white they call *śukra* [semen]; the name of the reddish variety is *mahārajas*; the *rajas* which resembles the coral tree in color stands in the seat of the genitals. The semen abides in the seat of the moon midway between the *ājñā cakra*[106] and the thousand-petaled lotus.[107] The union of the two is very rarely attained. The semen is Śiva, the *rajas* is the Śakti; the semen is the moon and the *rajas* is the sun; it is only by the union of the two that this exquisite body is attained." In the vocabulary of Indian mystical erotism, all

104 The number of *āsanas*, the text says (42), is considerable, but the four chief ones are the *siddha*, *bhadra*, *siṃha*, and *padma*. The list of the seven *cakras* (44 ff.) is that of the tantric treatises (see p. 241). Our text affirms (51) that there are 72,000 *nāḍīs*, of which only seventy-two are named in the scriptures; the most important are *iḍā*, *piṅgala*, and *suṣumṇā* cf. *Bṛhadāraṇyaka Upaniṣad*, II, 1, 9; *Praśna Upaniṣad*, III, 9.

105 The *khecarīmudrā* enjoyed an extraordinary celebrity in later yogico-tantric literature: by acquiring the ability to immobilize the *semen virile*, the adept gains immortality. See the texts reproduced by S. B. Dasgupta, *Obscure Religious Cults*, p. 278, n. 1. See also below, p. 408.

106 The frontal region.

107 I.e., the *sahasrāra*.

these terms have perfectly precise meanings. The chief consideration here is the "rupture of plane," the unification of the two polar principles (Śiva and Śakti), the transcending of all opposites, obtainable through a highly secret erotic practice, to which we shall return. But here we must note the marked experimental and tantric character of this Upaniṣad. It shows us that this current of erotic magic, which will later become so strong in the tantras, was not at first separated from yogic practices; that, from the beginning, these practices could have more than one value, could be accepted by and employed for various "paths."

The technical, experimental character of these Upaniṣads of the yogic group deserves to be emphasized. Here we no longer find the primacy of pure cognition, of the dialectic of the Absolute as the sole instrument of liberation. Here the identity *ātman-brahman* is no longer acquired by contemplation alone; it is realized experimentally, by means of an ascetic technique and a mystical physiology—in other words, by a process of transforming the human body into a cosmic body, in which the veins, the arteries, and the real organs play a decidedly secondary role in comparison with the "centers" and "veins" in which cosmic or divine forces can be experienced or "awakened." This tendency to concreteness and the experimental—even if "concreteness" here means the almost anatomical localization of certain cosmic forces—is peculiarly characteristic of the entire mystical trend of the Indian Middle Ages. Devotion, personal worship, and "subtle physiology" take the place of fossilized ritualism and metaphysical speculation. The road to liberation tends to become an ascetic itinerary, a technique not so difficult to learn as Vedāntic or Mahāyānic metaphysics.

"Brāhmanized" Magic and Yoga: the Ṛgvidhāna

Magicians, ascetics, and contemplatives continue to appear in the increasing corpus of ritual texts and commentaries. Sometimes there is no more than an allusion; as, for example, in the case of a certain class of black *śramaṇa*-magicians mentioned in the *Āpas-*

tamba-sūtra (2, IX, 23, 6–8): "Now they accomplish also their wishes merely by conceiving them. For instance, (the desire to) procure rain, to bestow children, second-sight, to move quick as thought, and other (desires) of this description." [108] Certain *siddhis* recur like a leitmotiv, especially the ability to fly through the air; a Brāhmaṇa of the *Sāmaveda*, the *Sāmavidhāna*, particularly concerned with magic, cites it among the "powers" (III, 9, 1). The *Ṛgvidhāna*,[109] a late but important collection—for its authors strain their ingenuity to exploit the Vedic *sūktas* for magical ends—declares that a special diet and particular rituals enable one to vanish, to depart from this world by flying through the air, to see and hear at great distances, like one standing in the highest place (III, 9, 2–3). This latter mystical experience has been attested in Arctic and north Asiatic shamanism.[110]

The *Ṛgvidhāna* discusses a great variety of magical, yogic, and devotional practices. This compilation perfectly illustrates the process of Hinduization of the Vedic tradition. In it we see the actual assimilation of practices that are non-Brāhmanic and very probably non-Āryan; all the technical details of magic, ecstasy, or contemplation are integrated and validated by citations from the Vedic scriptures. Praise of magic stands side by side with glorification of rituals and occult knowledge. By magic, one can force the supreme divinity to cause rain (II, 9, 2); by the power of meditation, one can burn an enemy (I, 16, 5); the appropriate rites will summon a *kṛtyā* (a female evil spirit) to rise from the water (II, 9, 3). Learning the sacred texts suffices to obtain the fulfillment of all desires (I, 7, 1). Certain rites enable one to remember one's former lives (II, 10, 1), a specifically yogic prodigy.[111]

Prāṇāyāma appears (I, 11, 5); it should be performed up to a hundred times (I, 12, 1), with mental repetition of the syllable *OṂ* (I, 12, 5). But it is with Chapter III (36 ff.) that the exposi-

108 Tr. Georg Bühler, *The Sacred Laws of the Āryas* (Sacred Books of the East, II), p. 157.

109 Ed. Rudolf Meyer; English tr. J. Gonda.

110 Eliade, *Shamanism*, pp. 61 ff., 225 ff., etc.

111 See above, p. 86.

tion of yogic technique properly begins. Yoga should be practiced at midnight, "when all beings are fast asleep" (36, 2); choosing a suitable spot, the yogin seats himself in an *āsana* position, "hands joined in homage" (36, 4)—for the meditation is made on Nārāyaṇa; cf. 36, 1—and eyes closed; he pronounces the syllable *OṂ* "in his heart" (36, 5); if he hears and perceives nothing, "if there is no more reflection on the subject of Yoga, the end is attained" (37, 1). As for *prāṇāyāma*, the yogin attempts to "raise" the *manas* above the navel, then above the heart, in order to "fix" it between the eyebrows (the "highest place") and finally in the skull, whence, still by force of breathing, he must make it pass down to the navel again (37, 2 ff.; 38, 1). The "highest place" belongs to Brahman. Through this yogic exercise, one finds the Self, becomes holy, and attains the highest state (*paramā;* 38, 2–4). Concentration (*dhāraṇā*) is realized by fixing the *manas* on the sun, fire, the moon, the tops of trees or mountains, the sea, etc. (38, 5; 39, 1). When the Brahman has been found in the skull, one can mount to the highest light, to the firmament; like the Supreme Spirit, the yogin becomes able to see his own Self (39, 3–4). But another text (41, 4) says that the "divine eye" can be obtained by magical formulas and oblations to fire; here we see the old position—the primacy of ritual magic—attempting to maintain its prestige.

All these yogic practices attested in the *Ṛgvidhāna* are already strongly colored with devotion. The text declares that even if the yogin does not attain the goal—the vision of the Self—he must not abandon *bhakti*, for Bhagavān "loves those who love him" (41, 1). Nārāyaṇa should be meditated upon as being in the center of the solar disk, and this already foreshadows the "visualization" of tantric iconography. Elsewhere it is said that Viṣṇu can be attained only through *bhakti* (42, 6). A previous passage (31, 3) cited the *pūjā* and gave details of the cult of the "imperishable Viṣṇu"; one must "fix the *mantras*" (*mantranyāsam*) "in one's own body and in that of the divinities" (32, 2). Another passage (30, 3–6) enumerates the organs in which one must "place" the sixteen stanzas (*sūkta*) of the famous hymn *Ṛg-Veda*, X, 90 (the *Puruṣa-*

sūkta): the first stanza in the left hand, the second in the right hand, and the other stanzas respectively in the two feet, the two knees, the two hips, the navel, the heart, the region of the throat, the two arms, the mouth, the eyes, and the skull. Now, if we bear in mind that the *Puruṣasūkta* sets forth that the universe was created by the sacrifice of the primordial Giant [112] (Puruṣa), the "ritual projection" (*nyāsa*) of its stanzas into the various parts of the body will result in identification both with the universe and with the gods (who are also believed to have issued from the sacrifice). *Nyāsa* will acquire an unexpected prestige in tantrism—furnishing one more illustration of the direction the great Hinduistic syntheses of the late period will take; the Vedic material will be integrated and revalorized in cult contexts more and more remote from the primordial tradition. The *Ṛgvidhāna* justifies everything—from vulgar erotic magic to Yoga and *bhakti*—by references to the Vedic scriptures. Later texts will no longer feel the need to justify themselves by the highest orthodox authority; the great Vedic gods will be partly forgotten. Both the *Puruṣasūkta* and the *sūkta* of Viṣṇu, the *Ṛgvidhāna* declares (III, 35, 1), lead to heaven; "and this is the highest meditation of Yoga." We do not know the exact date of this assertion; but, by that date, yogic technique had already been thoroughly incorporated into orthodoxy.

"Good" and "Evil" Ascetics and Contemplatives

We need not embark upon a history of the ascetic orders and mystical sects of India; to do so would be to go far beyond our subject. But it is important to show, on the basis of a definite text, the directions taken by the ascetics, yogins, and ecstatics. The most complete accounts that we have are several centuries later than Buddhism, and this must always be taken into consideration. But we have seen that ascetics and mystics were already numerous in Ṛg-Vedic times. Some classes of *munis*, *tapasvins*, and yogins, al-

112 The myth is Indo-European, but it has also been found among other ethnic groups, including some of the most archaic.

though documented only in comparatively late texts, probably go back to the protohistory of India.[113]

The *Vaikhānasasmārtasūtra*,[114] which can be dated in the fourth century of our era, but which contains far earlier material, furnishes us with a long list of ascetic "orders"; these are the various categories of hermits who retire to the forests, with or without wives. Four kinds of ascetics with wives are distinguished: (1) Audumbaras, who live on fruits, wild plants, or roots, practicing asceticism but retaining the *śrāmaṇaka* ritual fire; (2) Vairiñcas, who still perform the rituals (*agnihotra*, *śrāmaṇaka*, *vaiśvadeva*) but are "wholly absorbed in Nārāyaṇa" (theists, they have chosen the way of *bhakti*); (3) Vālakhilyas, recognizable by their matted hair and by their torn or bark clothing; (4) Phenapas, who are ecstatics (?*unmattaka*), sleep on the ground, live on "what falls to the ground," and practice the penance called *cāndrāyaṇa* (meals regulated in accordance with the waxing and waning of the moon); they "fix their thoughts on Nārāyaṇa and seek only deliverance." Of hermits without wives there are innumerable kinds; they have no names, but are referred to in accordance with their ascetic practices—those who live like pigeons, those who eat only what has been dried by the sun, etc. (VIII, 8). They resemble the fakirs of modern India—a proof of the extraordinary persistence of these practices. Another category is that of the ascetics who strive to gain liberation; this implies that the other hermits did not seek "liberation," but perhaps immortality, happiness, or yogic powers—except the Phenapas, who also *mokṣameva prārthayate* (VIII, 7, i.f.).

This category of hermits with soteriological tendencies is divided into four classes: (1) Kuṭīcakas (traveling from one famous monastery to another, where they swallow only eight mouthfuls; knowing the essentials of the Yoga "way," *yogamārgatattvajñā*, they seek deliverance); (2) Bahūdakas (who carry a "triple staff," wear red clothing, beg their food only at the houses of Brāhmans and other virtuous people, etc., and seek deliverance); (3) Haṃsas

113 See below, pp. 355 ff.

114 Ed. W. Caland; English tr. id.

(who may not remain more than a day and a night in a village, live on cow urine and dung, practice the *cāndrāyaṇa* fast, etc.); (4) Paramahaṃsas (VIII, 9, a). These last are the most interesting; they represent an extremely ancient, aboriginal, anti-Brāhmanic ascetic tradition and foreshadow certain "extremist" yogico-tantric schools. For they live under trees, in graveyards, or in deserted houses; go naked or wear clothing. In their view "there was no good and evil, no holiness or wickedness, or any other similar dualism." Indifferent to everything, they contemplated a ball of clay or of gold with the same placidity. Absorbed in the *ātman* (?*sarvātmānaḥ*), they accepted food from people of any caste.

In the text just summarized we may perhaps see an attempt at a brief classification of the ways leading to liberation. The Kuṭīcakas practice Yoga; the Paramahaṃsas, a kind of tantrism; the Bahūdakas and the Haṃsas, a "mystical way." Further on (VIII, 9, 6), the text refers to the two kinds of "renunciation of desires" (*niṣkāma*) or, rather, to two attitudes—"activity" and "inactivity." The *active* ascetic—resolved to end the circuit of lives by fortifying himself with the knowledge gained from Sāṃkhya and with Yoga practice [115]—obtains the eight *siddhis*. But these "miraculous powers" (*siddhi*), the text adds, are scorned by true *ṛṣis*. *Inactivity* consists in union, after death, between the individual soul and the *brahman* (*paramātman*). The soul then enters the highest light, which is situated above sensory knowledge and constitutes the permanent source of happiness. As we see, the conception is of a "mystical way," in which the individual soul abandons itself to the Supreme Soul, loses its "individuality," and obtains immortality, eternal bliss (*ānandāmṛta*).[116]

In respect to the various "practices of inactivity," the yogins are

115 The text is explicit: Sāṃkhya knowledge (*sāṃkhyajñāna*), and *prāṇāyāma*, *āsana*, *pratyāhāra*, *dhāraṇā*, yogic technical terms.

116 We can conclude that this "mystical way" is opposed to the "magical way" of Sāṃkhya-Yoga, which counseled meditation and sought for magical powers rather than for immortality.

divided into three categories: Sāraṇgas, Ekārṣyas, and Visāragas.[117] Each of these categories, in turn, is divided into several species. We do not know how far this classification corresponds to actual observations, but doubtless the groups of ascetics described by the *Vaikhānasasmārtasūtra* existed (some of them still exist), even if the relations between them were not precisely those given in the text. The Sāraṇgas comprise four species: (1) those who do not practice *prāṇāyāma* and the other yogic exercises, but live with the conviction "I am Viṣṇu" (hence they belong to one of the various currents that produced Viṣṇuism); (2) those who practice *prāṇāyāma* and the other exercises (they appear to follow an "orthodox" Yoga, related to that of the *Yoga-sūtras*); (3) those who follow the "right road," practicing the eight *aṇgas* of Yoga, but beginning with *prāṇāyāma* (i.e., omitting *yama* and *niyama*); (4) those who follow a "wrong road" (*vimārga*), practice a complete Yoga but go against God (the text is decidedly obscure; perhaps the reference is to an atheistic Yoga).

The Ekārṣya ascetics are of five kinds: (1) those who "go far" (*dūraga*) and who practice a cosmic meditation that is very close to tantrism (they attempt to gain union with Viṣṇu through "realization" of the cosmic forces latently present in the *piṇgalā* "vein"; the purpose of this meditation is to experience such states of consciousness as the cosmic-solar, lunar, etc.; the method is called *dūraga* because union with Viṣṇu is accomplished by passing through the cosmic circuit); (2) those who "do not go far" (*adūraga*), who experience the union of the individual soul with the Cosmic Soul directly; (3) those who "go through the middle of the brows" (*bhrūmadhyaga*), unite their soul with the Cosmic Soul by forcing the *prāṇa* back through the five regions (from the toes to the knees, from the knees to the anus, from the anus to the heart, from the heart to the palate, from the palate to the middle of the

117 The editor of the text, Caland, notes that these names of yogins are found nowhere else in Indian literature, and the Sanskrit commentary does not help us to understand them.

eyebrows) and making it return through the *piṅgalā;* (4) those who "are not devoted" (*asambhakta*) and who realize union with the Cosmic Soul through an experimental meditation—that is, by seeing it with their eyes, saluting it with their hands, etc. (despite their strange name, the *asambhaktas* are true mystical worshipers of the divinity); (5) those who "are attached" (*sambhakta*)

The Visāraga ascetics are innumerable and are so named because they "walk the wrong path." We are here undoubtedly confronted with a genuine variety of ascetics "of the left hand" (*vāmacārī*). To justify their origin, the text repeats an old explanation: Prajāpati invented "the doctrine of the Visāragas" in order to conceal the truth. The same explanation is found in other Indian texts to justify the existence of one or another immoral sect. However, as the *Vaikhānasasmārtasūtra* recognizes, these ascetics perform penances, know the Yoga technique, repeat the *mantras,* even practice certain meditations—but they "do not do this to unite themselves with the Cosmic Soul." They say that the Cosmic Soul "is in their heart." Some of them seek deliverance, at the same time declaring that "meditation is not necessary." Others say that union with the Cosmic Soul is accomplished through practicing the religious rites as they are described. But all these contradictory details do not make the Visāragas any the less heretical. Our text constantly calls them "those beasts of Visāragas," affirming that there is no liberation for them in this life and that they should under no circumstances be followed.

We have summarized the information given in the *Vaikhānasasmārtasūtra* in order to confirm the existence of certain ascetic and yogico-tantric sects long before the appearance of a tantric doctrine and literature. These are beliefs and practices whose roots go back to pre-Vedic times and whose continuity has never been broken in India, despite the fact that few documents mention them.[118]

118 Lists of ascetics and yogins occur rather often in the texts, but they are usually brief. (See Note III, 7.)

The Triumph of Yoga

Yoga and Hinduism

THE gradual spread of Yoga practice, regarded as an admirable way of salvation, can be traced both in juridico-theological literature and in the didactic and religious portions of the *Mahābhārata*. Yet it would be difficult to define the successive stages of this infiltration, which will finally result in the almost total conquest of Indian spirituality by Yoga. We shall say only that we are dealing with works whose composition lies in the period between the fourth century B.C. and the fourth century of our era. A fact of greater interest for us is the coincidence between this triumph of yogic practices and the irresistible upsurge of popular mystical devotion. For this planting of Yoga technique in the very heart of Hinduism took place at a moment of crisis for orthodoxy; that is, at the very moment when the latter validated the "sectarian" mystical movements en bloc. In the course of its expansion, Brāhmanism—like every victorious religion—was forced to accept a number of elements that had originally been foreign or even hostile to it. Assimilation of the forms in which autochthonous, pre-Āryan religious sentiment had found expression began very early, from the Vedic period (the god Śiva is an example). But this time—that is, at the beginning of the Indian Middle Ages (during the period that extends from the flowering of Buddhism to the *Bhagavad Gītā*)—assimilation assumes alarming proportions. We sometimes have the impression of a victorious revolution, before which Brāhman orthodoxy can only bow. What is called "Hinduism" dates from the still little-known period when the ancient Vedic pantheon was eclipsed by the enormous popularity of a Śiva, a Viṣṇu, or a Kṛṣṇa. There is no room here to study the causes of this profound and immense transformation. But let us note that one of its principal causes was precisely the need that the masses of the people felt for a more concrete religious experience, for a mystical devotion more easily accessible, more intimate, more personal. Now, the traditional (i.e., popular, "baroque," nonsystematic) practices of Yoga offered just this type of mystical experience; scorning rituals and theological science, they were based almost entirely on immediate, concrete data still hardly separated from their physiological substratum.

Naturally, this increasing infiltration of yogic techniques into orthodoxy did not take place without encountering a certain degree of resistance. From time to time voices were raised against the propaganda of the ascetics and "magicians," who claimed that neither final liberation (*mukti*) nor the "occult powers" (*siddhi*) could be gained except by adherence to their particular disciplines. Needless to say, this resistance appeared first in the official circles of orthodox Brāhmanism, made up of Vedāntist jurists and metaphysicians. Both groups adhered to the "golden mean" in respect to Yoga ascetic and contemplative techniques, which they considered to be exaggerated in some cases and contrary to the Vedāntic ideal in others. Manu writes: "If he keeps both his organs and his consciousness under subjection, he can attain his ends without further tormenting his body by Yoga." [1] Śaṇkara too writes in the same vein; Yoga, he warns, "leads to the acquirement of extraordinary powers," but "the highest beatitude cannot be obtained

1 *Smṛti*, II, 98; tr. G. Bühler, *The Laws of Manu*, p. 48. Gangānātha Jhā, *Manu-Smṛti: The Laws of Manu with the Bhāṣya of Medhātithi*, vol. I, pt. II, p. 363, following Medhātithi, translates *yogataḥ* "by careful means," but the commentators Nārāyaṇa and Nandana, followed by Bühler, give *yogataḥ* the meaning "by the practice of Yoga."

by the road of Yoga.'"[2] The true Vedāntist chooses purely metaphysical knowledge.

But reactions of this kind are sporadic. In fact, if the Vedāntic tradition continues to see Yoga practices only as a means for acquiring possession of magical powers or, at best, as a purification preliminary to true salvation, to which only metaphysical knowledge can lead, it nevertheless remains true that the majority of the juridico-theological treatises do in fact validate such practices and sometimes even praise them. The *Vasiṣṭha Dharma Śāstra*, for example, declares that "neither . . . through the daily recitation of the Veda, nor through offering sacrifices can the twice-born reach that condition which they attain by the practice of Yoga." [3] The magical and purifying power of this practice is incomparable: "If, untired, he performs three suppressions of his breath according to the rule, the sins which he committed during a day and a night are instantly destroyed." [4] And another theologico-juridic treatise, the *Viṣṇusmṛti*, confirms the miraculous value of yogic technique: "Whatever he meditates upon, that is obtained by a man: such is the mysterious power of meditation." It is true that the text immediately following contains the significant stipulation that the yogin's goal must be achieving final liberation, not enjoyment of the "powers" that his meditation will confer on him. "Therefore must he dismiss everything perishable from his thoughts and meditate upon what is imperishable only. There is nothing imperishable except Purusha. Having become united with him (through constant

2 Commentary on the *Vedānta-sūtras*, tr. G. Thibaut, *The Vedānta Sūtra. With Śaṅkara's Commentary* (Sacred Books of the East, XXXIV), I, 223, 298. For his part, Rāmānuja, without denying that one can "through the might of Yoga knowledge" know "everything that passes in the three worlds" and even attain to "direct intuition" of Brahman, affirms that "mystical concentration of the mind" must be maintained by *bhakti*, as in the *Bhagavad Gītā;* cf. G. Thibaut, tr., *The Vedānta Sūtra. With Rāmānuja's Commentary*, pp. 340, 273, 284.

3 XXV, 7; tr. G. Bühler, *The Sacred Laws of the Āryas* (Sacred Books of the East, XIV), p. 125.

4 Ibid., XXVI, 1; tr. Bühler, p. 126.

meditation), he obtains final liberation." [5] But this is precisely the counsel of the *Yoga-sūtras.*

Yoga in the Mahābhārata

It is only in connection with the latest in the series of additions to the *Mahābhārata* that we can justifiably refer to a complete Hinduization of yogic practices; for in this epic, whose success was considerable in nonsacerdotal circles, Yoga holds an important place. Recent studies [6] have elucidated the traces of Vedic mythology discernible in the principal personages, the Pāṇḍavas. But, begun as a heroic saga—and completed in that form probably between the seventh and sixth centuries B.C.—the *Mahābhārata* was subjected to countless interpolations. The first two centuries of our era are generally held to have been the period during which an immense number of mystico-theological, philosophical, and juridic texts were introduced into the poem—some in the form of complete units (e.g., Books XII, XIII), some as detached episodes. These various elements thus formed a veritable encyclopedia, markedly Viṣṇuist in tendency. One of the first portions added (in all probability before our era) was the *Bhagavad Gītā* (in Book VI); the most considerable additions occur in Book VII, the *Mokṣadharma;* and these are the books in which we find the most frequent allusions to Yoga and Sāṃkhya.[7]

But we must not forget that, although they were added late, these new portions contain traditions very much earlier than the dates at which they were interpolated. A sound chronology of the strata of the *Mahābhārata* is still only a probably illusory desideratum. The changes made in the text during the course of centuries can be seen in general outline, but few Indianists agree on the details. Nevertheless, the didactic and "sectarian" sections added to

5 XCVII, 11–14; tr. Julius Jolly, *The Institutes of Vishnu,* pp. 285–90.
6 By Stig Wikander and G. Dumézil; see Note IV, 1.
7 See Note IV, 1.

the poem are of incalculable value for the religious and philosophical history of India. On the one hand, many beliefs parallel to orthodox Brāhmanism and of undeniable antiquity here find open expression; on the other, it is here that we encounter the first organized and triumphant efforts of Indian theism. It was the *Bhagavad Gītā* that first formulated the identification of the Brahman of the Upaniṣads with Viṣṇu—a god who now becomes supreme—and with his earthly avatar, Kṛṣṇa. In the *Mokṣadharma*, as in the *Bhagavad Gītā* and other passages, there are also frequent allusions to Sāṃkhya and Yoga; but, as we shall see, these two disciplines are not valorized in their classic sense, as systematic *darśanas*.

Naturally, these constant additions injured the unity of the whole. Contradictions abound. The Vedas, for example, are usually regarded as the supreme authority (*pramāṇa*); but we also read that "the Veda is deceitful" (XII, 329, 6). Bhīṣma's words, inspired by Kṛṣṇa, have "an authority equal to the Vedas" (XII, 54, 29–30). "Grace" is put above *śruti* and scholastic learning (*tarka*), for it alone can illuminate "the secret and mysterious communication of truth" (XII, 335, 5). But in general, inference (*anumāna*) and scriptural revelation (*śruti*) are regarded as sufficiently proving the validity of a truth (XII, 205, 19, etc.). Hopkins has collected and classified an immense amount of material to illustrate the dogmas and beliefs recorded in the *Mahābhārata*, especially in its "pseudo-epic" portions. This composite and inadequately articulated mass is explained by the diversity of its authors, who often belonged to opposing schools; each attempted to impose his own religious conception. Nor must we forget that the composition of some books, especially the *Mokṣadharma*, perhaps continued for several centuries. It nevertheless remains possible to isolate the theoretical position of this pseudo-epic portion of the *Mahābhārata* with comparative precision: on the one hand, it reaffirms Upaniṣadic monism, colored by theistic experiences; on the other, it accepts any soteriological solution that does not explicitly contradict scriptural tradition.

In general, it is a literature of edification, which, without being of "popular" origin, is conceived so that it may reach all kinds of milieus. The last books attached to the *Mahābhārata* are, essentially, books of Viṣṇuist propaganda—a rather confused propaganda that seized on anything that gave it the opportunity to exalt Viṣṇu and Kṛṣṇa. And it is interesting to note that Yoga was freely utilized to support their exaltation. But in the *Mokṣadharma*, Yoga does not mean *cittavṛtti-nirodha*, as it does to Patañjali; it simply designates any practical discipline, just as the word Sāṃkhya is used to designate all metaphysical knowledge. The differences that opposed the classic Sāṃkhya system (which was atheistic) to the classic Yoga system (which was theistic) here become so blurred as almost to vanish.

Yoga and Sāṃkhya in the Mahābhārata

Asked by Yudhiṣṭhira to explain the difference between these two "paths," Bhīṣma answers: [8] "Sāṃkhya and Yoga each praises its own method as the best means [*kāraṇa*]. . . . Those who are guided by Yoga base themselves upon a direct perception [mystical in nature: *pratyakṣahetava*]; those who follow Sāṃkhya, upon traditional teachings [*śāstraviniścāyah*]. I consider both these teachings true. . . . If their instructions are rightly followed, they both lead to the highest end. They have in common purity, repression (of desires), and compassion for all beings; strict regard for oaths is common to both; but the opinions [*darśana*] are not the same in Sāṃkhya and in Yoga." [9]

The nonsystematic character of these two ways of salvation is obvious. Although, especially in the *Gītā* and the *Mokṣadharma*, we find technical terms such as *prakṛti, tattva, mahat*, etc., Sāṃkhya is nowhere presented as the method for distinguishing spirit from psychomental experience—which is the point of departure for Īśvarakṛṣṇa's system. In these texts Sāṃkhya means simply "true knowledge" (*tattva jñāna*) or "knowledge of the soul" (*ātma*

8 *Mahābhārata*, XII, 11,043 ff. 9 See Note IV, 2.

bhoda); in this respect it is closer to the Upaniṣadic positions. Not that we here have a mixture of Sāṃkhya and Vedānta ideas, as Hopkins thinks; it is simply a stage that is earlier than the Sāṃkhya and Vedānta systems. Nor is there any need to seek, in certain parts of the *Mahābhārata*, precise allusions to a theistic Sāṃkhya school, parallel to the atheistic *darśana* of Īśvarakṛṣṇa.

The *Mokṣadharma* (11,463) declares that the forerunners (*puraḥsarāḥ*) of the yogins are found in the Vedas (that is, in the Upaniṣads) and in Sāṃkhya. In other words, the "truth" discovered by the Upaniṣads and Sāṃkhya is accepted and assimilated by Yoga; for—whatever meaning it may be given—this latter term is applied above all to a spiritual technique. The *Bhagavad Gītā* goes even further and declares that "Children—not wise men [*paṇḍitāḥ*]—talk of Sāṃkhya and Yoga as distinct. One who pursues either well obtains the fruit of both. . . . He sees (truly) who sees the Sāṃkhya and Yoga as one." [10] This position is in perfect accord with the spirit of the *Bhagavad Gītā*. For, as we shall soon see, in that jewel of the *Mahābhārata* Kṛṣṇa tries to incorporate all ways of salvation into a single new spiritual synthesis.

Yoga Techniques in the Mahābhārata

In the *Mahābhārata* Yoga, in contrast to Sāṃkhya, designates any activity that leads the soul to Brahman and at the same time confers countless "powers." In the majority of cases this activity is equivalent to restraining the senses, asceticism, and various kinds of penance. Only occasionally does Yoga have the meaning that Kṛṣṇa gives it in the *Bhagavad Gītā*—"renunciation of the fruits of one's acts." This fluidity in the meanings of the word has been brought out by Hopkins in an exhaustive study.[11] "Yoga" sometimes means "method," [12] sometimes "activity," [13] "force," [14] "meditation," [15]

10 V, 4–5; tr. K. T. Telang, pp. 63–64.

11 "Yoga-Technique in the Great Epic."

12 E.g., *Bhagavad Gītā*, III, 3.

13 *Mokṣadharma*, 11,682.

14 Ibid., 11,675 ff.

15 Ibid., 11,691, etc.

or "renunciation" (*sannyāsa*),[16] etc. This variety of meanings corresponds to a real morphological diversity. If the word "yoga" *means* many things, that is because Yoga *is* many things. For the epic is the meeting place of countless ascetic and popular traditions, each with its own "Yoga"—that is, its particular mystical technique. The many centuries during which new episodes were interpolated allowed all these forms of "baroque" Yoga to find a place (and a justification), with the result that the epic was transformed into an encyclopedia.

In broad outline, we can distinguish three classes of data of possible interest to our study: (1) episodes involving asceticism (*tapas*), and revealing practices and theories closely related to Vedic *ascesis* but without references to Yoga, properly speaking; (2) episodes and discourses in which Yoga and *tapas* are synonymous and are both regarded as magical techniques; (3) didactic discourses and episodes in which Yoga is presented with a philosophically elaborated terminology of its own. It is especially the documents in this third category—most of them contained in the *Mokṣadharma*—that we regard as of interest, for they reveal some forms of Yoga that are inadequately documented elsewhere.

We find, for example, extremely ancient "magical" practices, which yogins use to influence the gods and even to terrorize them.[17] The phenomenology of this magical asceticism is archaic: silence (*mauna*), extreme torture (*ātīvatapas*), "desiccation of the body," are means employed not only by yogins but also by kings.[18] To move Indra (*ārirādhayiṣur devam*), Pāṇḍu stands on one foot for a day and thus obtains *samādhi*.[19] But this trance exhibits no yogic content; rather, it is a hypnosis provoked by physical means, and the relations between the man and the god remain on the level of magic. Elsewhere Yoga and pure asceticism, *tapas*, are confused.[20]

16 *Bhagavad Gītā*, VI, 2.

17 Cf. Hauer, *Die Anfänge der Yogapraxis*, pp. 98 ff. We have found similar examples among some of the wandering ascetics (see above, p. 136).

18 *Mahābhārata*, I, 115, 24; I, 119, 7 and 34.

19 Ibid., I, 123, 26.

20 E.g., ibid., XII, 153, 36.

Yatin (ascetic) and *yogin* become equivalent terms, and finally both come to designate any being "desirous of concentrating his mind" (*yuyukṣat*) and whose object of study is not the scriptures (*śāstra*), but the mystical syllable *OṂ*. There is little doubt that the "study of the syllable *OṂ*" designates techniques concerned with mystical audition, with repetition and "assimilation" of particular magical formulas (*dhāraṇī*), with incantation, etc.

But, whatever the method chosen, these practices are crowned by the acquisition of a force that our texts call the "force of Yoga" (*yoga-balam*). Its immediate cause is "fixation of mind" (*dhāraṇā*), which is obtained both by "placidity and equanimity" (the "sword" [21] of yogic equanimity) [22] and by progressively retarding the rhythm of respiration.[23] The latest interpolations in the *Mahābhārata* are full of mnemotechnic schemata and summaries of yogic practices. Most of them reflect the traditional clichés: "A yogin who, devoted to the great vow [*mahāvrātasamāhitaḥ*], skillfully fixes his subtle spirit [*sūkṣman ātman*] in the following places: navel, neck, head, heart, stomach, hips, eye, ear, and nose, quickly burning all his good and evil actions, were they like a mountain (in size), and seeking to attain the supreme Yoga, is released (from the snares of existence) if such be his will." [24]

Another text [25] magnifies the difficulty of these practices and draws attention to the danger that threatens him who fails: "Hard is the great path [*mahāpanthā*] and few are they who travel it to the end, but greatly guilty [*bahudoṣa*] is he called who, after entering the way of Yoga [*yogamārgam āsādya*], gives up his journey and turns back." This is the well-known danger inherent in all magical actions, which unleash forces capable of killing the magician if he is

21 Hopkins, *The Great Epic of India*, p. 181, gives some lists of the "five sins" that the yogin must "cut off." One of these lists (*Mahābhārata*, XII, 241, 3) names: sexual desire (*kāma*), wrath (*krodha*), greed (*lobha*), fear (*bhaya*), and sleep (*svapna*). There are many variants, for the theme of the "five sins" is very popular in India (it is also familiar to Buddhism: e.g., *Dhammapada*, 370).

22 *Mahābhārata*, XII, 255, 7.

23 Ibid., XII, 192, 13–14.

24 Ibid., XII, 301, 39 ff.

25 Ibid., V, 52 ff.

not strong enough to subdue them by his will and direct them in accordance with his desire. The yogin's ascetic practice has unleashed an impersonal and sacred force, similar to the energies released by any other magical or religious act.

The magical character of Yoga practices is also brought out on other occasions. One text, for example, explains that he who knows the most perfect carnal joys is not the Brāhman but the yogin; even on earth, in the course of his ascetic conditioning, the yogin is attended by luminous women, but in heaven all the pleasures he has renounced on earth will be his to enjoy with tenfold intensity.[26]

Yogic Folklore in the Mahābhārata

Hypnosis was well known; we have already referred to Vipulā,[27] who protected his master's wife by hypnotizing her.[28] Hypnotism is explained by "entering another's body," an extremely archaic belief, which has inspired innumerable tales and legends. The *ṛṣi* Uṣanas, master in Yoga, projects himself into the god of wealth, Kubera, and thus becomes master of all the god's treasures.[29] Another episode [30] relates how the ascetic Vidura, at the point of death, leaves his body leaning against the trunk of a tree and enters the body of Yudhiṣṭhira, who thus acquires all the ascetic's virtues. This is a motif belonging to the folklore of magic and especially exemplified in the countless stories of "entering a corpse." [31] Nor must we forget that, among the *siddhis* gained by yogins, Patañjali mentions the operation of "passing from one body into another" (*cittasya paraśarīrāveśaḥ*).[32] In nonsystematic texts, such as the added portions of the *Mahābhārata*, it is difficult to separate the

26 *Mahābhārata*, XIII, 107; cf. Hopkins, "Yoga-Technique," p. 366. Hauer, *Der Yoga als Heilweg*, p. 68, cites a similar passage: XII, 221.

27 Ibid., XIII, 40–41.

28 See above, p. 78.

29 *Mahābhārata*, XII, 290, 12.

30 Ibid., XV, 26, 26–29.

31 See Note IV, 3.

32 *Yoga-sūtras*, III, 38.

elements of magical folklore from the genuine yogic techniques.[33] Although Patañjali and all the representatives of classic Yoga considered the *siddhis* of no value toward deliverance, the "magical powers" acquired by the yogins have always made a deep impression on Indian audiences. Tantrism does not reject them; it even regards them as direct proof of man's gaining divinity. But the *siddhis* play no part in the *Bhagavad Gītā*.

The Message of the Bhagavad Gītā

The *Bhagavad Gītā*, one of the first substantial interpolations into Book VI of the *Mahābhārata*, gives Yoga a place of the highest importance. Naturally, the Yoga that Kṛṣṇa expounds and recommends in this masterpiece of Indian spirituality is neither the classic Yoga of Patañjali nor the arsenal of "magical" techniques that we have hitherto encountered, but a Yoga adapted to the Viṣṇuist religious experience—a method whose end is to gain the *unio mystica*. If we consider the fact that the *Bhagavad Gītā* represents not only the highest point of all Indian spirituality but also a very broad attempt at a synthesis, in which all the "paths" of salvation are validated and incorporated into Viṣṇuist devotion, the important place that the Kṛṣṇa of the *Gītā* accords to Yoga represents a real triumph for the yogic tradition. The strong theistic coloring that Kṛṣṇa gives it greatly assists us toward understanding the function performed by Yoga throughout Indian spirituality. Two conclusions follow from this observation: (1) Yoga can be understood as a mystical discipline whose goal is the union of the human and divine souls; (2) it is under this aspect—i.e., as "mystical experience"—that Yoga was understood and applied in the great popular "sectarian" trends, which are echoed in the *Mahābhārata* interpolations. There is no need to undertake a

33 Some passages refer to *samādhi*, but in the nonyogic sense of "arrange," "put in order"; "means for"; *apanītasya samādhiṃ cintaya*, "excogitate some arrangement of this evil" (XIII, 96, 12; Hopkins, "Yoga-Technique," p. 337).

detailed analysis of the *Bhagavad Gītā* here.[34] Broadly speaking, Kṛṣṇa reveals to Arjuna the "imperishable Yoga" (*yogam avyayam*). His revelations concern: (1) the structure of the universe; (2) the modalities of Being; (3) the ways leading to final liberation. But he is careful to add (IV, 3) that this "ancient yoga" (*purātanaḥ yogaḥ*), which is the "highest mystery," is not an innovation; he had already taught it to Vivasvat, who revealed it to Manu, who transmitted it to Ikṣvāku (IV, 1). "Coming thus by steps, it became known to royal sages. But that devotion was lost to the world by long (lapse of) time" (IV, 2).[35] Whenever order (*dharma*) languishes, Kṛṣṇa manifests himself (IV, 7)—that is, he reveals this timeless wisdom in a way appropriate to the respective "historical moment." In other words, if, as we shall see, historically the *Bhagavad Gītā* appears to be a new spiritual synthesis, it seems "new" only to the eyes of beings like ourselves, who are conditioned by time and history. This consideration applies to any Western interpretation of Indian spirituality; for, if we have the right to reconstruct the history of Indian documents and techniques, to attempt to determine the innovations that they contain, their evolution, and their successive modifications, we must not forget that, from the Indian point of view, the historical context of a "revelation" has only a limited importance; the "appearance" or "disappearance" of a soteriological formula on the plane of history can tell us nothing about its "origin." According to the Indian tradition, so steadfastly reaffirmed by Kṛṣṇa, the various "historical moments"—which are at the same time moments of the cosmic becoming—do not *create* doctrines, but only produce *appropriate formulas* for the timeless message. This amounts to saying that, in the case of the *Bhagavad Gītā*, its "innovations" are explained by the historical moment, which demanded precisely such a new and broader spiritual synthesis. In regard to the point that is of interest to us here—the meaning that the poem confers on yogic techniques—we have only to recall that the fundamental problem of the *Bhagavad Gītā* is to determine

34 See Note IV, 4.

35 Tr. Telang, p. 58.

whether *action* too can lead to salvation, or if *mystical meditation* is the only means of attaining it—in other words, the conflict between "action" (*karma*) and "contemplation" (*śama*). Kṛṣṇa attempts to solve the dilemma (which had obsessed Indian spirituality from the beginnings of the post-Vedic period) by showing that the two methods, previously opposed, are equally valid, it being possible for each individual to choose the method—be it action or be it knowledge and mystical contemplation—that his present karmic situation permits him to practice. It is here that Kṛṣṇa turns to "Yoga"—a Yoga that was not yet Patañjali's *darśana*, but that was equally far from being the "magical" Yoga referred to in other passages in the *Mahābhārata*.

Kṛṣṇa's Example

It could be said that the essence of the doctrine revealed by Kṛṣṇa is contained in the formula: "Understand Me and imitate Me!" For everything that he reveals regarding his own Being and his "behavior" in the cosmos and in history is to serve as model and example for Arjuna; the latter discovers the meaning of his historical life, and at the same time gains liberation, by understanding what Kṛṣṇa *is* and what he *does*. Indeed, Kṛṣṇa himself insists on the exemplary and soteriological value of the divine model: "Whatever a great man does, that other men also do. And people follow whatever he receives as authority" (III, 21).[36] And he adds, referring to himself: "There is nothing . . . for me to do in (all) the three worlds. . . . Still I do engage in action" (III, 23).[37] And he hastens to reveal the profound meaning of this activity: "For should I at any time not engage without sloth in action, men would follow in my path from all sides. . . . If I did not perform actions, these worlds would be destroyed, I should be the cause of universal confusion and of the end of created beings" (III, 23–24).[38]

36 Ibid., p. 54.

37 Ibid., pp. 54–55.

38 Ibid., p. 55 (modified).

Hence Arjuna must imitate Kṛṣṇa's behavior—that is, in the first place, he must continue to act, lest his passivity should contribute to "universal destruction." But, in order to act "as Kṛṣṇa acts," Arjuna must understand both the divinity's essence and his modes of manifestation. This is why Kṛṣṇa *reveals himself*—knowing God, man also knows the model that he must imitate. Kṛṣṇa begins by revealing that both Being and nonbeing reside in him and that the whole of creation—from the gods to minerals—descends from him (VII, 4–6; IX, 4–5; etc.). He is continually creating the world by the power of his *prakṛti* (IX, 8), but this perpetual activity does not fetter him (IX, 9); he is only the spectator of his own creation (IX, 10). Now, it is just this apparently paradoxical evaluation of activity (of *karma*) that constitutes the essential lesson of the Yoga that Kṛṣṇa reveals; by imitating God, who creates and sustains the world without participating in it, man will learn to do likewise. "A man does not attain freedom from action merely by not engaging in action; nor does he attain perfection by mere renunciation," for "nobody ever remains even for an instant without performing some action" (III, 4–5).[39] It is in vain that man restrains the activity of his senses; he who "continues to think in his mind about objects of sense"—that is, the generality of mankind—does not succeed in detaching himself from the world. Even if he abstains from action in the strict sense of the word, all his unconscious activity, provoked by the *guṇas* (III, 5), continues to fetter him to the world and keep him in the karmic circuit.

Condemned to action—for "action is better than inaction" (III, 8)—man must accomplish the acts prescribed for him—in other words, his "duties," the acts that are incumbent on him because of his particular situation. "One's own duty [*svadharma*], though defective, is better than another's duty [*paradharma*] well performed" (III, 35).[40] These specific activities are conditioned by the *guṇas* (XVII, 8 ff.; XVIII, 23 ff.). Kṛṣṇa more than once repeats that the *guṇas* proceed from him but do not fetter him: "I

39 Tr. Telang, pp. 52–53.

40 Ibid., p. 56.

am not in them, but they are in me" (VII, 21).[41] "The four-caste system was created by Me with distinction of strands [*guṇas*]; altho I am the door of this, know Me as one that eternally does no act" (IV, 13).[42] The lesson that man must learn from all this is: while accepting the "historical situation" created by the *guṇas* (and he must accept it, because the *guṇas* too derive from Kṛṣṇa), and acting in accordance with the necessities of that "situation," man must refuse to *valorize* his acts and thus accord his particular condition an *absolute value*. In other words, on the one hand he must deny ontological reality to any human "situation" (for only Kṛṣṇa is saturated with Being); on the other, he must not allow himself to enjoy the "fruits of his acts."

"Acts" and "Sacrifices"

In this sense, it may be said that the *Bhagavad Gītā* attempts to "save" all human acts, to "justify" all profane activity; for, by the very fact that he no longer enjoys their "fruits," man transforms his acts into *sacrifices*—that is, into transpersonal dynamisms contributing to the maintenance of cosmic order. Now, as Kṛṣṇa reminds Arjuna, only acts whose object is sacrifice do not fetter: "Therefore act, casting off all attachment" (III, 9). Prajāpati created sacrifice in order that the cosmos should be manifested and men should live and propagate (III, 10 ff.). But Kṛṣṇa reveals that man, too, can collaborate in the perpetuation of the divine work—not only by sacrifices, properly speaking (those which compose the Vedic cult), but *by all his acts*, of whatever nature. For him who engages in sacrifice, "all acts are destroyed" (IV, 23). This is to be understood as meaning that his activity no longer "fetters," creates no new karmic ties. It is in this sense that the various ascetics and yogins "sacrifice" their physiological and psychic activities: they *detach* themselves from these activities, give them a *transpersonal* value; and, doing so, "all of [them], conversant with

41 Cf. XIV, 5 ff., on the structure of the *guṇas*.

42 Tr. Franklin Edgerton, I, 45.

the sacrifice, have their sins destroyed by the sacrifice" (IV, 25–30).[43]

This transmutation of profane activities into rituals is made possible by Yoga. Kṛṣṇa reveals to Arjuna that the "man of action" can save himself—in other words, can escape the consequences of his participation in the life of the world—*while still continuing to act*. The "man of action" here means the man who cannot retire from secular life in order to accomplish his salvation through knowledge or mystical devotion. The only rule that he must follow is this: *he must detach himself from his acts and their results*—in other words, "renounce the fruits of his acts" (*phalatṛṣṇavairāgya*), *act impersonally*, without passion, without desire, as if he were acting by proxy, in another's stead. If he follows this rule strictly, his acts will no longer sow new karmic potentialities, will no longer keep him in subjection to the karmic circuit. "Forsaking all attachment to the fruit of action, always contented, dependent on none, he does nothing at all, though he engages in action" (IV, 20).[44]

The great originality of the *Bhagavad Gītā* lies in its insistence upon this "Yoga of action," which is realized by "renouncing the fruit of one's acts" (*phalatṛṣṇavairāgya*). This is also the reason for its unparalleled success in India. For henceforth every man may hope to be saved, by virtue of *phalatṛṣṇavairāgya*, even when, for all kinds of reasons, he must continue to participate in social life, to have a family, worries, to work, even to commit "immoral" acts (like Arjuna, who must kill his enemies in war). To act calmly, automatically, without being troubled by the "desire for the fruit," is to obtain a self-mastery and a serenity that probably only Yoga can bestow. As Kṛṣṇa teaches: while acting without restriction, one remains faithful to Yoga. This interpretation of Yoga technique, which presents it as an instrument permitting man to detach himself from the world while yet continuing to live and act in it, is characteristic of the magnificent synthetic effort of the author of the *Bhagavad Gītā*, which sought to reconcile all voca-

43 Tr. Telang, p. 62.

44 Ibid., p. 60.

tions (ascetic, mystical, active) as it had reconciled Vedāntic monism with Sāṃkhya pluralism. But at the same time, the fact that it could be so interpreted testifies to the extreme suppleness of Yoga—which thus once again proves that it can adapt itself to all religious experiences and satisfy all needs.

Yoga Technique in the Bhagavad Gītā

In addition to this Yoga within the reach of everyone, which consists in renouncing the "fruit of one's acts," the *Bhagavad Gītā* also briefly expounds a yogic technique in the strict sense, for the use of *munis* (VI, 11 ff.). Although morphologically (bodily postures, gazing at the tip of the nose, etc.) this technique resembles the one described by Patañjali, the meditation of which Kṛṣṇa speaks is different from that of the *Yoga-sūtras*. In the first place, *prāṇāyāma* is not mentioned in this context.[45] Secondly, yogic meditation in the *Gītā* does not achieve its supreme end unless the yogin concentrates on Kṛṣṇa.

"With soul serene and fearless, constant in his vow to keep the way of chastity [*brāhmacarī*], his mind firm and steadfastly thinking of Me, he must practice Yoga, taking Me for the supreme end. Thus, with his soul continually devoted to meditation and his mind under control, the yogin obtains the peace that dwells in Me and whose final boundary is *nirvāṇa*" (VI, 14–15).[46] The mystical devotion (*bhakti*) of which Kṛṣṇa is the object gives him an infinitely greater role than that which Īśvara played in the *Yoga-sūtras*. In the *Gītā*, Kṛṣṇa is the only goal; it is he who justifies yogic meditation and practice, it is upon him that the yogin "concentrates," it is through his grace (and in the *Gītā* the concept of

45 The *Gītā* (IV, 29; V, 27) refers to *prāṇāyāma*, but, rather than a yogic technique, it is here a substitutive meditation, an "interiorized ritual," such as is found in the period of the Brāhmaṇas and the Upaniṣads.

46 É. Senart translates this last verse: "the Yogin . . . attains the repose, the supreme peace, that has its seat in me" (*śāntiṃ nirvāṇaparamāṃ matsaṃsthām adhigacchati*). We have preferred to give a translation that, though freer, seems to us closer to the spirit of the text.

grace already begins to take form, foreshowing the luxuriant development that it will undergo in Viṣṇuist literature) that the yogin obtains the *nirvāṇa* that is neither the *nirvāṇa* of late Buddhism nor the *samādhi* of the *Yoga-sūtras*, but a state of perfect mystical union between the soul and its God.

A true yogin (*vigatakalmaṣaḥ*, "freed from the corruption" of good and evil) easily attains the infinite bliss (*atyantam sukham*) produced by contact with Brahman (*brahmasaṃsparśam*). This invoking of Brahman (VI, 28) in a text that is a vindication of Kṛṣṇa need not surprise us. In the *Bhagavad Gītā*, Kṛṣṇa is pure Spirit; the "great Brahman" is only the "womb" (*yoni*) for him (XIV, 3). "I am the father, the giver of the seed" (XIV, 4).[47] Kṛṣṇa is the "foundation of Brahman," as he is of immortality, of the imperishable, of eternal order and perfect happiness (XIV, 27). But although in this context Brahman is put in the "feminine" condition of *prakṛti*, his nature is spiritual. The *muni* attains him through Yoga (V, 6). The "infinite bliss" that results from union with Brahman allows the yogin to see "the soul [*ātman*] in all beings and all beings in the *ātman*" (VI, 29). And, in the following strophe, it is precisely the identification of the *ātman* of beings with Kṛṣṇa that provides the foundation for the mystical bond between the yogin and the God: "To him who sees me in everything and everything in me, I am never lost, and he is not lost to me. The devotee who worships me abiding in all beings, holding that all is one, lives in me, however he may be living" (VI, 30–31).[48] We find the same motif as that of the verse just cited (VI, 30) in the *Īśā Upaniṣad* (VI), which proves that the Upaniṣads contained theistic trends that they passed on to the *Gītā*, where they flowered so magnificently. Kṛṣṇa, the personal god and source of true mystical experiences (*bhakti*), is here identified with the Brahman of the purely speculative metaphysics of the earliest Upaniṣads.

Nevertheless, the *Gītā* reserves its highest praise not for the yogin completely detached from the pain and illusions of this

47 Tr. Telang, p. 107.

48 Ibid., p. 71.

world, but for him who regards another's pain and joy as his own (VI, 32). This is a leitmotiv of Indian mysticism, and particularly of Buddhist mysticism. The author of the *Bhagavad Gītā* bestows all his sympathy on him who practices this kind of Yoga. If he fails in this life, he will be reborn in a family of talented yogins, and, in another life, will succeed in accomplishing what he could not achieve in this (VI, 41). Kṛṣṇa reveals to Arjuna that the mere fact of having attempted the way of Yoga raises the yogin above the man who has confined himself to practicing the rites prescribed by the Vedas (VI, 44). Finally, Kṛṣṇa does not fail to say that, among the ways to salvation, the best and most commendable is the way of Yoga: "Yoga is higher than asceticism [*tapas*], higher even than knowledge [*jñāna*], higher than sacrifice" (VI, 46).[49]

The triumph of yogic practices is here complete. Not only are they accepted by the *Bhagavad Gītā*, the apogee of Indian spirituality; they are elevated to first place. It is true that this Yoga is purified from the last traces of magic (rigorous asceticism, etc.), and that the most important of its ancient techniques, *prāṇāyāma*, is reduced to a very minor role. It is true, too, that meditation and concentration here become instruments of an *unio mystica* with a God who reveals himself as a person. Nevertheless, the acceptance of yogic practices by the Viṣṇuist mystical and devotional trend [50] proves the considerable popularity of these practices as well as their universality in India. Kṛṣṇa's discourse amounts to a validation, for all Hinduism, of Yoga technique regarded as a purely Indian means of obtaining mystical union with a personal God. By far the greater part of the modern yogic literature published in India and elsewhere finds its theoretical justification in the *Bhagavad Gītā*.

49 Paraphrased.

50 See, for example, the role of Yoga in the very important "sect," the Pāñcarātras (Bhāgavatas), Note IV, 5.

Yoga Techniques in Buddhism

The Road to Nirvāṇa *and the Symbolism of Initiation*

DURING his period of study and asceticism, Śākyamuni had come to know both the doctrines of Sāṃkhya and the practices of Yoga. Arāḍa Kālāma taught a sort of preclassic Sāṃkhya at Vaiśālī, and Udraka Rāmaputra expounded the bases and goals of Yoga.[1] If the Buddha rejects the teaching of these two masters, it is because he has progressed beyond it. Naturally, the majority of the canonical texts allege an irreducible distance between the Enlightened One and his masters and contemporaries. This is a polemic position, which requires rectification. The Buddha himself proclaimed that he had "seen the ancient way and followed it." [2]

The "ancient," timeless way was that of liberation, of nondeath, and it was also the way of Yoga. As Émile Senart wrote as long ago as 1900, the Buddha did not repudiate the ascetic and contemplative traditions of India *in toto*; he completed them: "It was on the terrain of Yoga that the Buddha arose; whatever innovations he was able to introduce into it, the mold of Yoga was that in which his thought was formed." [3]

1 Cf. Aśvaghoṣa, *Buddhacarita*, XII, 17 ff.; id., *Saundarānanda*, XV–XVII; *Majjhima-nikāya*, I, 164 ff.

2 *Saṃyutta-nikāya*, II, 106. See other references in A. K. Coomaraswamy, *Hinduism and Buddhism*, pp. 45 ff.

3 "Bouddhisme et Yoga," *La Revue de l'histoire des religions*, XLII (1900), 348. On the relations between Yoga and Buddhism, see Note V, 1.

v. *Yoga Techniques in Buddhism*

The Awakened One is equally opposed to Brāhmanic ritualism and to exaggerated asceticism and metaphysical speculations. Hence he repeated and sharpened the criticisms already formulated against fossilized ritualism and excessive *ascesis* (*tapas*) by the Upaniṣadic contemplatives; but he also opposed the claim—principally represented by the classic Upaniṣads—that salvation could be gained only by the road of metaphysical knowledge. At first sight, the Buddha appears to reject Brāhmanic orthodoxy and the speculative tradition of the Upaniṣads no less than he does the countless marginal mystico-ascetic "heresies" of Indian society. Nevertheless, the central problem of Buddhism—suffering and emancipation from suffering—is the traditional problem of Indian philosophy. The Buddhist refrain, *sarvam dukham, sarvam anityam*, "all is painful, all is transient," can equally well be adopted by Sāṃkhya-Yoga and Vedānta (as in fact it was).

This seemingly paradoxical position, in which the Buddha opposed both orthodox doctrines and ascetico-contemplative disciplines yet at the same time adopted their premises and techniques, will be better understood if we consider that he set out to go beyond all the philosophical formulas and mystical rules current in his day, in order to deliver man from their dominance and to set him on the "way" to the Absolute. If he took over the pitiless analysis to which preclassic Sāṃkhya and Yoga submitted the notion of "person" and of psychomental life, it was because the "Self" had nothing to do with that illusory entity, the human "soul." But the Buddha went even further than Sāṃkhya and Yoga, for he declined to postulate the existence of a *puruṣa* or an *ātman*. Indeed, he denied the possibility of discussing any absolute principle, as he denied the possibility of having an even approximate experience of the true Self, so long as man was not "awakened." The Buddha likewise rejected the conclusions of Upaniṣadic speculation—the postulate of a *brahman*, a pure, absolute, immortal, eternal spirit identical with the *ātman*—but he did so because this dogma might satisfy the intellect and thus prevent man from awakening.

More careful examination shows that the Buddha rejected all contemporary philosophies and asceticisms because he regarded them as *idola mentis* interposing a sort of screen between man and absolute reality, the one true Unconditioned. That he had no intention of denying a final, unconditioned reality, beyond the eternal flux of cosmic and psychomental phenomena, but that he was careful to speak but little on the subject, is proved by a number of canonical texts. *Nirvāṇa* is the absolute in the highest sense, the *asaṃskṛta*—that is, what is neither born nor composed, what is irreducible, transcendent, beyond all human experience. "It were fruitless to maintain that *nirvāṇa* does not exist because it is not an object of knowledge.—Certainly, *nirvāṇa* is not known directly, as colors, sensation, etc., are known; it is not known indirectly, through its activity, as the sense organs are known. Yet its nature and its activity . . . are objects of knowledge. . . . The yogin enters into meditation . . . becomes conscious of *nirvāṇa*, of its nature, of its activity. When he emerges from contemplation, he cries: 'Oh! *nirvāṇa*, destruction, calm, excellent, escape!' Blind men, because they do not see blue and yellow, have no right to say that those who have sight do not see colors and that colors do not exist." [4] *Nirvāṇa* can be "seen" only with the "eye of the saints" (*ariya cakku*)—that is, with a transcendent "organ," which no longer participates in the perishable world. The problem for Buddhism, as for every other initiation, was to show the way and create the means by which this transcendent "organ" for revealing the unconditioned could be obtained.

We must remember that the Buddha's message was addressed to suffering man, to man caught in the net of transmigration. For the Buddha, as for all forms of Yoga, salvation could be gained only as the result of a personal effort, of a concrete assimilation of truth. It was neither a *theory* nor an escape into one or another kind of *ascetic effort*. "Truth" must be *understood* and at the same time

4 *Saṃghabhadra*, after L. de la Vallée Poussin, *Nirvāṇa*, pp. 73–74. Cf. Buddhagoṣa, *Visuddhimagga*, ed. C. A. F. Rhys Davids, p. 507: "One cannot say that a thing does not exist because fools do not perceive it."

known experimentally. Now, as we shall see, the two roads were attended by dangers; "understanding" ran the risk of remaining mere speculation, "experimental knowledge" might overwhelm ecstasy. But, for the Buddha, one can be "saved" only by attaining *nirvāṇa*—that is, by going beyond the plane of profane human experience and re-establishing the plane of the unconditioned. In other words, one can be saved only by *dying* to this profane world and *being reborn* into a transhuman life impossible to define or describe.

This is why the symbolisms of death, rebirth, and initiation persist in Buddhist texts. The monk must create a "new body" for himself, be "reborn," as in other initiations, after being "dead." The Buddha himself proclaims it: "Moreover, I have shown my disciples the way whereby they call into being out of this body [composed of the four elements] another body of the mind's creation [*rūpim manomayam*], complete in all its limbs and members, and with transcendental faculties [*abhinindriyam*]. It is just like a man who should draw a reed from its sheath—or a snake from its slough—or a sword from its scabbard,—recognizing that the reed, the snake, or the sword was one thing and the sheath, slough, or scabbard was another," etc.[5] The initiatory symbolism is obvious; the image of the snake and its cast skin is one of the oldest symbols of mystical death and resurrection, and occurs in the literature of Brāhmanism.[6] Ananda Coomaraswamy has shown that the Buddhist ordination continued the Vedic initiation (*dīkṣā*) and adhered to the schema of initiations in general. The monk gave up his family name and became a "son of Buddha" (*śākyaputto*), for he was "born among the saints" (*ariya*); so Kassapa, speaking of himself, said: "Natural Son of the Blessed One, born of his mouth, born of the Dhamma, fashioned by the Dhamma, and an heir of the Dhamma," etc.[7] The importance of the *guru* as initiatory master is

5 *Majjhima-nikāya*, II, 17; tr. Robert Chalmers, *Further Dialogues of the Buddha*, II, 10.

6 *Jaiminīya Brāhmaṇa*, II, 134, etc.

7 *Saṃyutta-nikāya*, II, 221; tr. Coomaraswamy. See Coomaraswamy, "Some Pāli Words" (*Harvard Journal of Asiatic Studies*, IV [1939], 144 ff.

no less great in Buddhism than in any other Indian soteriology.

The Buddha taught the way and the means of dying to the human condition, to bondage and suffering, in order to be reborn to the freedom, the bliss, and the unconditionality of *nirvāṇa.* But he hesitated to speak of that unconditionality, lest he should fail to do it justice. If he had attacked the Brāhmans and the *paribbājakas,* it was precisely because they talked too much about the inexpressible and claimed that they could define the Self (*ātman*). For the Buddha, "to maintain that the *ātman* exists, real, permanent, is a false view; to maintain that it does not exist is a false view." [8] But if we read what he says of the emancipated, the *nirvāṇa*-ized human being, we shall see that the latter in all respects resembles the non-Buddhist *jīvan-mukta,* the man "liberated while living." He is, "even in this life, cut off [*nicchāta*], *nirvāṇa*-ized [*nibbuta*], aware of happiness in himself, and lives with his soul identified with Brahman." [9] L. de la Vallée Poussin, who quotes this text, compares it with *Bhagavad Gītā,* V, 24: "He who finds no happiness nor joy nor light, except within, the yogin identified with Brahman, attains the *nirvāṇa* that is Brahman [*brahmanirvāṇam*]." From this we see in what sense the Buddha continues the Indian ascetico-mystical tradition; he believes in a "liberation in life," but he refuses to define it. "If the Buddha declines to explain himself on the subject of the Liberated Man, it is not because the saint does not exist, even in life, but because nothing definite can be said about the Liberated." [10] All that can be said of the *jīvan-mukta* (or, in Buddhist terminology, the *nirvāṇa*-ized) is that he is not of this world. "The Tathāgata can no longer be designated as being matter, sensations, ideas, volitions, knowledge; he is freed from these designations; he is deep, immeasurable, unfathomable, like the great ocean. One cannot say: 'He is,' 'He is not,' 'He is and he is not.' 'He neither is nor is not.' " [11] This is exactly the language of

8 Vasubandhu, cited in La Vallée Poussin, p. 107, n. 2.

9 *Aṅguttara-nikāya,* II, 206.

10 La Vallée Poussin, p. 112.

11 *Saṃyutta-nikāya,* IV, 374.

apophatic mysticism and theology; it is the famous *neti! neti!* of the Upaniṣads.

The Jhānas *and the* Samāpattis

To obtain the state of the unconditioned—in other words, to die completely to this profane, painful, illusory life and to be reborn (in another "body"!) to the mystical life that will make it possible to attain *nirvāṇa*—the Buddha employs the traditional yogic techniques, but correcting them by the addition of a profound effort to "comprehend" truth. Let us note that the preliminaries of Buddhist *ascesis* and meditation are similar to those recommended by the *Yoga-sūtras* and other classic texts. The ascetic should choose a retired spot (in the forest, at the foot of a tree, in a cave, in a graveyard, or even on a heap of straw in the open fields), assume the *āsana* position, and begin his meditation. "Putting away the hankering after the world, he abides with unhankering heart, and purifies his mind of covetousness. Putting away the canker of ill-will, he abides with heart free from enmity, benevolent and compassionate towards every living thing, and purifies his mind of malevolence. Putting away sloth and torpor, he abides clear of both; conscious of light, mindful and self-possessed, he purifies his mind of sloth and torpor. . . . Putting away doubt, he abides as one who has passed beyond perplexity; no longer in suspense as to what is good, he purifies his mind of doubt." [12]

Although containing "moral" elements, this meditation is not ethical in intent. Its purpose is to purify the ascetic's consciousness, to prepare it for higher spiritual experiences. Yogic meditation, as interpreted by the Buddha in some texts of the *Dīgha-nikāya*, definitely aims at "remaking" the ascetic's consciousness—that is, at creating for him a new "direct experience" of his psychic life and even of his biological life. Through all of his concrete actions—

12 *Udumbarikā Sīhanāda Suttanta, Dīgha-nikāya*, III, 49; tr. T. W. and C. A. F. Rhys Davids, *Dialogues of the Buddha*, III, 44. See also *Dialogues*, II, 327 ff.; *Vinaya Texts*, I, 119, etc.

gait, bodily posture, respiration, etc.—the ascetic must concretely rediscover the "truths" revealed by the Master; in other words, he turns all his movements and actions into pretexts for meditation. The *Mahā Sattipaṭṭhāna Suttanta*[13] specifies that the *bhikku,* after choosing a solitary spot for his meditation, should become conscious of all those physiological acts he had previously performed automatically and unconsciously. "Whether he inhale a long breath, let him be conscious thereof; or whether he exhale a long breath, let him be conscious thereof [etc.]. . . . Let him practice with the thought 'Conscious of my whole body will I inhale . . . will I exhale.' Let him practice with the thought 'I will inhale tranquillizing my bodily organism . . . I will exhale tranquillizing,' " etc.[14]

This procedure is not simply a *prāṇāyāma* exercise; it is also a meditation on the Buddhist "truths," a permanent experiencing of the unreality of matter.[15] For that is the purpose of this meditation—to assimilate the fundamental "truths" completely, to transform them into a "continual experience," to diffuse them, as it were, through the monk's entire being. For the same text of the *Dīgha-nikāya* (II, 292) later states: a *bhikku,* "whether he departs or returns, whether he looks at or looks away from, whether he has drawn in or stretched out [his limbs], whether he has donned under-robe, over-robe, or bowl, whether he is eating, drinking, chewing, reposing, or whether he is obeying the calls of nature . . . in going, standing, sitting, sleeping, watching, talking, or keeping silence, he knows what he is doing."[16]

13 *Dīgha-nikāya,* II, 327 ff. 14 Tr. Rhys Davids, *Dialogues,* II, 328.

15 We give the commentator's explanation of the text: "The yogin must ask himself: 'On what are these expirations and inspirations based? They are based on matter, and matter is the material body, and the material body is the four elements,' " etc. (H. C. Warren, *Buddhism in Translations,* p. 355, n. 1.) We have here, then, a meditation on the rhythm of respiration, setting out from an analytical understanding of the human body; a pretext for an understanding of the composite, "painful," and transitory nature of the body. This "understanding" sustains and justifies the meditation, for it reveals the insubstantiality of life and forces the ascetic to persevere in the way of salvation.

16 Tr. Rhys Davids, *Dialogues,* II, 329.

It is easy to comprehend the aim of this lucidity. Always, and whatever he may be doing, the *bhikku* must understand both his body and his soul, so that he may continually realize the fragility of the phenomenal world and the unreality of the "soul." The *Sumaṇgala Vilāsinī* commentary draws the following conclusion from this kind of meditation on the actions of the body: "They say it is a living entity that walks, a living entity that stands; but is there any living entity to walk or to stand? There is not." [17]

But this permanent attention to one's one life, this technique for destroying illusions created by a false conception of the "soul," are only the preliminaries. Real Buddhist meditation begins with experiencing the four psychic states called *jhānas* (cf. Skr. *dhyāna*).

We do not know exactly what meditational technique the Buddha chose and practiced. The same formulas are often used to express various contents. (We may recall the troublingly diverse meanings of the word *yoga* throughout all the Indian literatures.) It is, however, probable that at least a part of the meditational technique employed by the Buddha was preserved by his disciples and transmitted by the primitive ascetic tradition. How should so rich and coherent a corpus of spiritual exercises be lost, or how should it suffer mutilation, in a tradition in which the Master's direct teaching plays such an important part? But, according to the texts collected by Caroline Rhys Davids,[18] it is clear that the Buddha was a fervent *jhāin* and that he sought neither the Cosmic Soul (*brahman*) nor God (Īśvara) through the *jhāna* that he practiced, nor exhorted others to seek them. For him, *jhāna* was a means of "mystical" experimentation, a way of access to suprasensible realities, and not an *unio mystica*. This yogic experience prepared the monk for a "superknowledge" (*abhijñā*) whose final goal was *nirvāṇa*.

It is in the *Poṭṭhapāda-sutta* (10 ff.) [19] that the technique of

17 Warren, p. 358 n.

18 "Dhyāna in Early Buddhism," *Indian Historical Quarterly*, III (1927), 689–715.

19 *Dīgha-nikāya*, I, 182 ff.

Buddhist meditation was formulated, if not for the first time (which is highly probable), at least in the clearest fashion. We shall give several long extracts from this important text: "When he [the *bhikku*] has realized that these Five Hindrances [*nīvaraṇa*] [20] have been put away from within him, a gladness springs up within him, and joy arises to him thus gladdened, and so rejoicing all his frame becomes at ease, and being thus at ease he is filled with a sense of peace, and in that peace his heart is stayed. Then estranged from lusts, aloof from evil dispositions, he enters into and remains in the First Rapture [*jhāna*] . . . a state of joy and ease born of detachment [*vivekaja:* "born of solitude"], reasoning and investigation going on the while. Then that idea . . . of lusts, that he had before, passes away. And thereupon there arises within him a subtle, but actual, consciousness of the joy and peace arising from detachment, and he becomes a person to whom that idea is consciously present."

Then, "suppressing all reasoning and investigation, [the *bhikku*] enters into and abides in the Second Rapture [*jhāna*] . . . a state of joy and ease, born of the serenity of concentration [*samādhi*],[21] when no reasoning or investigation goes on, a state of elevation of mind, a tranquillization of the heart within. Then that subtle, but actual, consciousness of the joy and peace arising from detachment [*vivekaja*], that he just had, passes away. And thereupon there arises a subtle, but actual, consciousness of the joy and peace born of concentration. And he becomes a person conscious of that."

Then the *bhikku*, "holding aloof from joy, becomes equable; and, mindful and self-possessed, he experiences in his body that ease which the Arahats [*ārya*] talk of when they say: 'The man serene

20 According to *Dīgha-nikāya*, I, 71, the five *nīvaraṇas* are sensuality, malice, indolence of mind and body, agitation of mind and body, doubt. The lists differ. Compare the "five sins" in *Mahābhārata*, XII, 241, 3 ff. (Hopkins, *The Great Epic*, p. 181).

21 The *samādhi* of Buddhist texts, although an enstasis similar to that of the *Yoga-sūtras*, does not play the same role as it does in Patañjali's manual. *Samādhi* here seems to be a state preliminary to entrance into the way of *nirvāṇa*. See Note V, 2.

and self-possessed is well at ease.' And so he enters into and abides in the Third Rapture . . . [*jhāna*]. Then that subtle, but yet actual, consciousness, that he had just had, of the joy and peace born of concentration, passes away. And thereupon there arises a subtle, but yet actual, consciousness of the bliss of equanimity."

After that, the *bhikku*, "by the putting away alike of ease and of pain, by the passing away of any joy, any elation, he had previously felt, enters into and abides in the Fourth Rapture '. . . [*jhāna*] a state of pure self-possession and equanimity [*sati*], without pain and without ease.[22] Then that subtle, but yet actual, consciousness, that he just had, of the bliss of equanimity, passes away. And thereupon there arises to him a subtle, but yet actual, consciousness of the absence of pain, and of the absence of ease. And he becomes a person conscious of that." [23]

We shall not add further texts on the subject of these four *jhānas*.[24] The stages are quite clearly defined in the passages already given: (1) to purify the mind and the sensibility from "temptations"—that is, to isolate them from external agents; in short, to obtain a first autonomy of consciousness; (2) to suppress the dialectical functions of the mind, obtain concentration, perfect mastery of a rarefied consciousness; (3) to suspend all "relations" both with the sensible world and with memory, to obtain a placid lucidity without any other content than "consciousness of existing"; (4) to reintegrate the "opposites," obtain the bliss of "pure consciousness."

But the itinerary does not end here. The *jhānas* are followed by four other spiritual exercises, called *samāpattis*, "attainments," which prepare the ascetic for the final "enstasis." Despite the detailed description that the texts give of them, these "states" are

22 Physiologically, the fourth *jhāna* is characterized by the arrest of respiration, *assāsa-passāsa-nirodha;* Paul Oltramare, *La Théosophie bouddhique*, p. 364, n. 2.

23 *Dīgha-nikāya*, I, 182 ff.; tr. Rhys Davids, I, 247–49.

24 Cf. *Majjhima-nikāya*, I, 454 ff.; Vasubandhu, *Abhidharmakośa*, tr. L. de la Vallée Poussin, IV, 107; VIII, 161. Excellent analysis in Giulio Evola, *La Dottrina del risveglio*, pp. 220–25. On the pseudo *dhyānas*, see Note V, 3.

difficult to understand. They correspond to experiences too far removed not only from those of normal consciousness but also from the extrarational (mystical or poetic) experiences comprehensible to Occidentals. However, it would be wrong to explain them as hypnotic inhibitions. As we shall see, the monk's lucidity during the course of his meditation is constantly verified; in addition, hypnotic sleep and trance are obstacles with which Indian treatises on meditation are perfectly familiar and against which they constantly warn the aspirant. The four last *dhyānas* (in the terminology of asceticism, *samāpattis*) are described as follows: "And again . . . the *Bhikkhu*, by passing beyond the consciousness of form, by putting an end to the sense of resistance [*paṭigha*, the contact from which all sensation results], by paying no heed to the idea of distinction, thinking: 'The space is infinite,' reaches up to and remains in the mental state in which the mind is concerned only with the consciousness of the infinity of space. . . . And again . . . by passing quite beyond the consciousness of space as infinite, thinking: 'Cognition is infinite,' [he] reaches up to and remains in the mental state in which the mind is concerned only with the infinity of cognition [N.B., consciousness proves to be infinite as soon as it is no longer limited by sensory and mental experiences]. . . . And again, by passing quite beyond the consciousness of the infinity of cognition, thinking: 'There is nothing that really is,' [he] reaches up to and remains in the mental state in which the mind is concerned only with the unreality of things [*akiñcaññāyatana*, "nihility"]. Then that sense of everything being within the sphere of infinite cognition, that he just had, passes away. And there arises in him a consciousness, subtle but yet actual, of unreality as the object of his thought. And he becomes a person conscious of that." [25]

It would serve no purpose to comment on each of these stages, making use of the plentiful texts in the literature of later Buddhism, unless we were interested in reconstructing the psychology

25 *Dīgha-nikāya*, I, 183 ff.; tr. Rhys Davids, I, 249–50.

and metaphysics of Buddhist scholasticism.[26] But since what concerns us here is essentially the morphology of meditation, we shall proceed to the ninth and last *samāpatti.* "So from the time . . . that the Bhikkhu is thus conscious in a way brought about by himself [being in *dhyānā*, he cannot receive ideas from outside; he is *sakasaññī*], he goes on from one stage to the next . . . until he reaches the summit of consciousness. And when he is on the summit it may occur to him: 'To be thinking at all is the inferior state. 'Twere better not to be thinking. Were I to go on thinking and fancying,[27] these ideas, these states of consciousness, I have reached to, would pass away, but others, coarser ones, might arise. So I will neither think nor fancy any more.' And he does not. And to him neither thinking any more, nor fancying, the ideas, the states of consciousness, he had, pass away; and no others, coarser than they, arise. So he falls into trance." [28] Another text, of a later period, still more directly indicates the major importance of the ninth and last *samāpatti:* "Venerable monks, acquire the *samāpatti* that consists in the cessation of all conscious perception. The *bhikku* who has acquired it has nothing more to do." [29]

Yogins and Metaphysicians

It has been observed that these *dhyānas* and *samāpattis* have more than one point in common with the various stages of *samprajñāta* and *asamprajñāta samādhi* in classic Yoga. Indeed, the Buddhists themselves admitted that yogins and non-Buddhist ascetics could have access to the four *dhyānas* and the four "attainments" and even to the last, the *samāpatti* of "unconsciousness" (*asaṃjñisamāpatti*). However, they denied the authenticity of this ninth *samāpatti* when it was obtained by non-Buddhists; they believed that "the *samāpatti* of the destruction of consciousness and sensation"

26 See Note V, 4.

27 *Abhisaṃkhareyyaṃ,* perhaps "perfecting" or "planning out." (Rhys Davids' note.)

28 *Dīgha-nikāya,* I, 184; tr. Rhys Davids, I, 251.

29 Śāntideva, *Śikṣāsamuccaya,* ed. Cecil Bendall, p. 48.

(*saṃjñāveditanirodha samāpatti*) was a discovery of the Buddha's and constituted contact with *nirvāṇa*.[30] Now, if they forbade access to *nirvāṇa* to non-Buddhists, while still admitting the validity of their *jhānas*, this was undoubtedly because these "heretics" did not recognize the *truth* revealed by the Buddha. In other words, the unconditioned could not be reached solely by mystical meditation; the road leading to the unconditioned must be understood, otherwise the aspirant ran the risk of taking up his abode in one or another "heaven," while believing that he had attained *nirvāṇa*.

This brings us to the problem of "gnosis" and of the "mystical experience"—a problem that was destined to play a fundamental role in the history of Buddhism (but which remains of capital importance in the entire history of Indian spirituality). The two trends—that of the "experimentalists" (the *jhāins*), if we may so express ourselves, and that of the "speculatives" (the *dhammayogas*)—are two constants of Buddhism. The canonical texts very early tried to bring them into agreement. A *sūtra* of the *Aṅguttara-nikāya* (III, 355), to which L. de la Vallée Poussin has several times drawn our attention, says: "The monks who devote themselves to ecstasy [the *jhāins*] blame the monks who are attached to doctrine [the *dhammayogas*], and vice versa. On the contrary, they should esteem one another. Few, verily, are those who pass their time touching with their bodies [i.e., "realizing," "experiencing"] the immortal element [*amatā dhātu*; i.e., *nirvāṇa*]. Few, too, are they who see the deep reality [*arthapada*], penetrating it by *prajñā*, by intellect." The text emphasizes the extreme difficulty of the two "ways": gnosis, and experience through meditation. And rightly—for few, indeed, are they who have an *experience* of *nirvāṇa*; and no less few are they who "see" reality as it is and who—through that intellectual vision—conquer liberation. In the course of time, all means of approaching the Buddha by the way of "experience" will become equivalent; he who learns and understands the canon assimilates the "doctrinal body" of the Buddha; the pilgrim who

30 On all this, see La Vallée Poussin, "Musīla et Nārada" (*Mélanges chinois et bouddhiques*, V [1937]), pp. 210 ff.

visits a *stūpa* containing relics of the Enlightened One gains access to the mystical architectonic body of the same Buddha. But in the first stage of Buddhism, the problem that arose was the same problem that had arisen for Sāṃkhya-Yoga: which has the primacy, "intelligence" or "experience"?

There is sufficient evidence to prove that the Buddha always closely connected knowledge with a meditational experience of the yogic type. For him, knowledge was of little value so long as it was not "realized" in personal experience of it. As for meditational experience, it is the "truths" discovered by the Buddha that validated it. Take, for example, the statement: "The body is perishable." It is only by contemplating a corpse that one would assimilate this truth. But contemplation of a corpse would have no value for salvation if it did not rest upon a truth (*this* body is perishable; *all* bodies are perishable; there is no salvation except in the law of the Buddha, etc.). All the truths revealed by the Buddha must be tested in the yogic fashion—that is, must be meditated and experienced.

It is for this reason that Ānanda, the Master's favorite disciple, although unequaled in learning (according to the *Theragāthās*, v. 1024, he had learned eighty-two thousand of the Buddha's own *dhammas* and two thousand of those of his fellow disciples), was nevertheless excluded from the council; he was not an arhat—that is, he had not had a perfect "yogic experience." "As for the *sthavira* Ānanda, who has listened to, memorized, recited, and meditated upon all sorts of *sūtras*, his wisdom [*prajñā*] is vast, whereas his thought concentration [*citta saṃgraha*] is poor. Now, one must unite these two qualities in order to gain the state (that consists in) the destruction of impurities [arhatship]." [31] A famous text in the *Saṃyutta-nikāya* (II, 115) confronts Musīla and Nārada, each of them representing a particular degree of Buddhist perfection. Both possess the same knowledge, but Nārada does not consider

31 Nāgārjuna, *Mahāprajñāpāramitāśāstra*, tr. after E. Lamotte, *Le Traité de la grande vertu de sagesse*, I, 223. The Sanskrit original is lost, but the work has been preserved in several Chinese and Tibetan translations.

himself an arhat, since he has not himself experienced "contact with *nirvāṇa*." He puts it as follows: "It is just as if, friend, there were in the jungle-path a well, and neither rope nor drawer of water. And a man should come by foredone with heat, far gone with heat, weary, trembling, athirst. He should look down into the well. Verily in him would be the knowledge:—Water!—yet would he not be in a position to touch it." [32]

According to the *Aṅguttara-nikāya* (III, 355), the two methods—that of the "experimentalists" (the *jhāins*) and that of the "speculatives" (the *dhammayogas*)—are equally indispensable for obtaining arhatship. For the passions, the "impurities" (*kleśa*), are of two categories: "(1) *kleśas* of the intellect, 'views' [*dṛṣṭi*], 'errors,' aberration [*moha*]: belief in the 'I,' etc.; (2) *kleśas* of the emotions, which in our language are the 'passions'—that is, aversion and desire. To destroy 'errors' is not to destroy 'passions'; the fact that the ascetic has recognized the impermanent and harmful character of pleasant things does not prevent him from continuing to consider them pleasant and desiring them." [33] "Experience," then, is indispensable for salvation. But, on the other hand, the "experimental knowledge" given by the four *jhānas* and the *samāpattis* does not lead to *nirvāṇa* unless it is illuminated by "wisdom." Certain sources even hold that "wisdom" by itself can ensure gaining *nirvāṇa*, without any need for recourse to "yogic experiences." Harivarman, for example, believes that only "concentration" (*samādhi*) is necessary, to the exclusion of the other meditational exercises (*samāpatti*). There are arhats who have entered *nirvāṇa* without possessing any of the five *abhijñās* ("miraculous powers"), but no one has ever reached it without possessing the "knowledge of the disappearance of vices" (*āsravakṣaya*), which alone can confer sanctity. But Harivarman shows evidence of an antimystical, antiecstatic tendency,[34] which is also perceptible in other sources; ac-

32 *The Book of the Kindred Sayings*, tr. C. A. F. Rhys Davids and F. L. Woodward, II, 83. Cf. other texts in La Vallée Poussin, "Musīla et Nārada," pp. 191 ff.

33 La Vallée Poussin, "Musīla et Nārada," p. 193; cf. Lamotte, p. 213.

34 La Vallée Poussin, p. 206.

cording to the *abhidharma* doctrine, for example, the *prajñā-vimukta*, the "dry saint," he who is liberated by wisdom (*prajñā*), gains *nirvāṇa* in exactly the same way as does he who has had the experience of the *nirodhasamāpatti*.[35] It is easy to divine, in this defense of the "dry saint," a resistance, on the part of theologians and metaphysicians, to yogic excesses. We shall have occasion to return to this.

The "Miraculous Powers"

For the moment, let us note that the road to *nirvāṇa*—as, in classic Yoga, the road to *samādhi*—leads to the possession of "miraculous powers" (*siddhi*, Pāli *iddhi*). Now, for the Buddha (as, later, for Patañjali), this raised a new problem. On the one hand, the "powers" are inevitably acquired in the course of initiation, and, for that very reason, constitute valuable indications of the monk's spiritual progress; on the other hand, they are doubly dangerous, since they tempt the monk with a vain "magical mastery of the world" and, in addition, are likely to cause confusion in the minds of unbelievers. For the *iddhis* cannot be avoided; they, as it were, constitute the new experiential categories of the "mystical body" that the monk is engaged in creating for himself. The Buddhist monk, we must remember, like the Brāhmanizing or "heretical" yogin, must die to his earthly life in order to be reborn in an unconditioned state. Now, death to the profane condition is manifested, on the physiological, psychological, and spiritual planes, by a series of mystical experiences and magical powers, which announce nothing less than the adept's passage from the conditioned to freedom. The possession of the *iddhis* is not equivalent to deliverance; but these "miraculous powers" prove that the monk is in the process of deconditioning himself, that he has suspended the laws of nature, in whose cogs he was being crushed, condemned to suffer the karmic determinism forever. Consequently, the possession of *iddhis* is not harmful in itself; but the monk must be careful not to succumb to their temptation and, above all, must avoid exhibiting such

35 Ibid., p. 215.

powers before noninitiates. We shall soon see what reasons the Buddha found for forbidding the use and display of *siddhis*.

We remind the reader that the "miraculous powers" are one of the five classes of "superknowledges" (*abhijñā*), which are: (1) *siddhi*; (2) the divine eye (*divyacakśus*); (3) divine hearing (*divyaśrotra*); (4) knowledge of another's thought (*paracittajñāna*), and (5) recollection of previous existences (*pūrvanirvāsānusmṛti*). None of these five *abhijñās* (in Pāli, *abhiññā*) differs from the "powers" at the disposal of the non-Buddhist yogin.[36] Even the preliminaries of the meditation that makes it possible to obtain them are similar to those in non-Buddhist Yoga: mental purity, serenity, etc. "With his heart thus serene, made pure, translucent, cultured, devoid of evil, supple, ready to act, firm, and imperturbable, he applies and bends down his mind to the modes of the Wondrous Gift [*iddhi*]. He enjoys the Wondrous Gift in its various modes—being one he becomes many, or having become many becomes one again; he becomes visible or invisible; he goes, feeling no obstruction, to the further side of a wall or rampart or hill, as if through air; he penetrates up and down through solid ground, as if through water; he walks on water without breaking through, as if on solid ground; he travels cross-legged in the sky, like the birds on the wing; even the Moon and the Sun, so potent, so mighty though they be, does he touch and feel with his hand; he reaches in the body even up to the heaven of Brahmā. . . . With that clear Heavenly Ear surpassing the ear of men, he hears sounds both human and celestial, whether far or near. . . . Penetrating with his own heart the hearts of other beings, of other men, he knows them. . . . With his heart thus serene [etc.], he directs and bends down his mind to the knowledge of the memory of his previous temporary states."[37]

The same list of powers occurs in the *Akānkheya-sutta;* for each *iddhi*, a particular *jhāna* must be practiced. "If a priest [*bhikku*], O

36 See Note V, 5.

37 *Sāmaññaphala-sutta*, 87 ff. (*Dīgha-nikāya*, I, 78 ff.); tr. Rhys Davids (modified), I, 88–90.

priests, should frame a wish, as follows: 'Let me exercise the various magical powers,—let me being one become multiform, let me being multiform become one . . . and let me go with my body even up to the Brahma-world,' then must he be perfect in the precepts, bring his thoughts to a state of quiescence, practice diligently the trances, etc." [38] In this way, one gains clairaudience, divines what goes on in the heart of others, perceives previous existences, sees how beings pass from one state of existence to another, etc.

These lists of *siddhis* (= *iddhis*) are for the most part stereotyped, and they occur in all the ascetic and mystical literatures of India.[39] The yogins of the Buddha's time possessed such "mystical powers," and the Buddha did not question their genuineness any more than he doubted the genuineness of their yogic ecstasies. But the Buddha did not encourage his disciples to seek *siddhis*. The one true problem was deliverance, and the possession of "powers" entailed the danger that it might turn the monk away from his original goal, *nirvāṇa*. In reaction against contemporary excesses in mysticism and magic, the Buddha never failed to remind his hearers that the elements of the problem, together with its solution, were within man as man. "It is in this fathom-long carcase, friend, with its impressions and its ideas, that, I declare, lies the world, and the cause of the world, and the cessation of the world, and the course of action that leads to the cessation of the world." [40] For, if it was true that the monk must die to his profane condition in order that he might hope to attain the unconditioned, it was not less true that, if he let himself be tempted by the "miraculous powers," he ran the risk of fixing his abode in a higher mode of existence, the mode of gods and magicians—and of forgetting the final goal, integration of the Absolute. In addition, the possession of one or another "miraculous power" in no way furthered the propagation of the Buddhist message; other yogins and ecstatics

38 *Majjhima-nikāya*, I, 34 ff.; Warren, pp. 303–04.

39 See above, p. 85, the list preserved by Patañjali.

40 *Aṅguttara-nikāya*, II, 48; *Saṃyutta-nikāya*, I, 62; tr. C. A. F. Rhys Davids, I, 86.

could perform the same miracles. Even worse, one could obtain "powers" through magic, without undergoing any inner transformation. Nonbelievers could well suppose that what they witnessed was only the result of some magical charm. "Suppose that a [Buddhist] brother enjoys the possession, in various ways, of mystic power [*iddhi*]—from being one he becomes multiform, from being multiform he becomes one [etc.]. . . . And some believer, of trusting heart, should behold him doing so. Then that believer should announce the fact to an unbeliever. . . . Then that unbeliever should say to him: 'Well, Sir! there is a certain charm called the Gandhāra Charm. It is by the efficacy thereof that he performs all this.' . . . Well, Kevaddha! it is because I perceive danger in the practice of mystic wonders, that I loathe, and abhor, and am ashamed thereof." And if the Buddhist brother manifested the yogic power of divining the thoughts and feelings of others, etc., the unbeliever could say to him: " 'Sir! there is a charm called the Jewel Charm. It is by the efficacy thereof that he performs all this.' "[41] It is for this reason that the Buddha forbade the display of *siddhis:* "You are not, O *bhikkus*, to display before the laity the superhuman power of Iddhi. Whosoever does so shall be guilty of a *dukkata* [evil deed]."[42]

Knowledge of Previous Existences

Among the five (or six) superknowledges (*abhijñā*) a place is always given to the ability to remember one's former lives.[43] Like all the other *siddhis* and *abhijñās*, this mystical knowledge is also a part of the pan-Indian occult tradition: Patañjali lists it among the

41 *Kevaddha-sutta*, 4 ff. (*Dīgha-nikāya*, I, 212 ff.); tr. Rhys Davids, I, 277 f.

42 *Vinaya*, II, 112; *Vinaya Texts*, III, 81.

43 In other classifications this yogic prowess constitutes the first of the three sciences (*vidyā*) or the eighth of the "powers of wisdom" (*jñāna* or *prajñābala*). According to Buddhist scholasticism, the latter belong only to Buddhas, whereas the *abhijñās* and *vidyas* are attainable by others, too; cf. Paul Demiéville, "Sur la Mémoire des existences antérieures" (*Bulletin de l'École française d'Extrême-Orient*, XXVII [1927]), p. 283.

"perfections," [44] and the Buddha himself frequently admits that the *samaṇas* and Brāhmans are able to remember even a considerable number of their previous lives. "Some recluse [*samaṇa*] or Brāhman by means of ardor, of exertion, of application, of earnestness, of careful thought, reaches up to such rapture of heart that, rapt in heart, he calls to mind his various dwelling-places in times gone by—in one birth, or in two, or three, or four, or five, or ten, or twenty, or thirty, or forty, or fifty, or a hundred, or a thousand, or in several hundreds or thousands . . . of births—to the effect that 'There I had such and such a name, was of such and such a lineage and caste, lived on such and such food, experienced such and such pains and pleasures, had such and such a span of years. And when I fell from thence, I was reborn in such and such a place under such and such a name, in such and such a lineage. . . . And when I fell from thence, I was reborn here.' Thus does he recollect, in full detail both of condition and of custom, his various dwelling-places in times gone by. And he says to himself: 'Eternal is the soul; and the world, giving birth to nothing new, is steadfast as a mountain peak, as a pillar firmly fixed.' " [45]

But the Buddha refuses to accept the philosophical conclusions drawn by the *samaṇas* and Brāhmans from their remembrance of their former lives—the eternity of the Self and the world. More precisely, he declines to draw any conclusion from it: "Now of these, brethren, the Tathâgata knows that these speculations thus arrived at, thus insisted on, will have such and such a result, such and such an effect on the future condition of those who trust in them. That does he know, and *he knows also other things far beyond . . . and having that knowledge he is not puffed up*, and thus untarnished he has, in his own heart, realised the way of escape from them." [46] The Buddha's refusal to discourse on the metaphysical consequences that might be drawn from one or another supra-

44 *Yoga-sūtras*, III, 18.

45 *Dīgha-nikāya*, I, 13 ff.; tr. Rhys Davids, I, 27 f.; cf. also *Dīgha*, III, 108 ff.

46 Ibid., I, 16–17; tr. Rhys Davids, I, 29 (italics ours).

normal experience is a part of his teaching; he will not let himself be drawn into idle discussions of the ultimate reality. In the text just cited, the *samaṇas* and Brāhmans postulated the "eternity" of the world and the Self, because they had found the same world and the same Self a hundred thousand existences previously. Now, this was not a necessary conclusion, for the *samaṇas* and Brāhmans always recalled an *existence in time*—and the problem for the Buddha, the problem of Yoga, was precisely "emergence from time," entrance into the unconditioned; observations made within the infinite cycle of transmigrations provided no data for any deductions as to the "reality" whose beginning had been beyond the karmic cycle.

Like the *samaṇas* and Brāhmans, the Buddhist monks attempted to recollect their earlier lives. "With heart thus steadfast, clarified and purified . . . it was thus that I applied my heart to the knowledge which recalled my earlier existences. I called to mind my divers existences in the past,—a single birth, then two . . . [and so on, to] a hundred thousand births, many an aeon of disintegration of the world, many an aeon of its redintegration." [47] As we see, it is the same superknowledge, whether among the Buddhists or among the non-Buddhists. "In what does this knowledge consist? The texts do not tell us: they show how the heretics derive the notion of eternity from their knowledge of their former lives, but what conclusion the Buddhists draw from the same knowledge will not be stated until the *abhidharma* literature comes into existence. It seems, then, that in the early *sūtras* the memory of former existences is still conceived in the spirit of Yoga, simply as a form of supernatural knowledge." [48] From the *Mahāvibhāṣā* on, what a Buddhist monk can gain from this superknowledge is stated: it is disgust with impermanence. And the same opinion is held by Vasubandhu in his *Abhidharmakośa*.[49]

But it would seem that this late justification by Buddhist scho-

47 *Majjhima-nikāya*, I, 22 ff.; tr. Chalmers, *Further Dialogues*, I, 15. Cf. other texts, Demiéville, p. 284.

48 Demiéville, p. 292.

49 Ibid., pp. 292 ff.

lasticism is incorrect; it is, rather, proof of the triumph of the "speculatives" over the "experimentalists," of theory over yogic mysticism. As for the use to which the Buddha put knowledge of former lives, if we lack precise statements on the subject, the canonical texts afford allusions enough for us to orient ourselves. Thus, for a beginning, let us recall that the Buddha attached great importance to *memory* as such; the gods lose their divine condition and fall from their heavens when "their memory is troubled." [50] Even more: inability to remember *all* of one's former existences is equivalent to metaphysical ignorance. Buddha enlarges on the case of the gods who fall from their heavens because of their defective memories. Some, having become men, withdraw from the world, practice asceticism and meditation, and, by virtue of their yogic exercises, become able to remember their former existences, but not *all* of them,[51] in other words, they do not remember the *beginning* of their series of lives—and, because of this "forgetting," they have a false view of the eternity of the world and the gods. The Buddha, then, set a very high value on the ability to remember previous lives. This mystical ability made it possible to reach the "beginning of time"—which, as we shall see in a moment, implied "emerging from time."

Ānanda or other disciples "remembered their births" (*jātiṃ saranti*), were among the "rememberers of their births" (*jātis-sāra*). Coomaraswamy has shown [52] that the epithet *jātissaro* [53] suggests Agni's epithet, *Jātavedas*, for Agni too "knows all births" (*viśva veda janimā*) [54] and is the "All-knower" (*viśvavit*).[55] Vāmadeva, author of a famous Ṛg-Vedic hymn, said of himself: "Being now in the womb [*garbhe nu san*], I have known all the births of the gods." [56] "Thus spake Vāmadeva, lying in the

50 *Dīgha-nikāya*, I, 19.

51 Ibid.

52 "Recollection, Indian and Platonic," *Journal of the American Oriental Society* Supplement, III (Apr.–June, 1944), 1–18.

53 *Milinda Pañha*, 78, etc.

54 *Ṛg-Veda*, VI, 15, 13.

55 Ibid., III, 29, 7, etc.

56 Ibid., IV, 27, 1. According to the *Garbha Upaniṣad* (III, 4), memory of uterine life is lost at birth.

womb." [57] Kṛṣṇa "knows all his births." [58] Hence, for Brāhmanism as for the Buddha, *memory* (in short, *knowledge*) was a "divine" and most precious faculty; "he who knows," "he who recollects," proves that he is "concentrated"; distraction, forgetfulness, ignorance, "fall," are causally connected situations and modes of behavior.

The scholastic Buddhist texts give us some details of the technique employed. "It is the faculty that consists in retracing in memory the days, months, and years until one arrives at one's time in the womb and finally at one's past lives: one existence, ten, a hundred, a thousand, ten thousand, a *koṭi* of existences. The great arhats and the Pratyeka Buddhas can even remember back through 80,000 great *kalpas*. The great Bodhisattvas and the Buddhas remember an unlimited number of *kalpas*." [59] According to the *Abhidharmakośa* (VII, 123), "the ascetic who wants to remember his earlier lives begins by grasping the character of the thought that has just perished; from this thought he proceeds back, considering the immediately successive states of his present existence, to the thought of his conception. When he remembers a moment of thought in the intermediate existence [*antarābhava*], *abhijñā* is realized." [60]

The procedure, then, consists in starting from a particular moment, the nearest to the present moment, and traveling through time backward (*patiloman*, Skr. *pratiloman*, "against the fur"), in order to arrive *ad originem*, when the first life "burst" into the world, setting time in motion; thus one reaches the paradoxical moment beyond which time did not exist because nothing was yet manifested. The meaning and the end of this yogic technique, which consists in unrolling time in reverse, are perfectly clear. Through it the practitioner obtains the true superknowledge, for he not only succeeds in re-cognizing all his former lives, but he reaches the very "beginning of the world"; proceeding backward against the stream, one must necessarily come to the point of

57 *Aitareya Āraṇyaka*, II, 5.

58 *Bhagavad Gītā*, IV, 5.

59 Lamotte, p. 332.

60 Ibid., p. 332, n. 2.

departure, which, in the last analysis, coincides with the cosmogony, with the first cosmic manifestation. To relive one's past lives is equivalent to understanding them, and, in a certain measure, to "burning" one's "sins"—the sum, that is, of the acts performed under the domination of ignorance and transmitted from life to life by the law of *karma*. But there is something still more important: One arrives at the beginning of time and one finds nontime, the eternal present that preceded the temporal experience begun by the first fallen human life. In other words, one "touches" the non-conditioned state that preceded man's fall into time and the wheel of existences. This is as much as to say that, setting out from any moment of temporal duration, one can succeed in *exhausting* that duration by traveling through it in the reverse direction, and will finally reach nontime, eternity. But to do so was to transcend the human condition and enter *nirvāṇa*. This is what led the Buddha to declare that he alone had re-cognized all his former existences, whereas the arhats, while they knew a large number of their past lives, were far from knowing them all; as to the *samaṇas* and Brāhmans, they hastened, as we have seen, to formulate certain philosophical theories on the reality of the world and the Self, instead of penetrating deeper into the past and beholding the dissolution of all these "realities" (for the one true reality, the Absolute, could not be formulated in the language of the current philosophies).

It is easy to see the importance of this memory of former lives for the yogic technique whose aim was to emerge from time. But Buddha did not claim that this was the only means. According to him, it was perfectly possible to get beyond time—that is, to abolish the human condition—by taking advantage of the "favorable moment" (*kṣaṇa*), by obtaining "instantaneous illumination" (the *eka-kṣanābhisambodhi* of the Mahāyānist writers), which "broke time" and allowed "egress" from it by a rupture of planes.[61]

61 See Eliade, *Images and Symbols*, pp. 81 ff. The reader will certainly have noted the correspondence between the yogic technique for recollecting former lives and the psychoanalytical method of reconstituting and, through a corrected understanding, assimilating one's memories of earliest childhood.

The Paribbājakas

In the days of the Buddha there were countless groups of wandering ascetics, yogins, and "sophists." Some of these groups had existed from post-Vedic times.[62] It was a period of luxuriant spiritual vitality—together with monks and mystics, we find dialecticians, formidable magicians, and even "materialists" and nihilists, the forerunners of the Cārvākas and the Lokāyatas. About most of them we know little more than their names. Their doctrines receive fragmentary mention in the Buddhist and Jaina texts; but since both the Buddhists and the Jainists combated them, they are usually distorted and ridiculed. However, it is probable that among these monks and wandering ascetics (*paribbājaka*, Skr. *parivrājaka*) there were strong personalities, teachers of bold and revolutionary doctrines.

The Buddhist texts contain several lists of dialecticians and wandering ascetics contemporary with the Buddha; the best known is the one preserved in the *Sāmaññaphala-sutta*,[63] which summarizes the views of six famous *samaṇas*. Each is described as "head of a community" (*gaṇācariyo*), famous "founder of a sect" (*titthakāno*), respected as a saint (*sādhusammato*), venerated by many people, and advanced in age. Pūraṇa Kassapa seems to have preached the uselessness of action; Makkhali Gosāla, the head of the Ājīvikas, maintained a strict determinism, and we shall have occasion to return to him. Ajita Kesakambala professed a materialism very like that of the Cārvākas; Pakudha Kaccāyana, the pereniality of the seven "bodies"; Sañjaya Velaṭṭhaputta, an obscure agnosticism; and the Nigaṇṭha Nāṭaputta, probably skepticism. We find allusions to the doctrines of the "heretics" in other Buddhist texts, especially in the *Majjhima-nikāya* (I, 513 ff.), *Saṃyutta-nikāya* (III, 69), *Aṅguttara-nikāya* (III, 383 ff.); the last also gives a list of ten religious orders contemporary with the

62 See above, p. 138.

63 *Dīgha-nikāya*, I, 47 ff.

Buddha (III, 276–77), but we know almost nothing about their spiritual techniques.

In general, the majority of the "heretical" groups shared with the Buddha and Mahāvīra the same critical attitude toward the traditional values of Brāhmanism; they rejected the revealed character of the Vedas and the doctrine of sacrifice, as they did the metaphysical speculations of the Upaniṣads. In addition, some of them (Makkhali Gosāla, for example) showed an interest in the structures of organic life and the laws of nature—an interest unknown before this time.

A distinction might perhaps be made between the pure ascetics (*tāpasa*) and the dialecticians (*paribbājaka*); the latter did not practice any severe mortifications. The *Aṅguttara-nikāya* mentions two classes of *paribbājakas: aññatitthyia paribbājakas* and *brāmana paribbājakas;* the latter chiefly discussed *samdittika dhammā* (problems connected with material reality), while the former applied themselves to transcendental problems.

Buddha had several encounters with *paribbājakas* of these two classes. With one such, Poṭṭhapāda, he argued on the soul; with another, Nigrodha, on the value of the ascetic life; with a third, Ajita, on the "states of consciousness" (*pañcasatāni cittaṭṭhānāni*), etc. The texts that record these conversations emphasize the Buddha's answers rather than the doctrines and customs of the *paribbājakas.* At least we know that, although criticizing Brāhmanic institutions, they led lives of considerable austerity, and that they practiced *prāṇāyāma,* which once again proves the pan-Indian character of Yoga techniques.

From the allusions in the Pāli texts, we can sometimes identify certain specific mortifications. Thus, for example, in the *Kassapa-Sīhanāda-sutta,* Kassapa mentions ascetics who remain constantly standing, others who sleep on spikes, on a board, or on the ground, others who eat the dung of cows, etc. (probably in order to remain in permanent penitence, for the Hindus attribute a purifying power to these substances).[64] Each of these ascetics bears the name of the

64 *Dīgha-nikāya,* I, 167 ff.; tr. Rhys Davids, I, 231 ff.

particular mortification he practices. In this exacerbated penitence, we can recognize the same trend toward absolute asceticism that is still to be found in modern India. Probably the spiritual experience of the ascetics was extremely rudimentary, and the value they attributed to penitence was purely magical. We have no information as to their techniques, if they had any.

In the *Udumbarikā Sīhanāda Suttanta*, the Buddha reproaches the *paribbājakas* with being infatuated with their own asceticism, despising other men, believing that they have gained their end and boasting of it, having an exaggerated idea of their abilities, etc.[65] This text proves that severe asceticism was also sometimes practiced by wandering ascetics, though in general it is characteristic of "those of the forest" (*tāpasa*). The Buddha's opinion of the ascetics is made clear in the *Kassapa-Sīhanāda-sutta*, where he tells Kassapa that what characterizes the true *samaṇa* (recluse) or *brāhmaṇa* is not his outward appearance, his penitence, or his physical mortification, but inner discipline, charity, self-mastery, a mind emancipated from superstitions and automatisms, etc.[66]

Makkhali Gosāla and the Ājīvikas

Among the "heads of communities" and "founders of sects," Maskarin (Makkhali) Gosāla, the head of the Ājīvikas, stands out in somber majesty. A former disciple, and later the adversary, of Mahāvīra, he was regarded by the Buddha as his most dangerous rival. Attacked and vilified to the utmost by the Buddhists and Jainas, the practices and doctrines of the Ājīvikas are hard to reconstruct. The Ājīvika canon comprised a complex system of philosophy, but except for a few citations in books by its opponents, nothing of it has survived. Yet the Ājīvika movement had a long history; preceding Buddhism and Jainism by several generations, it did not disappear until the fourteenth century. Gosāla did not claim to have founded the Ājīvika order; according to a Jaina text,

65 Ibid., III, 43 ff.; tr. Rhys Davids, III, 39 ff.

66 Ibid., I, 169 ff.; tr. Rhys Davids, I, 234 ff.

the *Bhagavatī Sūtra*, he held that he was the twenty-fourth *tīrthaṇkara* of his epoch, and the names of some of his legendary predecessors have come down to us. The etymology of the word *ājīvika* remains obscure; A. F. R. Hoernle explains it by the root *ājīva*, "mode of life, or profession, of any particular class of people," [67] but it could equally well derive from the expression *ā jīvāt*, "as long as life," alluding to a fundamental doctrine of the sect, the necessity of passing through a vast number of existences before obtaining liberation.

What distinguished Gosāla from all his contemporaries was his rigorous fatalism. "Human effort is ineffective" (*n'atthi purisakāra*)—such was the essence of his message, and the cornerstone of his system is contained in a single word: *niyati*, "fatality," "destiny." According to the summary of his doctrine in the *Sāmaññaphala-sutta* (53), Gosāla believed that "there is . . . no cause, either ultimate or remote, for the depravity of beings; they become depraved without reason and without cause. There is no cause . . . for the rectitude of beings; they become pure without reason and without cause. . . . [There is no such thing as] one's own acts, or . . . the acts of another, or . . . human effort. There is no such thing as power or energy, or human strength or human vigor. All animals . . . creatures . . . beings . . . souls are without force and power and energy of their own. They are bent this way and that by their fate, by the necessary conditions of the class to which they belong, by their individual nature." [68] In other words, Gosāla was in revolt against the pan-Indian doctrine of *karma*. According to him, every being must pursue its cycle through 8,400,000 *mahākalpas*, at the end of which time liberation came spontaneously, without effort. To the Buddha, this implacable determinism was criminal; hence he attacked Makkhali Gosāla more often than he did any other of his contemporaries; he regarded the *niyati* doctrine as the most dangerous of all.

67 "Ājīvikas," *Encyclopaedia of Religion and Ethics*, ed. James Hastings, I, 259.

68 Tr. Rhys Davids, I, 71.

As the disciple and companion of Mahāvīra for several years, Gosāla practiced asceticism, obtained magical powers, became the head of the Ājīvikas. He was known as taciturn (*Saṃyutta-nikāya*, I, 66, says that he had "abandoned speech"), and the fragments of his biography preserved in Buddhist and Jaina texts seem to show that, like others, Gosāla was a powerful magician. He kills one of his disciples with his "magical fire." [69] And his death (probably between 485 and 484 B.C.) was the result of a curse pronounced on him by Mahāvīra after the two had engaged in a tournament of magic.

Initiation into the Ājīvika order had the archaic nature of initiations into traditional mystery societies. A reference in the commentary on the *Tittira Jātaka* (III, 536–43) [70] shows that the neophyte was obliged to burn his hands by holding a hot object. A passage in the commentary on the *Dhammapada* (II, 52) [71] reveals another initiatory rite; the candidate was buried up to the neck, and his hairs were pulled out one by one. The Ājīvikas went completely naked—a usage that antedated the appearance of Mahāvīra and Makkhali Gosāla. Like all ascetics, they begged their food and followed very strict rules of diet; many of them ended their lives by starving themselves to death.[72] Nevertheless, the Buddhists and Jainas cast doubt on their asceticism; the former accused them of worldliness,[73] the latter of unchastity. If we can believe Mahāvīra, Makkhali Gosāla held that it was not a sin for an ascetic to have intercourse with a woman.[74] These accusations very probably originated in polemics; on the other hand, it must not be forgotten that, in India, sexual practices have always been used both to gain magical powers and to conquer a state of bliss by force.

Nothing has come down to us regarding the Ājīvikas' spiritual techniques. It is true that Makkhali Gosāla holds an original posi-

69 A. L. Basham, *History and Doctrines of the Ājīvikas*, p. 60.

70 Ibid., p. 104.

71 Ibid., p. 106.

72 Ibid., pp. 127 ff.

73 Ibid., p. 123.

74 Hermann Jacobi, tr., *Gaina Sûtras* (Sacred Books of the East, XLV), p. 411; cf. other accusations of immorality, ibid., p. 245, 270 ff.

tion in the horizon of Indian thought. His deterministic conception led him to study natural phenomena and the laws of life; he proposed a classification of living beings in accordance with the number of their senses, and outlined a doctrine of the transformations in nature (*pariṇāmavāda*), based on accurate observations of the periodicity of vegetable life. But all this does not explain the Ājīvikas' popular success and their survival for two millenniums. The doctrine of *niyati* offered nothing to attract people in general. We must suppose that the sect had its own ascetic tradition and its own secrets for meditation, and that it was this esoteric heritage that accounted for its survival. The supposition is supported by references to a sort of *nirvāṇa*, comparable to the supreme heaven of other mystical schools (for *niyati* was not annulled).[75] In any case, about the tenth century the Ājīvikas, like the whole of India, adopted *bhakti* and ended by merging with the Pāñcarātras.[76]

Metaphysical Knowledge and Mystical Experience

Tension between the partisans of *knowledge* and the partisans of *yogic experience* can be traced throughout the history of Buddhism. Toward the beginning of our era, a third group entered the dispute —the partisans of *bhakti*. The attribution of soteriological value to faith in the Buddha (really in the *dhamma* revealed by the Buddha) is not entirely absent from the canonical texts. "All who have but faith in me and love for me, have heaven as their destiny." [77] For "faith is the seed . . . faith is in this world the best property for a man." [78] With time, and especially in response to the pressure of popular religious experiences, mystical devotion will become markedly important. The Boddhisattvas, the Amitābha, Avalokiteśvara, and Mañjuśrī Buddhas, the innumerable celestial Buddhas,

75 Basham, p. 261.

76 Ibid., pp. 280 ff. On the Ājīvikas, see Note V, 6; on the Pāñcarātras, Note IV, 5.

77 *Majjhima-nikāya*, I, 142; tr. Chalmers, I, 100.

78 *Sutta Nipāta*, 76, 181; tr. V. Fausbøll, pp. 12, 30.

are creations of *bhakti*. Buddhism is no exception to the general trend of Indian spirituality. The process will be facilitated by homologies between the several "bodies of the Buddha," by the growing importance of *mantras*, above all by the triumph of tantrism.[79]

For the moment, we shall confine our considerations to the tension between the "philosophers" and the "disciples of Yoga." Particularly interesting is Vasubandhu's vast encyclopedia, the *Abhidharmakośa*. It contains more than one unmistakable reference to the value of "ecstasy" in obtaining *nirvāṇa*.[80] But, even when he is discussing Yoga, Vasubandhu tries to rationalize mystical experiences, to interpret them in terms of the school; not that he denies the value of "yogic ecstasy," but, writing on the *abhidharma*, the "supreme *dharma*," he is determined to remain on the plane of "philosophy." For this kind of "supreme knowledge" is supposed to achieve the same result as yogic practice. The *abhidharma* set out to demonstrate the fluidity and, in the last analysis, the unreality of the external world and of all experience that partook of it; for "reality" so called was in fact only a succession of instantaneous and evanescent events. Now, for the "speculatives," clear, thorough, and pitiless analysis of "reality" was a means of salvation, for it destroyed the world by reducing its apparent solidity to a series of momentary appearances. Hence, he who understood the ontological unreality of the various "composite" universes—physical, vital, psychic, mental, metaphysical, and so on—at the same time entered the transcendental plane of the Absolute, the unconditioned and incomposite, and could attain deliverance.

Buddhaghoṣa's *Visuddhimagga*, "Way of Purity," the fullest and most learned treatise on meditation produced by Hīnayāna Buddhism (*c.* the middle of the fifth century of our era), shows the same orientation. The stages of meditation are classified, explained, justified by canonical texts, interpreted "rationally." Naturally, all the traditional motifs of Indian asceticism and medi-

79 See below, pp. 200 ff.

80 E.g., II, 43; VI, 43; VIII, 33, etc.

tation are present: lists of *siddhis,*[81] meditation on the impurities of the body,[82] the spiritual profit to be gained from oral description of the elements composing the human body,[83] transfiguration by fixing thought on the Buddha,[84] concentration on the rhythm of respiration,[85] and so on. But it is clear that Buddhaghoṣa's principal aim is to justify all these practices, to make them comprehensible, almost "logical." The last chapter of his long work is entitled "On the Advantages of Developing Understanding," and one section of it [86] is devoted to showing that ecstasy (*nirodha,* "arrest of states of consciousness") can be attained through the intellect alone.

In the other direction, we have the Yogācāra school, which flourished after the fifth century, and which reaffirms the necessity for the yogic experience; to destroy the phenomenal (i.e., the "profane") world and regain the unconditioned, it is easier to "withdraw to the center of oneself" through meditation and ecstasy than to undertake to annihilate the world through analysis! But the Yogācāras did not renounce philosophy; as a "philosophical school," they expounded their point of view with all the traditional scholastic armory.

All Buddhist monks who practiced Yoga used various objects to fix their attention. These were the *kasiṇas,* which functioned as supports for meditation and were known long before Buddhism.[87] There are several references to them in the *Visuddhimagga.*[88] These *kasiṇas* will play an extremely important role in tantrism. Any object, any phenomenon, can serve as a *kasiṇa:* the light coming

81 Ed. C. A. F. Rhys Davids, pp. 175 ff., especially pp. 373–406.

82 Ibid., p. 241.

83 Ibid., p. 243.

84 Ibid., p. 144.

85 Ibid., pp. 272 ff.

86 Ibid., pp. 703–09.

87 On *kasiṇas,* see C. A. F. Rhys Davids, ed., *A Buddhist Manual of Psychological Ethics* (*Dhammasangaṇi*), p. 43, n. 4; p. 47, n. 2; S. Z. Aung and C. A. F. Rhys Davids, eds., *The Compendium of Philosophy* (*Abidhammattha-saṇgaha*), p. 54; La Vallée Poussin, *Bouddhisme: Études et matériaux,* pp. 94 ff.

88 Cf. ed. C. A. F. Rhys Davids, pp. 118 ff.: the earth, p. 170; water, p. 172; colors, p. 173; light, p. 174, etc.

through the crack of door in a dark place, a jar of water, a lump of earth, etc. Through meditation, the practitioner obtains perfect coincidence between his thought and the object—that is, he unifies the mental flux by suspending every other psychic activity. This technique will later become popular both in Ceylon and Tibet.

We possess an extremely important, if obscure, text on the Buddhist Yoga centering upon *kasiṇas;* it is the book known as *The Yogāvacara's Manual of Indian Mysticism as Practised by Buddhists.*[89] The state of the text leaves much to be desired, thus increasing the difficulty of understanding it. The *Manual* is by an unknown author, but the date of its composition can be fixed as roughly between the sixteenth and seventeenth centuries. It is written in Pāli and Singhalese, and the suggestion has been made that its very late appearance might be connected with the arrival in Ceylon of Buddhist monks from Siam, summoned by King Vimala Dharma Surya (1684–1706) to rekindle the spiritual life of the Buddhist monasteries in the island.[90] As we have it, schematic and obscure, it is more a list of technical formulas than a manual properly speaking. The *yogāvacara* practitioner undoubtedly received oral instruction; the text was only a mnemonic aid. It is true that the majority of Indian texts on meditation have the same appearance of being schematic summaries and that the real technical initiation was transmitted and preserved orally; but the *Manual* is excessively hermetic. T. W. Rhys Davids and Caroline Rhys Davids have attempted to explain it as far as possible. The translator, Woodward, mentions a *bhikku,* Doratiyāveye, who was still living in Ceylon in 1900 and who had received the *yogāvacara* technique directly from his *guru.* He refused to practice it, for fear of attaining *nirvāṇa* at once; for, being a Boddhisattva, he still had many lives to live on earth. But he initiated one of his disciples into the practice, and the disciple went insane and died. Hence, according to Woodward, there is no one left alive in Ceylon who

89 Ed. T. W. Rhys Davids under the above title and tr. F. L. Woodward under the title *Manual of a Mystic.*

90 See Woodward, *Manual,* pp. 145 ff.

knows these practices, and the obscurities of the text remain insoluble. The structure of the *yogāvacara* technique is comprehensible, but unfortunately what would be of the greatest interest, precise details of the various meditations, remains unknown.

The chief peculiarity of the technique is a complicated meditation on the "elements." The ascetic seats himself in the yogic posture (*āsana*) and begins *prāṇāyāma* by concentrating on the phases of breathing—that is, by "understanding," by "entering into," each inhalation and exhalation. He then says: "With eye-consciousness I look down on the tip of my nose, with thought-consciousness fixed on the indrawal and the outbreathing, I fix my thought-form in my heart and prepare myself with the word *Arahan, Arahan.*" The Singhalese commentary adds: "When he has thus fixed his thought, alert and keen-minded, two images appear, first a dim, then a clear, one. When the dim image has faded away, and when the clear image, cleansed of all impurities, has entered his whole being, then, entering the threshold of the mind, the element of heat appears. In this, the Ecstasy has the color of the morning star, the Preamble is golden-colored, the Access is colored like the young sun rising in the East. Developing these three thought-forms, of the element of heat, withdrawing them from the tip of the nose, he should place them in the heart and then in the navel." [91]

Despite its seeming obscurity, the text is intelligible. The initiate must meditate, one after the other, on the "elements" fire, water, earth, air. Each meditation comprises, in addition to the preliminaries, three stages: entrance (access), preamble, and ecstasy. Each stage has its corresponding "color"—that is, the ascetic experiences the sensation of a particular light that at once verifies and stimulates his meditation. But he had obtained these "mental forms" by concentrating on the tip of his nose; he must now make them pass from this "center" to the centers corresponding to the heart and the navel. Having concluded the meditation on the element "heat" (*tejodhātu*), he undertakes the meditation on the element "water," more precisely, on cohesion (*apodhātu*, for

91 Ibid., p. 8.

the essential virtue of water is cohesion). The preliminaries to the meditation proper are exactly the same. The "colors" experienced through this meditation on the element "water" are: the color of the full moon for the ecstasy, the color of the lotus for the preamble, the color of a yellow flower for the entrance. In the following meditation, on the *vāyodhātu* (the element "air," expressing mobility), the color of the ecstasy is that of the noonday sun; the color of the preamble, orange; that of the entrance, indigo. And so on. In each meditation the "colors" thus obtained by concentration on the tip of the nose must be put in the two "centers" mentioned above. Each meditation has its corresponding "rapture": meditation on the *tejodhātu*, "momentary rapture" (*khanikā-pīti*); meditation on the *apodhātu*, "flooding rapture" (*okkantika-pīti*); meditation on the *vāyodhātu*, "transporting rapture" (*ubbega-pīti*), etc.

After successively accomplishing the meditations on the elements, the initiate attempts the meditation on the four elements together, then in the reverse order, etc. The *Manual* contains whole series of meditations—on respiration,[92] on happiness, on the five *jhānas*, on repulsive things, on the *kasiṇa*, on the parts of the body, on the four higher states (*brahmavihara*), on the ten forms of knowledge, etc. Each of these meditations is, in turn, divided into several stages, and each stage is related to a color or employs a color belonging to the meditations on the elements.

What distinguishes the *Manual* is the preponderant importance given to chromatic sensations; each meditation is accomplished and verified by the initiate's obtaining a color.[93] In addition, he continues to work on his chromatic sensations themselves; he removes them a hand's-breadth from his body, then a league, and even "as far as Mount Meru"; he fixes them in particular "centers," etc. The role that the *Manual* attributes to the "centers" leads us to

92 Disciplining the respiratory rhythm "was held by our Blessed Lord to be the chief aim of meditation," the Singhalese commentator writes (Woodward, p. 67).

93 "Colors" and "lights" play a significant part in some tantric meditational experiences.

suspect some tantric influence, although erotic elements are completely absent; mystical physiology is reduced to the "centers" and to visual experiences (auditory experiences play a much smaller part). However this may be, the "experimental" nature of these meditations is obvious; here dogmas and truths are subjects of experiments, they are "entered into," they create concrete "states." The mind's cry for "happiness" [94] is the leitmotiv. Even "grace" plays a part; at the beginning of each meditation, the ascetic invokes the Buddha, casts himself on his grace; the *guru* (*bhante*) is also invoked, etc.

T. W. Rhys Davids noted that the *Manual* contained 1344 meditations (112 mental states each exercised in twelve different ways and creating an equal number of "experiences"). The position of the body changes with each meditation—which excludes the possibility of a hypnotic trance. In some meditations eight pieces of wood are stuck to a candle at intervals of an inch. Each stage of the meditation continues during the time that it takes for one section of the candle to be consumed. When the flame touches the wood, the wood falls, the noise rouses the ascetic from his meditation, forcing him to change his position. These constant changes are probably intended to avoid possible hypnotic sleep, or the prolongation of one stage of meditation to the detriment of another. In any case, they offer the monk a permanent method of verification and greatly aid him in preserving his lucidity.

An interesting detail of mystical technique is what we might call "creation of the milieu necessary for meditation"—that is, the concrete value acquired by the image of the *kasiṇa* (*uggahanimitta*). The ascetic projects its image before him with such force that he can meditate on it as if he were in the presence of the real object that it signifies. Such exercises in meditation "without an object" (*nirmitta*) are frequently employed in almost all types of Indian mysticism.

This too-brief summary of some forms of yogic meditation in late Buddhism will help us to understand the immense success of

94 E.g., Woodward, p. 96, etc.

tantrism. For the importance that they accord to concrete supports for meditation (*kasiṇa*), to the "elements" and their "images," to the "centers" and "colors," etc., is of value to our study in more than one respect. In the first place, it expresses the effort made to anchor all meditational experiences in the concrete. Concentration is rendered possible by intensively reducing consciousness of the reality of the world; but this does not make the fragment isolated for concentration any the less *real*, and it is "assimilated" as such, more particularly in so far as it concentrates and, to a certain degree, represents the reality of the whole world. It is true that the function of these external supports always remains secondary, that the experience takes place within consciousness itself. But in India, to work on one's consciousness is not to isolate oneself from the real, nor to lose oneself in dreams and hallucinations; on the contrary, it is to make direct contact with life, to force one's way into the concrete. To meditate is to rise to planes of reality inaccessible to the profane.

During the first centuries of our era, all "contacts" with the Buddha are homologized; whether one assimilates the Awakened One's message—that is, his "theoretical body" (the *dharma*)—or his "physical body," present in the *stūpas*, or his "architectonic body," symbolized in temples, or his "oral body," actualized by certain formulas—each of these paths is valid, for each leads to transcending the plane of the profane. The "philosophers" who "relativized" and destroyed the immediate "reality" of the world, no less than the "mystics" who sought to transcend it by a paradoxical leap beyond time and experience, contributed equally toward homologizing the most difficult paths (gnosis, asceticism, Yoga) with the easiest (pilgrimages prayers, *mantras*). For in this "composite" and conditioned world, one thing is as good as another; the unconditioned, the Absolute, *nirvāṇa*, is as distant from perfect wisdom and the strictest asceticism as it is from repetition of the Blessed One's name, or homage to his relics, or the recitation of a *mantra*. All these procedures, and many more, are only means of approaching the inaccessible, the transcendent, the inexpressible.

Strictly speaking, this evolution of Buddhist thought is not too discordant with the spirit of the Enlightened One's message. The Buddha had refused to discuss the Absolute. He had contented himself with pointing out the way to reach it, and that way necessarily led through *dying to the profane condition;* the unconditioned was beyond experience—that is, in the last analysis, beyond unregenerate life. The "path" was equivalent to an initiation—death and mystical resurrection, rebirth to another mode of being. One could, then, try to *die to the profane world* by taking any "sector" of it as starting point. He, that is, who, circumambulating a temple, realized that he was entering a transphysical universe sanctified by the symbolism of the Buddha, annihilated profane experience as successfully as did a monk who "withdrew into himself" by means of the *jhānas* and *samāpattis,* or as did a philosopher who realized the unreality of the world through logical demonstration. In all these cases, the seeker renounced *this world,* transcended profane experiences, already participated in a transhuman mode of existence. It was not yet *nirvāṇa,* the unconditioned—but it was a spiritual exercise teaching how to "emerge from the world," it was a step forward in the long process of Buddhist initiation, which, like all initiations, killed the neophyte in order to resuscitate him to another mode of being.

Now, in the course of time, methods of transcending the profane condition multiplied and tended to become "easy"—that is, within everyone's reach. This explains the overwhelming success of tantrism. But its success had, in turn, been prepared by the pressure of laymen within the Buddhist community and by the invasion of various forms of popular spirituality into both Hinduism and Buddhism. Moreover, all this had been foreseen in Buddhist tradition—which, here as elsewhere, carried on the traditions of Brāhmanism. Buddhism knew that it "would degenerate," that the world would become increasingly dense, obscure, sinful, and that the "way of the Buddha" would become unrealizable; this was only the pan-Indian doctrine of cosmic cycles and of hastened degeneration in the last *yuga.* Hence it is that tantrism finally imposed itself as pre-eminently the message of the *kali-yuga.*

Yoga and Tantrism *

Approximations

IT IS not easy to define tantrism. Among the many meanings of the word *tantra* (root *tan*, "extend," "continue," "multiply"), one concerns us particularly—that of "succession," "unfolding," "continuous process." *Tantra* would be "what extends knowledge" (*tanyate, vistāryate, jñānam anena iti tantram*). In this acceptation, the term was already applied to certain philosophical systems.[1] We do not know why and under what circumstances it came to designate a great philosophical and religious movement, which, appearing as early as the fourth century of our era, assumed the form of a pan-Indian vogue from the sixth century onward. For it was really a vogue; quite suddenly, tantrism becomes immensely popular, not only among philosophers and theologians, but also among the active practitioners of the religious life (ascetics, yogins, etc.), and its prestige also reaches the "popular" strata. In a comparatively short time, Indian philosophy, mysticism, ritual, ethics, iconography, and even literature are influenced by tantrism. It is a pan-Indian movement, for it is assimilated by all the great Indian religions and by all the "sectarian" schools. There is a Buddhist tantrism and a Hindu tantrism, both of considerable proportions. But Jainism too accepts certain tantric methods (never those of the "left hand"), and strong tantric influences can be seen in Kashmirian

1 *Nyāya-tantreṣu*, etc.

Śivaism, in the great Pāñcarātra movement (*c.* 550), in the *Bhāgavata Purāṇa* (*c.* 600), and in other Viṣṇuist devotional trends.

According to Buddhist tradition, tantrism was introduced by Asaṇga (*c.* 400), the eminent Yogācāra master, and by Nāgārjuna (second century A.D.), the brilliant representative of the Mādhyamika and one of the most famous and mysterious figures in medieval Buddhism. But the problem of the historical origins of Buddhist tantrism is still far from being solved.[2] There is reason to suppose that the Vajrayāna ("Diamond Vehicle"), the name under which Buddhist tantrism is generally known, appeared at the beginning of the fourth century and reached its apogee in the eighth. The *Guhyasamāja-tantra*, which some scholars attribute to Asaṇga, is probably the earliest Vajrayānic text and certainly the most important.

In principle, the Buddhist tantras are divided into four classes: *kriya-tantras*, *caryā-tantras*, *yoga-tantras*, and *anuttara-tantras*, the first two being concerned with rituals and the others with yogic procedures for attaining supreme truth. In fact, however, nearly all tantric texts include ritual matter as well as yogic instruction and passages of philosophy. According to Tibetan tradition, the four classes of tantras are related to the principal human types and temperaments: the *kriya-tantra* texts are suitable for Brāhmans and, in general, for all those whose cast of mind is ritualistic; the *caryā-tantras* are for businessmen, and so on.

It is noteworthy that tantrism developed in the two border regions of India—in the Northwest, along the Afghan frontier, in western Bengal, and especially in Assam. On the other hand, according to Tibetan tradition, Nāgārjuna was a native of Andhra, in southern India—that is, in the heart of the Dravidian region. From all this we may conclude that, especially at first, tantrism developed in provinces that had been but little Hinduized, where the spiritual counteroffensive of the aboriginal inhabitants was in full force. For the fact is that tantrism served as the vehicle by

2 See the summary of progress in Note VI, 1.

which a large number of foreign and exotic elements made their way into Hinduism; it is full of names and myths of peripheral divinities (Assamese, Burmese, Himālayan, Tibetan, to say nothing of the Dravidian gods), and exotic rites and beliefs are clearly discernible in it. In this respect, tantrism continues and intensifies the process of Hinduization that began in the post-Vedic period. But this time the assimilation extends not to aboriginal Indian elements alone, but also to elements outside of India proper; the "tantric country" par excellence is Kāmarūpa, Assam. We must also reckon with possible Gnostic influences, which could have reached India by way of Iran over the Northwest frontier. For more than one curious parallel can be noted between tantrism and the great Western mysterio-sophic current that, at the beginning of the Christian era, arose from the confluence of Gnosticism, Hermetism, Greco-Egyptian alchemy, and the traditions of the Mysteries.

Since our chief concern is with the application of yogic disciplines to tantric *sādhana* ("realization"), we are obliged to neglect certain important aspects of tantrism. Let us note, however, that, for the first time in the spiritual history of Āryan India, the Great Goddess acquires a predominant position. Early in the second century of our era, two feminine divinities made their way into Buddhism: Prajñāpāramitā, a "creation" of the metaphysicians and ascetics, an incarnation of Supreme Wisdom, and Tārā, the epiphany of the Great Goddess of aboriginal India. In Hinduism the Śakti, the "cosmic force," is raised to the rank of a Divine Mother who sustains not only the universe and all its beings but also the many and various manifestations of the gods. Here we recognize the "religion of the Mother" that in ancient times reigned over an immense Aegeo-Afrasiatic territory and which was always the chief form of devotion among the autochthonous peoples of India. In this sense, the irresistible tantric advance also implies a new victory for the pre-Āryan popular strata.

But we also recognize a sort of religious rediscovery of the mystery of woman, for, as we shall see later, every woman becomes the incarnation of the Śakti. Mystical emotion in the presence of the mystery of generation and fecundity—such it is in part. But it is also recognition of all that is remote, "transcendent," invulnerable in woman; and thus woman comes to symbolize the irreducibility of the sacred and the divine, the inapprehensible essence of the ultimate reality. Woman incarnates both the mystery of creation and the mystery of Being, of everything that *is*, that incomprehensibly becomes and dies and is reborn. The schema of the Sāṃkhya philosophy is prolonged on both the metaphysical and the mythological planes: Spirit, the "male," *puruṣa*, is the "great impotent one," the motionless, the contemplative; it is Prakṛti that works, engenders, nourishes. When a great danger threatens the foundations of the cosmos, the gods appeal to the Śakti to avert it. A well-known myth thus accounts for the birth of the Great Goddess. A monstrous demon, Mahiṣa, threatened the universe and even the existence of the gods. Brahmā and the whole pantheon appealed to Viṣṇu and Śiva for help. Swollen with rage, all the gods put forth their energies in the form of fire darting from their mouths. The flames joined into a fiery cloud, which finally took the form of a goddess with eighteen arms. And it was this goddess, Śakti, who succeeded in crushing the monster Mahiṣa and thus saved the world. As Heinrich Zimmer remarks, the gods "had returned their energies to the primeval Shakti, the One Force, the fountain head, whence originally all had stemmed. And the result was now a great renewal of the original state of universal potency." [3]

We must never lose sight of this primacy of the Śakti—in the last analysis, of the Divine Woman and Mother—in tantrism and in all the movements deriving from it. It is through this channel that the great underground current of autochthonous and popular spirituality made its way into Hinduism. Philosophically, the rediscovery of the Goddess is bound up with the carnal condition of Spirit in the *kali-yuga*. Thus the tantric writers present the doctrine

3 *Myths and Symbols in Indian Art and Civilization*, ed. Joseph Campbell, p. 191.

as a new revelation of timeless truth, addressed to the man of this "dark age" in which the spirit is deeply veiled under the flesh. The doctors of Hindu tantrism regarded the Vedas and the Brāhmanic tradition as inadequate for "modern times." Man, they held, no longer possessed the spiritual spontaneity and vigor that he enjoyed at the beginning of the cycle; he was incapable of direct access to truth; [4] he must, then, "stem the current," and, to do so, he must set out from the basic and typical experiences of his fallen condition—that is, from the very sources of his life. This is why the "living rite" plays such a decisive role in tantric *sādhana;* this is why the "heart" and "sexuality" serve as vehicles for attaining transcendence.

For the Buddhists the Vajrayāna similarly constituted a new revelation of the Buddha's doctrine, a revelation adapted to the greatly diminished possibilities of "modern man." The *Kālacakra-tantra* tells how King Sucandra went to the Buddha and asked him for the Yoga that could save the men of the *kali-yuga.* In answer, the Buddha revealed to him that the cosmos is contained in man's own body, explained the importance of sexuality, and taught him to control the temporal rhythms by disciplining respiration—thus he could escape from the domination of time. The flesh, the living cosmos, and time are the three fundamental elements of tantric *sādhana.*

From this follows a first characteristic of tantrism—its antiascetic and, in general, antispeculative attitude. "Donkeys and other animals wander about naked, too. Does that make them yogins?" [5] Since the body represents the cosmos and all the gods, since liberation can be gained only by setting out from the body, it is important to have a body that is healthy and strong.[6] In some tantric schools, contempt for asceticism and speculation is accompanied by complete rejection of all meditation; liberation is pure spontaneity. Saraha writes: "The childish Yogins like the Tīrthikas and others

4 *Mahānirvāṇa-tantra,* I, 20–29, 37–50.

5 *Kulārṇava-tantra,* V, 48.

6 See below, p. 227.

can never find out their own nature. . . . One has no need of Tantra or Mantra, or of the images or the Dhāraṇīs—all these are causes of confusion. In vain does one try to attain Mokṣa by meditation. . . . All are hypnotised by the system of the *jhānas* (meditation), but none cares to realise his own self." [7] Again, another Sahajīyā author, Lui-pā, writes: "What use is meditation? Despite meditation, one dies in pain. Give up all complicated practices and the hope of obtaining *siddhis*, and accept the void [*śūnya*] as your true nature."

Viewed from outside, then, tantrism would seem to be an "easy road," leading to freedom pleasantly and almost without impediments. For, as we shall presently see, the *vāmacārīs* expect to attain identification with Śiva and Śakti through ritual indulgence in wine, meat, and sexual union. The *Kulārṇava-tantra* (VIII, 107 ff.) even insists that union with God can be obtained only through sexual union. And the famous *Guhyasamāja-tantra* categorically affirms: "No one succeeds in attaining perfection by employing difficult and vexing operations; but perfection can be gained by satisfying all one's desires." [8] The same text adds that sensuality is permitted (one may, for example, eat any kind of meat, including human flesh),[9] that the tantrist may kill any kind of animal, may lie, steal, commit adultery, etc.[10] Let us not forget that the aim of the *Guhyasamāja-tantra* is rapid arrival at Buddhahood! And when the Buddha reveals this strange truth to the countless assembly of the Bodhisattvas, and they protest, he points out that what he is teaching them is nothing but the *bodhisattvacaryā*, the "conduct of a Bodhisattva." For, he adds,[11] "the conduct of the passions and attachments [*rāgacaryā*] is the same as the conduct of a Bodhisattva [*bodhisattvacaryā*], that being the best conduct [*agracaryā*]." In other words: all contraries are illusory, extreme evil coincides with extreme good. Buddhahood can—within the

7 Dasgupta, *Obscure Religious Cults*, pp. 64–65.

8 Ed. B. Bhattacharyya, p. 27.

9 Ibid., p. 26, etc.

10 Ibid., pp. 20, 98, 120 ff.

11 Ibid., p. 37.

limits of this sea of appearances—coincide with supreme immorality; and all for the very good reason that only the universal void *is*, everything else being without ontological reality. Whoever understands this truth (which is more especially the truth of the Mādhyamika Buddhists, but to which other schools subscribe, at least in part) is saved—that is, becomes a Buddha.

But the "easiness" of the tantric path is more apparent than real. Certainly, the metaphysical ambiguity of the *śūnya* encouraged and, in sum, justified many excesses among the *vāmacārīs* (for example, the "tantric orgies"). But aberrant interpretations of dogma appear in the history of all mystical cults. The fact is that the tantric road presupposes a long and difficult *sādhana*, which at times suggests the difficulties of the alchemical *opus*. To return to the text just quoted, the "void" (*śūnya*) is not simply a "non-being"; it is more like the *brahman* of the Vedānta, it is of an adamantine essence, for which reason it is called *vajra* (= diamond). "*Śūnyatā*, which is firm, substantial, indivisible and impenetrable, proof against fire and imperishable, is called *vajra*." [12] Now, the ideal of the Buddhist tantrika is to transform himself into a "being of diamond"—in which, on the one hand, he is at one with the ideal of the Indian alchemist, and, on the other, renews the famous Upaniṣadic equation *ātman* = *brahman*. For tantric metaphysics, both Hindu and Buddhist, the absolute reality, the *Urgrund*, contains in itself all dualities and polarities, but reunited, reintegrated, in a state of absolute Unity (*advaya*). The creation, and the becoming that arose from it, represent the shattering of the primordial Unity and the separation of the two principles (Śiva-Śakti, etc.); in consequence, man experiences a state of duality (object-subject, etc.)—and this is suffering, illusion, "bondage." The purpose of tantric *sādhana* is the reunion of the two polar principles within the disciple's own body. "Revealed" for the use of the *kali-yuga*, tantrism is above all a practice, an act, a realization (= *sādhana*). But although the revelation is addressed to all, the tantric path includes an initiation that can be performed only by

12 *Advayavajra-saṃgraha*, ed. H. Shāstri, p. 37.

a *guru;* hence the importance of the master, who alone can communicate the secret, esoteric doctrine, transmitting it "from mouth to ear." Here, too, tantrism shows striking similarities to the antique Mysteries and the various forms of Gnosticism.

Iconography, Visualization, Nyāsa, Mudrās

In tantric *sādhana,* iconography plays a role that, though of the greatest importance, is difficult to define in a few words. To be sure, divine images are "supports" for meditation, but not in exactly the sense of the Buddhist *kasiṇas.*[13] Tantric iconography represents a "religious" universe that must be entered and assimilated. This "entrance" and "assimilation" are to be understood in the direct meaning of the terms: in meditating on an icon, one must first "transport" oneself to the cosmic plane ruled by the respective divinity, and then assimilate it, incorporate into oneself the sacred force by which the particular plane is "sustained" or, as it were, "created." This spiritual exercise comprises emerging from one's own mental universe and entering the various universes governed by the divinities. Certainly, even such a preliminary exercise, the first step toward the interiorization of iconography, cannot be performed without yogic discipline, without *dhārāṇa* and *dhyāna.* Nevertheless, to understand the meaning of an icon, to extract its symbolism, is not yet tantric *sādhana.* The complete operation includes several stages, the first of which is to "visualize" a divine image, to construct it mentally or, more precisely, to project it on a sort of inner screen through an act of creative imagination. There is no question here of the anarchy and inconsistency of what, on the level of profane experience, is called "imagination"; no question of abandoning oneself to a pure spontaneity and passively receiving the content of what, in the language of Western psychology, we should term the individual or collective unconscious; it is a question of awakening one's inner forces, yet at the same time maintaining perfect lucidity and self-control.

13 See above, p. 193.

Yoga practice makes it possible for the *sādhaka* to undertake such exercises. The traditional iconographic canon must be respected—that is, the aspirant must visualize what has been "seen" and prescribed and codified by the masters, not what his personal imagination might project. When a tantric text describes the way to construct a mental image of a divinity, we seem to be reading a treatise on iconography. A passage from the *Satantra-tantra*, cited by Kṛṣṇānanda in his *Tantrasāra*,[14] expounds the visualization of Durgā. The goddess is like a black mountain, her face is terrifying, she is embraced by Śiva and wears several wreaths of skulls around her neck; her hair hangs loose and she is smiling. Not a single detail is omitted—neither the snake (*nāga*) that serves her as sacred thread, nor the moon on her forehead, the thousands of dead hands about her hips, the bleeding mouth and bloodstained body, the two infant corpses in place of earrings, etc.

The visualization of a divine image is followed by a more difficult exercise—identification with the divinity it represents. A tantric proverb says that "one cannot venerate a god unless one is a god oneself" (*nadevo devam arcayet*). To identify oneself with a divinity, to become a god oneself, is equivalent to awakening the divine forces that lie asleep in man. This is no purely mental exercise. Nor, by the same token, is the final goal sought through visualization manifested in terms of mental experience, even though, in sum, the goal is a Mahāyānic dogma—the discovery of the universal void, of the ontological unreality of the universe and its "gods." But in tantric Buddhism, to *realize* the *śūnya* for oneself is no longer an intellectual operation; it is not the communication of an "idea," it is *experiencing* "truth."

We present a tantric *sādhana* for the visualization of the goddess Candamahāroṣaṇa. The disciple begins by imagining that his own heart contains a solar *maṇḍala* (red in color), resting on an eight-petaled lotus; from the center of the *maṇḍala* rises the syllable *hum*, in black. From this syllable countless rays of light traverse

14 The text is given by Rāmaprasād Chanda, *The Indo-Āryan Races*, pt. 1, p. 137.

immense spaces, and on the rays are the *guru*, all the Buddhas, the Bodhisattvas, and the goddess Candamahāroṣaṇa. After having honored them and confessed his sins, after seeking refuge in the threefold Buddhist truth, etc., the disciple offers himself to redeem the crimes of others and vows to attain supreme illumination. He then meditates on the four virtues, becomes conscious that "this world is without a self of its own, without subject, without object," and meditates on absolute emptiness, repeating the formula: "My adamantine essence is knowledge of the void." Then he imagines the syllable *hum* resting on the pommel of a sword arising from the first black syllable *hum*. The beams radiating from this second syllable draw all the Buddhas and cause them to enter it. The disciple meditates on Candamahāroṣaṇa, visualizing her as having emerged from this second syllable *hum*. Then, in the heart of the goddess, he imagines a sword bearing the syllable *hum*, and in the center of this third syllable he visualizes another Candamahāroṣaṇa seated on a syllable *hum*, etc. Thus he arrives at identification with the goddess.[15]

The void is realized by creating a cascade of universes; the disciple creates them, using a graphic sign as starting point, peoples them with gods, then destroys them. These cosmogonies and theogonies succeed one another in his own heart; it is in images that he discovers universal emptiness. Similar exercises occur in medieval Jaina Gnosticism, for Jainist *dhyāna* was also influenced by tantrism. Sakalakīrti (fifteenth century) recommends the following meditation in his *Tattvārthasāradīpikā:* the yogin should imagine a vast sea of milk, calm and waveless, and in the midst of the sea a lotus as vast as Jambudvīpa (India), with a thousand petals and bright as gold. He should imagine himself sitting on a throne in the center of its pericarp—serene, without desires or hate, ready to conquer his enemy, *karma*. This is the first *dhāraṇā*. The yogin should then imagine a shining sixteen-petaled lotus as existing in his navel. On its petals are inscribed the four vowels,

15 *Sādhanamālā*, ed. B. Bhattacharyya, I, 173 ff. On tantric iconography, see Note VI, 2.

with *aṃ* and *aḥ*, and the great *mantra arhan* shines in the center of its pericarp. Then he should imagine a mass of smoke rising from the letter *r* of the word *arhan*, then sparks, then finally flame will dart out and spread farther and farther until it has completely burned the lotus of the heart, which is the product of the eight *karmas* and hence has eight petals. This exercise forms part of the second meditation, called *āgneyi dhāraṇā*. Next comes the *mārūti dhāraṇā*, during which the yogin visualizes a violent storm scattering the ashes of the lotus. Then he imagines rain falling and washing away the ashes that cover his body (this is the fourth *dhāraṇā*, *vāruṇī*). Finally, he should imagine himself identified with the God, freed from the seven elements, seated on his throne, shining like the moon, and worshiped by the gods.[16]

The *Tattvārthasāradīpikā* also contains instructions for the various *dhyānas*, in connection with a mental liturgy that is tantric in structure. The aspirant imagines lotuses as existing in certain parts of his body, with different numbers of petals, each inscribed with a letter or mystical syllable. The Jaina *sādhaka* also makes use of *mantras*, which he murmurs while visualizing them as inscribed on the lotus of his body.[17] But the practices of tantric Yoga are also attested much earlier in Jaina literature. Śubhadra's *Jñānārṇava* (*c.* A.D. 800) includes several chapters on Yoga, as well as long discussions of *āsana*, *prāṇāyāma*, *maṇḍala*, and the four *dhyānas* and *dhāraṇās* that we have just summarized after the *Tattvārthasāradīpikā*. Like Buddhism and Hinduism, Jainism had its wave of enthusiasm for tantrism, though without the latter's implications of sexual mysticism; however, it shows a greater interest in the ascetic techniques and *siddhis* that were part of the most archaic Indian tradition, which Jainism took over.[18]

In connection with tantric iconography, mention must be made of *nyāsa*, the "ritual projection" of divinities into various parts of the body, a practice of considerable antiquity but one that tantrism

16 R. G. Bhāndārkar, *Report on the Search for Sanskrit Manuscripts*, pp. 110 ff.

17 Ibid., pp. 111–12.

18 See Note VI, 3.

revalorized and enriched. The disciple "projects" the divinities, at the same time touching various areas of his body; in other words, he homologizes his body with the tantric pantheon, in order to awaken the sacred forces asleep in the flesh itself. Several kinds of *nyāsas* are distinguished, according to their degree of interiorization,[19] for in some cases the divinities and their symbols are "put" into the various organs of the body by a pure act of meditation. The brief treatise entitled *Hastapūjāvidhi* [20] recommends, for example, a meditation in which the fingers of the left hand are identified with the five cosmic elements and the five tutelary divinities, while at the same time five mystical syllables, "colored white, yellow, red, black, and green respectively," are "imposed" on the fingernails; the syllables represent the five Tathāgatas: Vairocana, Amitābha, Akṣobhyā, Ratnasambhava, and Amoghasiddhi.

Dependent to some extent upon iconography—for they originally imitated the postures and gestures of the Buddhas—are the *mudrās*, a word that has a great many meanings (seal, gesture, finger posture, etc.), one of them erotic.[21] In the tantric liturgy, *mudrā* is susceptible of several interpretations, the most frequent being the realization of certain states of consciousness by hieratic gestures and postures, more precisely by the echo aroused in the deepest strata of the human being upon his rediscovering the "message" hidden in every archetypal gesture. For Haṭha Yoga, *bandha* or *mudrā* designates a position of the body in which the disciple practices *prāṇāyāma* and concentration in order to "immobilize" the *semen virile*.[22] But we should always bear in mind that

19 See, for example, *Mahānirvāṇa-tantra*, II, 40, etc.

20 Ed. and tr. L. Finot, "Manuscrits sanskrits de Sādhana's retrouvés en Chine," *Journal asiatique*, CCXXV (1934), 54–56, 69–71.

21 See below, p. 408.

22 On the *mūlabandha*, see *Haṭhayogapradīpikā*, III, 61–63; *Gheraṇḍa Saṃhitā*, III, 14–17; *Śiva Saṃhitā*, IV, 64–66; on the *mahābandha*, see *Śiva Saṃhitā*, IV, 37–42; *Haṭhayogapradīpikā*, III, 19–21; *Gheraṇḍa Saṃhitā*, III, 18–20; on *mudrās*, see ch. III of the *Gheraṇḍa Saṃhitā;* on one of the most important, the *śakticālanā-mudrā*, see *Haṭhayogapradīpikā*, III, 114–18. *Śiva Saṃhitā*, IV, 22 ff., list of *mudrās* and description of the most important ones. Cf. also Alain Daniélou, *Yoga: the Method of Re-integration*, pp. 40 ff.

tantric *sādhana* is closely connected with a liturgical complex in which images, gestures, and sounds all play their parts together.[23]

Mantras, Dhāraṇīs *

The value of "mystical sounds" was known as early as the Vedic period. From the time of the *Yajur-Veda*, *OṂ*, the *mantra* par excellence, enjoyed universal prestige; it was identified with *brahman*, with the Veda, with all the great gods; Patañjali [24] held that it expressed Īśvara. It would serve no purpose here to summarize the various speculations on Vāc (the Word), on the creative value of ritual formulas.[25] We shall only observe that certain tantric *mantras* are already to be found in the Brāhmaṇas.[26] But it was tantrism especially, Buddhistic as well as Śivaistic, that raised the *mantras* and *dhāraṇīs* to the dignity of a vehicle of salvation (*mantrayāna*).[27]

Several aspects must be distinguished in the universal vogue of the sacred formula—a vogue that, on the one hand, led to the highest speculations on "mystical sounds," and, on the other, to the Lamaistic prayer wheel. First of all, we must take into consideration the inevitable "popular success" of such a method, of the apparent ease with which salvation, or at least merit, could be gained, simply at the cost of repeating *mantras* or *dhāraṇīs*. We shall not dwell on this popularization and degradation of a spiritual technique; it is a familiar phenomenon in the history of religions, and, in any case, it is not its popular success that will teach us the secret of the *mantrayāna*. The practical value and philosophic importance of *mantras* rest upon two orders of facts: first, the yogic function of the phonemes used as "supports" for concentration; second—and this is the peculiarly tantric contribution—the elabo-

23 For the various meanings of *mudrā*, see Note VI, 4.

24 *Yoga-sūtras*, I, 27.

25 *Aitareya Brāhmaṇa*, X, 3, 1; XIII, 11, 7, etc.

26 E.g., *khaṭ*, *phaṭ*, etc.: *Āpastamba*, XII, 11, 10, etc.

27 For texts and critical bibliographies, see Note VI, 5.

ration of a gnostic system and an interiorized liturgy through revalorization of the archaic traditions concerning "mystical sound."

The *dhāraṇī*, literally "she who upholds or encloses," was already employed in Vedic times as a "support" and "defense" for concentration (*dhārāṇa*); hence, the additional names *kavaca* and *rakṣa*, "protection," "breastplate." For the common man, *dhāraṇīs* are talismans; they protect against demons, diseases, and spells. But for the ascetics, the yogins, the contemplatives, *dhāraṇīs* become instruments for concentration, whether they follow the rhythm of *prāṇāyāma* or are mentally repeated during the phases of respiration. In some instances, we divine the meaning of mutilated words (*amale*, *vimale*, *hime*, *vame*, *kale*, etc., which express ideas of purity, snow, etc.; *cchinde*, which suggests tearing, cutting up, etc.), but the great majority of them are bizarre and unintelligible phonemes: *hrīṃ*, *hrāṃ*, *hrūṃ*, *phaṭ*, etc. As *dhāraṇīs* were probably employed and refined during meditations directed by *prāṇāyāma*, phonetic invention, necessarily limited to a certain number of syllables, was compensated for by the profound inner echo that such "mystical sounds" awakened. In any case, whatever the historical origin of *dhāraṇīs* may have been, they certainly had the value of a secret, initiatory language. For these sounds revealed their message only during meditation. For the uninitiated, *dhāraṇīs* remained unintelligible; their meaning did not belong to rational language, to the language that serves to communicate ordinary experiences. A *dhāraṇī*, a *mantra*, yielded their meanings only when they had been spoken in accordance with the rules and assimilated—that is, discovered, "awakened." This process will be better understood when we come to the underlying metaphysics of the *mantrayāna*.

Phonemes discovered during meditation probably expressed states of consciousness "cosmic" in structure and hence difficult to formulate in secular terminology. Experiences of this kind were already known in the Vedic period, although the few documents by which they have been transmitted to us seldom contain more than allusions, particularly in the form of images and symbols. It is a definitely archaic spiritual technique that here confronts us; some "cosmic ecstasies" of the shamans are expressed by unintelligible phonetic inventions, which sometimes result in the creation of a secret language.[28] These are experiences, then, that are in some measure bound up with the discovery of language and that, by this ecstatic return to a primordial situation, shatter diurnal consciousness. All of the tantric yogin's effort is expended upon reawakening this primordial consciousness and rediscovering the state of completeness that preceded language and consciousness of time. In tantrism, the tendency toward a rediscovery of language to the end of a total revalorization of secular experience is shown especially by its employment of secret vocabularies.[29]

Dhāraṇīs, like *mantras*, are learned from "the master's mouth" (*guruvaktrataḥ*); they are, then, something quite different from the phonemes that make up secular language or that can be learned from books—they have to be "received." But once received from the master's mouth, *mantras* have unlimited powers. A tantric text of the first rank, the *Sādhanamālā*, does not hesitate to ask: "What is there that cannot be accomplished by *mantras* if they are applied in accordance with the rules?" [30] One can even gain Buddhahood.[31] The *lokanātha mantra*, for example, can absolve the greatest sins,[32] and the *ekajatā mantra* is so powerful that, as soon as the disciple utters it, he is safe from all danger and achieves the sanctity of the Buddha.[33] All *siddhis* of any description—from success in love to achieving salvation—are obtained through these mystical formulas. Supreme knowledge itself can be acquired directly, without study, by proper utterance of certain *mantras*. But the technique is difficult; uttering the *mantra* is preceded by a purification of thought; the practitioner must concentrate on each of the letters composing the *mantra*, avoid fatigue, etc.[34]

28 See Eliade, *Shamanism*, pp. 96 ff.

29 See below, p. 249.

30 Ed. Bhattacharyya, II, 575.

31 Ibid., p 270.

32 Ibid., p. 31.

33 Ibid., p. 262.

34 Ibid., p. 10.

The unlimited efficacy of *mantras* is owing to the fact that they *are* (or at least, if correctly recited, *can become*) the "objects" they represent. Each god, for example, and each degree of sanctity have a *bīja-mantra*, a "mystical sound," which is their "seed," their "support"—that is, their very *being*. By repeating this *bīja-mantra* in accordance with the rules, the practitioner appropriates its ontological essence, concretely and directly assimilates the god, the state of sanctity, etc. Sometimes an entire metaphysics is concentrated in a *mantra*. The 8000 stanzas of a voluminous Mahāyāna treatise, the *Aṣṭasāhasrikā-prajñā-pāramitā*, were summarized in a few stanzas, which constitute the *Prajñā-pāramitā-hṛdaya-sūtra;* this short text was reduced to the few lines of the *Prajñā-pāramitā-dhāraṇī*, which in turn was concentrated into a *Prajñā-pāramitā-mantra;* finally, the *mantra* was reduced to its "seed," the *bīja-mantra: praṃ.*[35] Thus one could master the whole of *Prajñā-pāramitā* metaphysics by murmuring the syllable *praṃ.*

Yet we have here no "summary" of the *Prajñā-pāramitā;* we have direct and total assimilation of the "truth of the universal void" (*śūnyatā*) under the form of a "goddess." For the entire cosmos, with all its gods, planes, and modes of being , is manifested in a certain number of *mantras:* the universe *is* sonorous, just as it *is* chromatic, formal, substantial, etc. A *mantra* is a "symbol" in the archaic sense of the term—it is simultaneously the symbolized "reality" and the symbolizing "sign." There is an occult correspondence between the *mantra's* mystical letters and syllables (the *mātṛkās*, "mothers," and the *bījas*, "seeds") and the subtle organs of the human body on the one hand and, on the other, between those organs and the divine forces asleep or manifested in the cosmos. By working on the "symbol," one awakens all the forces that correspond to it, on all the levels of being. Between the *mantrayāna* and tantric iconography, for example, there is perfect correspondence; for each plane and each degree of sanctity has its corresponding image, color, and letter. By meditating on the color or the mystical sound that represents it, the disciple enters

35 B. Bhattacharyya, *An Introduction to Buddhist Esoterism*, p. 56.

into a particular modality of being, absorbs or incorporates a yogic state, a god, etc. The "supports" are homologizable; he can set out from any one of them, employ any "vehicle" (images, *mantrayāna*, etc.) in order to assimilate the ontological modality or the divine manifestation that he wishes to acquire. Between these many planes there is continuity, but it is a mystical continuity—that is, it can be realized only in certain "centers." In the tantric conception, the cosmos appears as a vast fabric of magical forces; and the same forces can be awakened or organized in the human body, through the techniques of mystical physiology.

When Vasubandhu, in his *Bodhisattvabhūmi*,[36] wrote that the true meaning of the *mantras* lay in their absence of meaning, and that by meditating on their nonmeaning one came to understand the ontological unreality of the universe, he was translating into the terms of his own philosophy an experience whose profound value escaped him or did not interest him. For, if it is true that repeating *mantras* annuls the "reality" of the secular world, this is only a first mental step, an indispensable prerequisite to reaching a deeper "reality." All indefinite repetition leads to the destruction of language; in some mystical traditions, this destruction appears to be the condition for further experiences.

Excursus: D͟hikr *

The similarities between the yogico-tantric technique and the Moslem *d͟hikr*, or incessant repetition of the name of God, were observed long ago. In a recent study, L. Gardet has described the varieties of *dhikr* in detail, at the same time examining its relations with *japa-yoga* and the *nembutsu* of Zen.[37] We must emphasize the mystical physiology assumed by the practice of *d͟hikr;* there are references to "centers" and subtle organs, to a certain inner vision of the human body, to chromatic and acoustic mani-

36 Ed. Unrai Wogihara, pp. 272 ff., quoted by S. B. Dasgupta, *An Introduction to Tantric Buddhism*, p. 66.

37 See Note VI, 6.

festations accompanying the various stages of the experience, etc. Respiratory discipline and ritual enunciation play an essential role; the process of concentration is not unlike the yogic method. The problem of historical contacts and reciprocal influences between India and Islam is not yet solved. Although constant repetition of the name of God is attested in the Koran, and although *dhikr* is highly esteemed by all the Ṣūfīs, it is probable that the regulation of bodily postures and breathing techniques is owing, at least in part, to Indian influences; we know that such influences were definitely exerted after the twelfth century (instructions for the physiological side of ecstasy, etc.).

In presenting the following texts, we have no intention of expounding the theology and technique of *dhikr;* we merely wish to emphasize its similarities to the morphology of tantric yoga. According to Ibn 'Iyāḍ, the practitioner "begins the recitation from the left side (of the chest), which is as it were the niche containing the lamp of the heart, source of spiritual light. He pursues it by proceeding from the lower part of the chest to the right side and following the right side upward. He continues by returning to the original position." [38] According to Muḥammad al-Sanūsī, "the positions to be assumed . . . consist in squatting on the ground, legs crossed, arms extended around the legs, head bowed between the two knees, and eyes closed. One raises the head, saying *lā ilāh* during the time that passes between the head's reaching the level of the heart and its position on the right shoulder. One is careful to clear one's mind of everything that is not God. When the mouth reaches the level of the heart, one carefully articulates the invocation *illā*. . . . And one says *Allāh* opposite the heart, more forcefully." [39] The chosen formula is repeated as many times as possible, "in order that all counting may cease, once continuity of prayer is established." [40] The respiratory rhythm and the rhythm of the verbal repetition are in accord. A twelfth-century text (referring to the earliest known collective *dhikr*) prescribes: the breath is "emitted above the left breast (to empty the heart); then the word *lā* is exhaled from the navel (against the sexual demon); then *ilāha* is uttered on the right shoulder, and *illā* at the navel; finally *Allāh* is strongly articulated in the empty heart." [41]

38 Tr. after Gardet, p. 654.
39 Ibid., pp. 654–55.
40 Ibid., p. 656.
41 Tr. after L. Massignon, quoted in Gardet, p. 658.

A modern author, Sheikh Muḥammad Amīn al-Kurdī (d. 1914), gives more precise details of the relations between the breath, the "centers" of the subtle body, and the mystical syllables, during *dhikr*. We give the following passage from his *Tanwīr al-qulub*, after the translation by Jean Gouillard: [42] "Let the *dhakīr* hold his tongue tightly against the soft palate, and, after inhaling, let him hold his breath. Then let him begin enunciating with the word *lā*, imagining it to be placed under his navel; from there let him draw the word toward the middle of the subtle centers, where the center called the 'most hidden' lies, and then draw it on until it reaches the point corresponding to the subtle center of the 'logical (or reasonable) soul'; this center is symbolically situated in the first region of the brain, called the 'chief.' Then let the *dhakīr* proceed to articulate the word *'ilāha*, beginning by imagining the phonetic element called *hamzah* (represented in the transliteration by the apostrophe) in the brain; from thence let him make it descend to the right shoulder, so that it will flow toward the point corresponding to the subtle center called the 'spirit.' Finally let the *dhakīr* proceed to pronounce *'illā-Lhāh*, imagining himself to be making the *hamzah* of *'illā* set out from the (right) shoulder and drawing it on toward the 'heart,' on which the *dhakīr* will strike with the final word *Allāh* (represented in the foregoing transliteration without the *A* because of the elision caused by joining these two elements of the formula); the force of the held breath will thus strike the 'little black point of the heart,' making its effect and warmth pass out into the rest of the body, so that the warmth will burn all the corrupted parts of the body, while its pure parts will be illuminated by the light of the name *Allāh*."

The preceding passages treat of the "*dhikr* of the tongue," the interiorized oral liturgy. There are two higher stages, the "*dhikr* of the heart" and the "intimate" (*sirr*) *dhikr*. It is particularly during the stage of "*dhikr* of the heart" that visual phenomena (luminosity, colors) [43] are manifested; the "*dhikr* of the tongue" provokes concomitant auditory phenomena. [44] In the "intimate *dhikr*," duality is abolished. "Not through fusion, it is true, as in the Indian ambient, for conceptualization of the divine transcendence remains, but in a line felt as a 'disappearance' of the subject in its very being." [45] The state attained is that of *fanā'*, "annihilation." The concomitant luminous phenomena increase. This time, "the

42 *Petite Philocalie*, pp. 332–33. 43 Cf. Gardet, p. 671.
44 Ibid., p. 667. See Note III, 6, on "mystical sounds."
45 Ibid., p. 675.

fires of *dhikr* are not extinguished, its lights do not flee. . . . Still thou seest lights rising, others descending; the fires about thee are clear, very hot, and they flame." [46] All this suggests the photic experiences of Yoga, tantrism, and shamanism.[47]

Maṇḍala *

A ritual peculiar to the tantric liturgy consists in constructing the *maṇḍala*. Literally, the word means "circle"; the Tibetan translations render it sometimes by "center," sometimes by "that which surrounds." It is, in fact, a quite complex design, comprising a circular border and one or more concentric circles enclosing a square divided into four triangles; in the center of each triangle, and in the center of the *maṇḍala* itself, are other circles containing images of divinities or their emblems. This iconographic schema is susceptible of countless variations; some *maṇḍalas* look like labyrinths, other like palaces with ramparts, towers, gardens; we find floral patterns side by side with crystallographic structures, and sometimes the diamond or the lotus blossom seems to be discernible.

The simplest *maṇḍala* is the *yantra*, employed by Hinduism (literally, "object serving to hold," "instrument," "engine"); it is a diagram "drawn or engraved on metal, wood, skin, stone, paper, or simply traced on the ground or on a wall." [48] Its structure may be regarded as the linear paradigm of the *maṇḍala*. A *yantra*, that is, is composed of a series of triangles—nine in the *śrīyantra*, four apex up, five apex down—surrounded by several concentric circles, which are framed in a square with four "doors." The triangle pointing down symbolizes the *yoni*—that is, the Śakti; the triangle pointing up designates the male principle, Śiva; the central point (*bindu*) signifies the undifferentiated Brahman. In other words, the *yantra* is an expression, in terms of linear symbolism, of the cosmic manifestations, beginning with the primordial unity.

46 Ibn 'Aṭā' Allāh, tr. after Gardet, p. 677.

47 See below, p. 334.

48 Louis Renou, *L'Inde classique*, p. 568.

The *maṇḍala* employs the same symbolism and develops it on planes that, though different, are homologizable. Like the *yantra*, the *maṇḍala* is at once an image of the universe and a theophany—the cosmic creation being, of course, a manifestation of the divinity. But the *maṇḍala* also serves as a "receptacle" for the gods. In Vedic India the gods descended into the altar—which proves continuity between the tantric liturgy and the traditional cult. In the beginning, every altar or sacred site was regarded as a privileged space, separated from the rest of the territory; in this qualitatively different space, the sacred manifested itself by a rupture of planes permitting communication among the three cosmic zones—heaven, earth, subterranean region. Now, this conception was extremely widespread, existing beyond the frontiers of India and even of Asia; the symbolism of royal cities, temples, towns, and, by extension, every human habitation was based upon such a valorization of the sacred space as the center of the world and hence the site of communication with heaven and hell.

Tantrism employs this archaic symbolism, but incorporates it into new contexts. It is by a study of the symbolism of the *maṇḍala*, as interpreted in the texts, and by a description of the tantric ritual of initiation, that we can best become acquainted with the revalorizations imposed by tantrism.[49] The border of a *maṇḍala* consists of a "barrier of fire," which at once prohibits access to the uninitiate and symbolizes the metaphysical knowledge that "burns" ignorance. Next comes a "ring of diamond"; now, diamond is the symbol of the highest consciousness, *bodhi*, illumination. Immediately within the "ring of diamond" is a circle, around which eight cemeteries, symbolizing the eight aspects of disintegrated consciousness, are represented; this iconographic motif of cemeteries is principally found in *maṇḍalas* dedicated to terrible divinities. Next comes a ring of leaves, signifying spiritual rebirth. In the center of this last circle is the *maṇḍala* proper, also called "palace" (*vimana*)—that is, the place where the images of the gods are set.

Royal symbolism plays an important part in the construction and

49 For texts and critical bibliographies, see Note VI, 7.

ritual of the *maṇḍala.* In India as elsewhere, sovereignty is related to the sacred. The Buddha is the *cakravartin* par excellence, the cosmocrat. The ceremony that is performed within the *maṇḍala* (to which we shall return in a moment) is, in fact, an *abhiṣeka*—that is, a ritual of royal consecration, a baptism by water; [50] the images of the Buddha set in the various circles of the *maṇḍala* wear royal diadems, and before entering the *maṇḍala* the disciple is given the insignia of royalty by his master. The symbolism here is easy to understand: the disciple is assimilated to the sovereign because he rises above the play of cosmic forces; [51] he is autonomous, wholly free. Spiritual freedom—and this is true not only of India—has always been expressed by sovereignty.

At the periphery of the construction there are four cardinal doors, defended by terrifying images called "guardians of the doors." Their role is twofold. On the one hand, the guardians defend consciousness from the disintegrating forces of the unconscious; on the other, they have an offensive mission—in order to lay hold upon the fluid and mysterious world of the unconscious, consciousness must carry the struggle into the enemy's camp and hence assume the violent and terrible aspect appropriate to the forces to be combated.[52] Indeed, even the divinities inside the *maṇḍala* sometimes have a terrifying appearance; they are the gods whom man will encounter after death, in the state of *bardo.* The guardians of the doors and the terrible divinities emphasize the initiatory character of entrance into a *maṇḍala.* Every initiation presupposes passing from one mode of being to another, but this ontological change is preceded by a shorter or longer series of "ordeals" that the candidate must successfully undergo. The typical initiatory ordeal is the "struggle with a monster" (in the literal sense of the word in military initiations). On the tantric plane, the monsters represent the forces of the unconscious, arising from the

50 One of the most important tantric texts on initiation into a *maṇḍala* is entitled *Sekoddeśaṭīkā*—that is, "Commentary on the Treatise of Baptism." Its author is Naḍapāda (Nāropā).

51 Giuseppe Tucci, *Teoria e pratica del maṇḍala,* p. 51.

52 Ibid., p. 65.

universal "void"; the candidate must conquer the fear that they arouse. Now, as has often been shown, the size and terrible appearance of the monsters encountered in initiation are nothing but a creation of "initiatory fear."

This aspect of initiation discloses certain similarities of structure between the *maṇḍala* and the labyrinth. Many *maṇḍalas* are, in fact, clearly labyrinthine in design. Among the ritual functions of the labyrinth, two in particular are of interest to us: first, the labyrinth symbolized the beyond, and whoever entered it as a part of initiation realized a *descensus ad inferos* ("death" followed by "resurrection"); secondly, it represented a "system of defense," both spiritual (against evil spirits and demons, forces of chaos) and material (against enemies). Since the city, like the temple or the palace, constituted a "center of the world," it was by labyrinths or walls that it was defended, not only against invaders but also against maleficent forces, against the "spirits of the desert" who attempted to return "forms" to the amorphous state from which they originated. Viewed in this light, the functions of the *maṇḍala*—like that of the labyrinth—would be at least twofold. On the one hand, entrance into a *maṇḍala* drawn on the ground is equivalent to an initiation; on the other, the *maṇḍala* "defends" the disciple against any destructive force and at the same time helps him to concentrate, to find his own "center." This last function will become more clearly apparent when we discuss tantric *sādhana.*

The liturgy comprises a number of rites. The ground on which the *maṇḍala* is to be drawn is carefully selected. It must be smooth, without stones and grass; in other words, it is homologized with the transcendent plane. This already indicates the spatio-temporal symbolism of the *maṇḍala*—the disciple is to enter an ideal, transcosmic plane. "Flat ground" is well known to be the image of paradise or of any other transcendent plane; whereas orographic variations signify creation, the appearance of forms and time. The *maṇḍala* can, then, be regarded as a symbol of paradise. Several paradise symbols are evident in it. First, there is the resemblance between the pantheon that is an integral part of the *maṇḍala* and the paradises of Buddhist imagination (Sukhāvatī, Abhirati, Tuṣita, Trayastriṃśa, etc.), in the center of which the Supreme God sits in his royal pavilion in the midst of a park with lakes, flowers, and birds, and surrounded by other divinities.[53] But the Buddhist paradise is only a variant of the Indian paradise, whose earliest image is Uttarakuru, the Northern Country, regarded as the seat of the blessed.[54] According to Buddhist texts, Uttarakuru, the Golden Land, shines day and night and enjoys four qualities: the ground is level, there is absolute calm, it is pure, and its trees bear no thorns. Rice grows without being sown, as it did on earth in the golden age.[55]

The paradisal symbolism of the *maṇḍala* is also apparent in another element—the expulsion of demons. The ground is purified from demons by an invocation to the earth goddess, she who had been called upon by the Buddha in the night at Bodhgayā. In other words, the Buddha's exemplary gesture is repeated and the ground is magically transformed into a "diamond land," the diamond, as we have seen, being the symbol of incorruptibility, of absolute reality. All this implies abolishing time and history and returning *in illo tempore*, to the exemplary moment of the Buddha's Illumination. And abolishing time is known to be a paradisal syndrome.

After these preparations, the *maṇḍala* is drawn by means of two cords; the first, which is white, is used to trace its outer limits; the second is composed of threads of five different colors. The diagram can also be made with colored rice powder. Vases filled with precious or aromatic substances, fillets, flowers, branches, etc., are set in the triangles for the "descent" of the gods. The disciple is initiated on an auspicious day and in a place close to the sea or a river.

53 Tucci, "Buddhist Notes," *Mélanges chinois et bouddhiques*, IX (1951), 196.

54 Already in *Aitareya Brāhmaṇa*, VIII, 23; Tucci, "Buddhist Notes," p. 197.

55 On Uttarakuru, see the bibliography compiled by Tucci, "Buddhist Notes," p. 197, n. 1. The classic description of the golden age according to the Buddhists is found in the *Mahāvastu* (I, 338 ff.). On the other Hindu and Buddhist paradises and their relation with Yoga, see below, p. 416.

The night before the ceremony, he goes to sleep in the position of "the Buddha entering *nirvāṇa*" (the "lion posture"—i.e., lying on the right side, with the head resting on the right hand); in the morning he tells his *guru* what he dreamed, and the initiation cannot take place unless the *guru* considers the dream auspicious.

The ceremony proper begins with a series of purifications and consecrations. The *Sekoddeśaṭīkā* gives numerous details: the *guru* purifies the disciple's organs with *mantras* (*U* on the forehead, *I*, *A*, *R*, *AN* on the genitals); he also purifies the objects to be used in the ritual, especially the vases, sets the "triumphal pot" (*vijaya-kalaśa*) in the middle of the *maṇḍala* and honors it with perfumes and incense; then he crowns the disciple, who is dressed in white, with a garland of flowers. The disciple draws a small *maṇḍala*, decorated with flowers and gold, around his master's feet to do him reverence; then offers himself to him, together with a girl who must, if possible, be a member of his immediate family. The *guru* puts five drops of ambrosia (that is, five sacred substances) on his tongue, with the appropriate *mantras*, and consecrates the incense with other *mantras*. He then brings on "possession by the furious god" (*krodāveśa*), a rite peculiar to the initiation recorded in the *Sekoddeśaṭīkā*. The disciple repeats certain *mantras* and inhales vigorously, whereupon Vajrapāṇi, the angry god, takes possession of him, and he begins to sing and dance, imitating the traditional gestures of wrathful divinities. This rite allows the forces of the unconscious to invade the disciple, who, by confronting them, "burns" all fear and timidity. Then, chiefly by *mudrās*, he invokes the five peaceful divinities, the Śaktis of the five Tathāgatas, and becomes calm again. If the possession continues too long, the *guru* touches his forehead with a flower consecrated by the *mantra OṂ A H Hūm*. Then he blindfolds the disciple and puts a flower in his hand; the disciple throws it into the *maṇḍala*, and the section into which it falls reveals the divinity who will be especially favorable to him during his initiation.

Entrance into the *maṇḍala* resembles every "march toward the center." (It has been shown that ritual circumambulation of a *stūpa* or temple, *pradakṣiṇa*, and ascending the successive terraces of great religious monuments both indicate a "march toward the center.") Since the *maṇḍala* is an *imago mundi*, its center corresponds to the infinitesimal point perpendicularly traversed by the *axis mundi;* as he approaches its center, the disciple approaches the "center of the world." In fact, as soon as he has entered the *maṇḍala*, he is in a sacred space, outside of time; the gods have already "descended" into the vases and insignia. A series of meditations, for which the disciple has been prepared in advance, help him to find the gods in his own heart. In a vision, he sees them all emerge and spring from his heart; they fill cosmic space, then are reabsorbed in him. In other words, he "realizes" the eternal process of the periodic creation and destruction of worlds; and this allows him to enter into the rhythms of the cosmic great time and to understand its emptiness. He shatters the plane of *saṃsāra* and enters a transcendent plane; this is the "great mystery" of Mahāyānic and tantric Buddhism, the "complete reversal" (*parāvṛtti*), the transformation of *saṃsāra* into the absolute, which can also be obtained by other techniques.[56]

Drawn on cloth, the *maṇḍala* serves as a "support" for meditation; the yogin uses it as a "defense" against mental distractions and temptations. The *maṇḍala* "concentrates," it makes the meditating yogin invulnerable to external stimuli; the analogy with the labyrinth that safeguards against evil spirits or enemies is easy to see. By mentally entering the *maṇḍala*, the yogin approaches his own "center," and this spiritual exercise can be understood in two senses: (1) to reach the center the yogin re-enacts and masters the cosmic process, for the *maṇḍala* is an image of the world; (2) but since he is engaged in meditation and not in ritual, the yogin, starting from this iconographic "support," can find the *maṇḍala* in his own body. We must never lose sight of the fact that the tantric

56 Professor Tucci interprets this mysterious process as an integration of the unconscious, obtained by taking possession of its symbols (*Maṇḍala*, p. 23). Now, since the "unconscious" is nothing but cosmic consciousness, "stored consciousness' (*ālayavijñāna*), its integration would, in Jung's psychology, be what he terms integration of the collective unconscious.

universe is made up of an endless series of analogies, homologies, and symmetries; starting from any level, one can establish mystical communication with the others, in order finally to reduce them to unity and master them.

Before studying the process of introducing the *maṇḍala* into the yogin's own body, let us briefly discuss similar designs from outside the Indo-Tibetan realm. Various cultures have been found to possess a number of figures based on circles, triangles, and labyrinths, and connected with religious worship; this is particularly evident in the case of magical circles and initiatory labyrinths. Maṇḍalic in character, too, are the ritual drawings made by certain North and South American tribes to represent the various phases of the creation of the universe. They need not be studied here. We shall only emphasize that these *maṇḍalas* are usually constructed in connection with the curing of disease. And this brings us to another class of *maṇḍalas*, discovered by C. G. Jung in the paintings executed by some of his patients. According to the author of the hypothesis of the collective unconscious, these *maṇḍalas* represent structures of the deep psyche. Hence they play a role in that central process of the unconscious which Jung terms the process of individuation. Jung proposed his hypothesis after observing the following fact: in the dreams and visions of a number of his patients, *maṇḍalas* appeared when the process of individuation was about to reach a successful conclusion. Hence the spontaneous image of the *maṇḍala* corresponded to a spiritual victory, in the sense that a portion of the collective unconscious—that immense zone of the psyche which was threatening the integrity of the person—was assimilated and integrated by consciousness.

The spontaneous rediscovery of *maṇḍalas* by the unconscious raises an important problem. We may well ask if the "unconscious" is not in this case trying to imitate processes by which "consciousness" (or, in some cases, the "transconscious") [57] seeks to obtain completeness and conquer freedom. For this unconscious discovery

57 We put all these terms in quotation marks because, in this context, they are not taken solely in their psychological sense.

of an initiatory schema does not stand alone; it is known that all the great mystical symbolisms are spontaneously rediscovered in dreams, in hallucinations, and even in pathological ecstasies. Experiences and symbols of ascent, of the "march toward the center," of the descent into hell, of death and resurrection, of initiatory ordeals, and even the complex symbols of alchemy, have all been recorded in one or another of these states. To a certain degree, we may speak of a "mimicking imitation," using the term in its strict sense—imitation of behavior and gestures, but without the integral experience of the implied contents.

The yogin can discover the *maṇḍala* in his own body, and then the liturgy is interiorized—that is, is transformed into a series of meditations on the various "centers" and subtle organs.

Praise of the Body: Haṭha Yoga

In tantrism, the human body acquires an importance it had never before attained in the spiritual history of India. To be sure, health and strength, interest in a physiology homologizable with the cosmos and implicitly sanctified, are Vedic, if not pre-Vedic, values. But tantrism carries to its furthest consequences the conception that sanctity can be realized only in a "divine body." The Upaniṣadic and post-Upaniṣadic pessimism and asceticism are swept away. The body is no longer the source of pain, but the most reliable and effective instrument at man's disposal for "conquering death." And since liberation can be gained even in this life, the body must be preserved as long as possible, and in perfect condition, precisely as an aid to meditation.[58] As we shall see later, Indian alchemy propounds a similar goal.

In the *Hevajra-tantra*, the Buddha (Bhagavān) proclaims that, without a perfectly healthy body, one cannot know bliss. This is an adage that is insistently repeated in tantric and Sahajīyā literature. Saraha puts it in his figurative style: "Here (within this body) is the Ganges and the Jumnā . . . here are Prayāga and Benares—here

58 Cf. *Gheraṇḍa Saṃhitā*, I, 8.

the sun and the moon. Here are the sacred places, here the *Pīṭhas* and the *Upa-pīṭhas*—I have not seen a place of pilgrimage and an abode of bliss like my body." The Buddha himself is hidden in the body, Saraha adds.[59]

We can distinguish at least two orientations, different yet convergent, in this emphatic valuation of the human body and its possibilities: (1) there is the importance accorded to the *total experience of life* as constituting an integral part of *sādhana*, and this is the general position of all tantric schools; (2) there is, in addition, the will to master the body in order to transmute it into a divine body, and this is especially the position of Haṭha Yoga. Such a mastery must begin modestly, on the basis of an accurate knowledge of the organs and their functions. For "How can the Yogīs who do not know their body (as) a house of one column (with) nine doors, and (as presided over by) five tutelary divinities, attain perfection (in Yoga)?" [60] But perfection is always the goal, and, as we shall soon see, it is neither athletic nor hygienic perfection. Haṭha Yoga cannot and must not be confused with gymnastics. Its appearance is linked with the name of an ascetic, Gorakhnāth, founder of an order, the Kānphaṭa Yogīs. He is supposed to have lived in the twelfth century, perhaps even earlier. All that we know about Gorakhnāth is distorted by a sectarian mythology and a profuse magical folklore,[61] but facts that may be considered reliable warrant the supposition that he was in close relation with the "Diamond Vehicle." In any case, as we shall see, the Haṭha Yoga treatises refer to sexual practices advocated by Buddhist tantrism.

Gorakhnāth is credited with the authorship of a treatise no longer extant, entitled *Haṭha Yoga*, and of a text that has come down to us, the *Gorakṣa Śataka*. A commentary on this latter, the *Gorakṣa Paddhati*, explains the word *haṭha* (lit., "violence," "vio-

59 Texts cited and tr. Dasgupta, *Obscure Religious Cults*, pp. 103 ff.

60 *Gorakṣa Śataka*, 14; tr. G. W. Briggs, *Gorakhnāth and the Kānphaṭā Yogīs*, pp. 287–88.

61 See below, p. 303.

lent effort") by *ha* = sun and *ṭha* = moon; the union of moon and sun forming Yoga. (According to other texts, *ha-ṭhau* = *sūrya-candrau* = *prāṇapānau.*) We shall later see that this interpretation perfectly accords with tantric doctrine. The Kānphaṭas called their particular discipline Haṭha Yoga, but the term soon came to be the collective designation for the traditional formulas and disciplines that made it possible to attain to perfect mastery of the body. In any case, in one way or another the Haṭha Yoga treatises stem from the literature composed by or fathered upon the Gorakhnātha yogīs. We possess a large number of texts,[62] but, aside from the *Gorakṣa Śataka*, only three are of interest for the present study: (1) the *Haṭhayogapradīpikā* (by Svātmārāma Svāmin, probably of the fifteenth century; uses and reproduces a number of stanzas from the *Gorakṣa Śataka*); (2) the *Gheraṇḍa Saṃhitā* (by a certain Gheraṇḍa, a Vaiṣṇavite of Bengal; abundantly reproduced in the *Haṭhayogapradīpikā*); (3) *Śiva Saṃhitā* (longer than the two preceding—contains 517 stanzas—and more elaborated philosophically; tantric yoga strongly colored by Vedānta). Of these three texts, the oldest appears to be the *Haṭhayogapradīpikā*, which itself, according to tradition, is based on the lost *Haṭha Yoga*.[63]

Buddhist influences are easily discernible. The *Haṭhayogapradīpikā* even employs the Mādhyamika vocabulary (e.g., the term *śūnya*), and the first verse of the *Śiva Saṃhitā* has a strong Buddhist coloring (*ekamjñānam nityamādhyantaśūnyam* . . .). Vedānta is mixed with Yoga, but philosophical justification has a very small place[64] in these brief treatises, which are almost

62 Briggs, pp. 251 ff.

63 Fitz-Edward Hall, *A Contribution Towards an Index to the Bibliography of the Indian Philosophical Systems*, p. 15. For editions and translations of Haṭha Yoga texts, see Note VI, 8.

64 The following will serve as examples of the underlying "theory." Suffering is universal; it is present even in the heavens (*Śiva Saṃhitā*, I, 29). Man must renounce the fruits of his actions (ibid., I, 30), vices and virtues (I, 32), etc. The universe originates from *caitanya* (I, 49) and Māyā (I, 64), for Īśvara wished to create the world, but from his desire was born *avidyā*, mother of the false universe (I, 69), etc.

entirely devoted to technical formulas. The states of consciousness corresponding to the various exercises are mentioned only rarely and in a rudimentary way. It is the physics and physiology of meditation that are the chief concern of these writers. Thirty-two *āsanas* are described in the *Gheraṇḍa Saṃhitā*, and fifteen in the *Haṭhayogapradīpikā*; the *Śiva Saṃhitā* mentions eighty-four *āsanas*, but discusses only four of them. The magical and hygienic value of the *āsanas* is stressed: some of them strengthen health and "conquer death," others confer *siddhis*.[65] The repeated assurances "destroys old age and death" and "conquers death" (*mṛtyum jayati*) illustrate the real meaning and final orientation of all these techniques. The *Gheraṇḍa Saṃhitā* devotes five stanzas to *pratyāhāra*, whereas *prāṇāyāma* receives ninety-six stanzas and the *mudrās* one hundred. We shall presently see, however, that certain physiological details mentioned in connection with respiratory discipline are not without interest.

Haṭha Yoga accords great importance to preliminary "purifications," of which it distinguishes six kinds: *dhāutī*, *basti*, *neti*, *nauli*, *trāṭaka*, *kapāla bhāti*.[66] The most commonly employed are the first two. The *dhāutīs* (lit., "cleansings") are divided into several classes and subclasses: "internal cleansings," cleaning the teeth, the rectum, etc.[67] The most effective is *dhāutī karma:*[68] a long piece of cloth is swallowed and left for some time in the stomach.[69] *Basti* comprises cleansing the large intestine and the rectum,[70] which is performed by anal suction.[71] *Neti* consists in cleansing the nasal fossae by threads inserted into the nostrils.[72] To practice *nauli* one

65 For example, *padmāsana* destroys any sickness (*Gheraṇḍa Saṃhitā*, II, 8), *muktāsana* and *vajrāsana* confer "miraculous powers" (ibid., II, 11–12), *mṛtāsana* calms agitation of mind (II, 19), and *bhujaṅgāsana* awakens the *kuṇḍalinī* (II, 42–43).

66 *Haṭhayogapradīpikā*, II, 22.

67 *Gheraṇḍa Saṃhitā*, I, 13–44.

68 *Haṭhayogapradīpikā*, II, 24.

69 See also Bernard, *Haṭha Yoga*, pp. 15 ff.

70 *Haṭhayogapradīpikā*, II, 26–28; *Gheraṇḍa Saṃhitā*, I, 45–49.

71 Cf. Bernard, pp. 17 ff.

72 *Haṭhayogapradīpikā*, II, 29–30; *Gheraṇḍa Saṃhitā*, I, 50–51.

executes energetic and complex movements of the stomach and intestines; [73] the *Gheraṇḍa Saṃhitā* (I, 52) calls this exercise *laulikī yoga*.[74] *Trāṭaka* consists in gazing steadily at a small object until the eyes fill with tears.[75] *Kapāla bhāti* comprises three variations of "purification" of the nasal fossae (*vāmakrama, vyutkrama,* and *śitkrama*): [76] water is drawn in through the nostrils and expelled through the mouth, etc.

The texts repeatedly emphasize that these "purifications" are of great value for the yogin's health, that they prevent affections of the stomach, the liver, etc.,[77] and there would seem to be little doubt that this is true. Detailed instructions are given for diet,[78] social behavior (the yogin should avoid journeys, morning baths, the presence of sinful men and of women).[79] As might be expected, "practice" (*abhyāsa*) plays a decisive role; [80] nothing can be obtained without "practice"—which, by the way, is also a leitmotiv of tantrism. On the other hand, if the yogin "realizes" Haṭha Yoga, there are no sins or crimes that cannot be blotted out (killing a Brāhman or a fetus, violating the *guru's* bed, etc., are all crimes nullified by the *yonimudrā*).[81] Praise of the magical efficacy of a perfectly accomplished act is as old as India.

Prāṇāyāma destroys sins and confers the eighty-one *siddhis*,[82] but this exercise is used chiefly to purify the *nāḍīs*.[83] Each new stage in the discipline of respiration is accompanied by physiological phenomena. In general, sleep, excretions, and urine diminish.[84] During the first stage of *prāṇāyāma* the yogin's body breaks out

73 *Haṭhayogapradīpikā*, II, 33–34.
74 Cf. Bernard's experiences, pp. 21 ff.
75 *Haṭhayogapradīpikā*, II, 31–32; *Gheraṇḍa Saṃhitā*, I, 53–54.
76 *Gheraṇḍa Saṃhitā*, I, 56–60.
77 Ibid., I, 15–16, etc.
78 *Haṭhayogapradīpikā*, I, 58, 59, 62; *Gheraṇḍa Saṃhitā*, V, 17, etc.
79 *Haṭhayogapradīpikā*, I, 62, 66, etc.
80 Cf. *Śiva Saṃhitā*, IV.
81 *Gheraṇḍa Saṃhitā*, III, 43–44.
82 *Śiva Saṃhitā*, III, 51–52; *Gheraṇḍa Saṃhitā*, V, 1–2.
83 *Śiva Saṃhitā*, III, 26; *Haṭhayogapradīpikā*, II, 4–9, 11, 20, 44.
84 *Śiva Saṃhitā*, III, 40.

into perspiration; [85] during the second stage he trembles; during the third he "hops about like a frog"; and in the fourth he rises into the air.[86] According to Theos Bernard's personal experiences,[87] all these manifestations except the last correspond to states really undergone during the practice of Haṭha Yoga *prāṇāyāma*. In any case, they are unimportant symptoms, recorded by the texts only because they serve as objective verifications of the success of a practice.

Far more important are the real "powers" obtained by the yogins, especially their astonishing ability to control the neurovegetative system and the influence they are able to exercise on their cardiac and respiratory rhythms. We shall not discuss this important problem here. It will suffice to mention that, according to Dr. Charles Laubry and Dr. Thérèse Brosse, the Haṭha yogins extend the control normally exercised over the striated muscles to the nonstriated muscles. This would explain both the pumping and expulsion of liquids by the urethra or the rectum and the arrest of seminal emission (and even the "return of semen"!), an exercise of the utmost importance in "left-hand" tantrism. Some of these "powers" will perhaps receive a different physiological explanation. In the case of the pumping and expulsion of liquids by the urethra, Dr. Jean Filliozat believes that the phenomenon can be explained by insufflation of air into the bladder. He bases his opinion on a passage from the *Haṭhayogapradīpikā* (III, 86): "With a good tube, carefully and gently make an insufflation into the thunderbolt cavity [*vajra* = urethral meatus] by a current of wind." The Sanskrit commentary gives some details of the operation: "One has a rod made, of lead, smooth, and fourteen fingerbreadths long, and one practices introducing it into the urethra. The first day one inserts it one fingerbreadth. The second day, two fingerbreadths. . . . And so on, increasing progressively. When the in-

85 *Haṭhayogapradīpikā*, II, 12–13; *Śiva Saṃhitā*, III, 40.
86 *Śiva Saṃhitā*, III, 41; cf. *Gheraṇḍa Saṃhitā*, V, 45–57.
87 *Haṭha Yoga*, p. 32.

sertion is twelve fingerbreadths, the urethral canal is cleansed. One has a similar rod made, with a curved section two fingerbreadths long and an orifice above, and one should insert it twelve fingerbreadths. One should place the curved section of two fingerbreadths outside, orifice up. Then one takes a blowpipe like a jeweler's blowpipe for blowing flame and one inserts the end of it into the two-fingerbreadth-long curved section with the orifice, at the top of the tube introduced twelve fingerbreadths into the urethra, and one then performs the insufflation. In this way, the cleansing of the canal is properly accomplished. Then one should practice absorbing water by the urethra." [88]

After translating this important text, Dr. Filliozat adds: "However, inflation of the bladder with air is not indispensable for all yogins practicing vesical suction. We ourselves observed one of them performing without a preliminary injection of air. If such an injection had taken place out of our presence, it would have had to be made more than a half-hour earlier, for the yogin performed several other exercises during that period of time, before vesical suction. More accurate observations than those which it has yet been possible to make are necessary." [89]

It would appear, then, that there are several Haṭha-yogic methods of obtaining the same results. Hence we are justified in supposing that some yogins specialized in physiological techniques, but that the majority of them followed the age-old technique of "mystical physiology." For, although the Hindus have elaborated a complex system of scientific medicine, nothing obliges us to believe that the theories of mystical physiology were developed in dependence upon this objective and utilitarian medicine or at least in connection with it. "Subtle physiology" was probably elaborated on the basis of ascetic, ecstatic, and contemplative experiences expressed in the same symbolic language as the traditional cosmology

88 J. Filliozat, "Les Limites des pouvoirs humains dans l'Inde," *Études carmélitaines* (1953), pp. 23–38.

89 Ibid., p. 33.

and ritual. This does not mean that such experiences were not *real;* they were perfectly real, but not in the sense in which a physical phenomenon is real. The tantric and Haṭha-yogic texts impress us by their "experimental character," but the experiments are performed on levels other than those of daily secular life. The "veins," the "nerves," and the "centers" that we shall presently discuss no doubt correspond to psychosomatic experiences and are related to the deep life of the human being, but it does not seem that the "veins" and similar terms designate anatomical organs and strictly physiological functions. Several attempts have been made to locate these "veins" and "centers." H. Walter,[90] for example, thinks that in Haṭha Yoga *nāḍī* means "vein"; he identifies *iḍā* and *piṅgalā* with the carotid (*laeva* and *dextra*) and *brāhmarandhra* with the *sutura frontalis.* It has, furthermore, become usual to identify the "centers" (*cakra*) with their plexuses; *mūlādhāra cakra* is supposed to be the sacral plexus; *svādhisṭhāna*, the prostatic plexus; *maṇipūra*, the epigastric plexus; *anāhata*, the pharyngeal plexus; *ājñā cakra*, the cavernous plexus.[91] But careful reading of the texts suffices to show that the experiences in question are transphysiological, that all these "centers" represent yogic states—that is, states that are inaccessible without preliminary spiritual *ascesis.* Purely psychophysiological mortifications and disciplines are not enough to "awaken" the *cakras* or to penetrate them; the essential and indispensable factor remains meditation, spiritual "realization." Thus, it is safer to regard "mystical physiology" as the result and the conceptualization of experiments undertaken from very remote times by ascetics and yogins. Now, we must not forget that the yogins performed their experiments on a "subtle body" (that is, by making use of sensations, tensions, and transconscious states inaccessible to the uninitiate), that they became masters of a zone infinitely greater than the "normal" psychic

90 "Svātmārāma's *Haṭhayogapradīpikā* (*Die Leuchte des Haṭhayoga*) aus dem Sanskrit übersetzt," pp. iv, vi, ix.

91 See Note VI, 8.

zone, that they penetrated into the depths of the unconscious and were able to "awaken" the archaic strata of primordial consciousness, which, in other human beings, are fossilized.

The body thus built up in the course of time by the Haṭha yogins, tantrists, and alchemists corresponded in some measure to the body of a "man-god"—a concept that, we know, has a long prehistory, both Indo-Āryan and pre-Āryan. The tantric theandry was only a new variant of the Vedic macranthropy. The point of departure for all these formulas was of course the transformation of the human body into a microcosmos, an archaic theory and practice, examples of which have been found almost all over the world and which, in Āryan India, had already found expression from Vedic times. The "breaths," as we have seen, were identified with the cosmic winds [92] and with the cardinal points.[93] Air "weaves" the universe,[94] and breath "weaves" man [95]—and this symbolism of weaving developed in India into the grandiose concept of cosmic illusion (Māyā) and elsewhere into the concepts of the "life thread" and of fate as spun by certain goddesses.[96] When the Vedic sacrifice is "interiorized," the body becomes a microcosmos.[97] The spinal column is identified with Mount Meru—that is, with the cosmic axis. This is why, according to Buddhist symbolism, the Buddha could not turn his head but had to turn his entire body, "like an elephant"; his spinal column was fixed, motionless, as is the axis of the universe. According to tradition, the Merudaṇḍa is made of a single bone—which indicates its ideal, nonanatomical character. One tantric text declares that Sumeru is located in the body itself; the cavern of the mountain is assimilated to supreme truth.[98] The aspirant "realizes" the anthropocosmos through a yogic meditation: "Imagine the central part [or spinal column] of thy body to be Mount Meru, the four chief limbs to be the Four

92 *Atharva Veda*, XI, 4, 15.
93 *Chāndogya Upaniṣad*, III, 13, 1–5.
94 *Bṛhadāraṇyaka Upaniṣad*, III, 7, 2.
95 *Atharva Veda*, X, 2, 13.
96 See Eliade, *Images and Symbols*, pp. 114 ff.
97 Cf. *Vaikhānasasmārtasūtra*, II, 18.
98 Kāṇhupāda, *Dohākoṣa*, 14.

Continents, the minor limbs to be the Sub-Continents, the head to be the worlds of the *Devas*, the two eyes to be the Sun and Moon," etc.[99]

Tantric *sādhana* makes use of this archaic cosmophysiology. But all these images and all these symbols presupposed a mystical experimentation, the theandry, the sanctification of man through ascetic and spiritual disciplines. In these disciplines sensory activities were magnified in staggering proportions as the result of countless identifications of organs and physiological functions with cosmic regions, stars and planets, gods, etc. Haṭha Yoga and tantra transubstantiated the body by giving it macranthropic dimensions and assimilating it to the various "mystical bodies" (sonorous, architectonic, iconographic, etc.). For example, a Javanese tantric treatise, the *Sang hyang kamahāyānikan*, to which Stutterheim and P. Mus have drawn attention,[100] identifies each somatic element of the human body with a letter of the alphabet and a part of the architectonic monument, *stūpaprāsāda* (which, in turn, is assimilated to the Buddha and the cosmos). Several "subtle bodies" are here superimposed: the sonorous body, the architectonic body, the cosmological body, the mystico-physiological body (for the homology refers not to the organs of ordinary life, but to the *cakras*, the "centers"). This multilayered homologization must be "realized"; but as a result of the yogic experience, the physical body becomes "dilated," "cosmicized," transubstantiated. The "veins" and "centers" mentioned in the texts refer first of all to states realizable only through an extraordinary amplification of the "sensation of the body."

The Nāḍis: Iḍā, Piṅgalā, Suṣumṇā

The body—both the physical and the "subtle"—is made up of a certain number of *nāḍīs* (lit., "conduits," "vessels," "veins," or "arteries," but also "nerves") and of *cakras* (lit., "circles,"

99 W. Y. Evans-Wentz, *Tibetan Yoga and Secret Doctrines*, pp. 324–25.
100 Cf. Paul Mus, *Barabuḍur*, I, 66 ff.

"disks," but usually translated "centers"). Simplifying slightly, we could say that the vital energy, in the form of "breaths," circulates through the *nāḍīs* and that the cosmic energy exists, in a latent state, in the *cakras*.

There are many *nāḍīs:* "like the large and small *nāḍīs* spreading through an *aśvattha* leaf, they cannot be counted." [101] Some figures have, however, been proposed: 300,000,[102] 200,000,[103] 80,000,[104] but especially 72,000.[105] Among them, seventy-two are of particular importance. Not all of these have names. The *Śiva Saṃhitā* speaks of fourteen, the majority of the texts enumerate ten: *iḍā, piṅgalā* (or *piṅglā*), *suṣumṇā, gāndhārī, hastijihvā, pūsā, yaśasvinī, ālambuṣā, kūhūś,* and *śaṃkhinī.*[106] These *nāḍīs* terminate respectively in the left nostril, the right nostril, the *brāhmarandhra,* the left eye, the right eye, the right ear, the left ear, the mouth, the genital organ, and the anus.[107]

The most important of all these *nāḍīs,* those which play an essential role in all yogic techniques, are the first three: *iḍā, piṅgalā,* and *suṣumṇā.* We shall later review some names applied to *iḍā* and *piṅgalā,* and the extremely complex system of homologies that has been elaborated around them. For the moment, let us note a few of the synonyms for the *suṣumṇā: brahmanāḍī,*[108] *mahāpatha* (the "Great Way"), *śmaśāṇa* (the cemetery), *śāmbhavī* (=Durgā), *madhyamārga* (the "Middle Way"), *śaktimārga* (the way of Śakti).[109] Their symbolism will become clear later.

The descriptions of the *nāḍīs* are usually brief; clichés and stereotyped formulas abound, and we shall see that the "secret language" makes them even more difficult to understand. We cite one of the

101 *Triśikhibrāhmaṇopaniṣad,* 76.

102 *Śiva Saṃhitā,* II, 14; *Gorakṣa Śataka,* 13.

103 *Gorakṣa Paddhati,* 12.

104 *Triśikhibrāhmaṇopaniṣad,* 67.

105 *Haṭhayogapradīpikā,* IV, 8, etc.

106 *Gorakṣa Śataka,* 27, 28; some of the names differ in other lists; cf., for example, *Triśikhibrāhmaṇopaniṣad,* 70–75.

107 *Gorakṣa Śataka,* 29–31; but there are variants: according to other texts, some of the *nāḍīs* reach the heels.

108 *Haṭhayogapradīpikā,* II, 46.

109 Ibid., III, 4.

fundamental texts on the mystical structure of the *suṣumṇā:* "In the space outside the Meru,[110] placed on the left and the right, are the two Shirās,[111] Shashī[112] and Mihira.[113] The Nā*d*ī Su*sh*um*n*ā, whose substance is the threefold Gu*n*as,[114] is in the middle. She is the form of Moon, Sun, and Fire;[115] Her body, a string of blooming Dhūstūra[116] flowers, extends from the middle of the Kanda[117] to the Head, and the Vajrā inside Her extends, shining, from the Me*dh*ra[118] to the Head.

"Inside Her[119] is Chitri*n*ī, who is lustrous with the lustre of the Pra*n*ava[120] and attainable in Yoga by Yogīs. She (Chitri*n*ī) is subtle as a spider's thread, and pierces all the Lotuses which are placed within the backbone, and is pure intelligence.[121] She (Chitri*n*ī) is beautiful by reason of these (Lotuses) which are strung on her. Inside her (Chitri*n*ī) is the Brahma-nā*d*ī,[122] which extends from the orifice of the mouth of Hara[123] to the place beyond, where Ādi-deva[124] is.

"She[125] is beautiful like a chain of lightning and fine like a

110 The spinal column. (This and the following seventeen notes are by the translator of the text, Arthur Avalon [Sir John Woodroffe].)

111 I.e., Nā*d*īs.

112 Moon—that is the feminine, or Shakti-rupa Nā*d*ī I*d*ā, on the left.

113 Sun, or the masculine Nā*d*ī Pinggalā, on the right.

114 Meaning either the Gu*n*as, Sattva, Rajas, and Tamas; or, as "strings," the Nā*d*ī Su*sh*um*n*ā with the Nā*d*ī Vajrā inside it, and the Nā*d*ī Chitri*n*ī within the latter.

115 That is, as Chitri*n*ī, Vajri*n*ī, and Su*sh*um*n*ā.

116 *Dhatura fastuos.*

117 The root of all the Nā*d*īs. Kanda = Bulb.

118 Penis.

119 That is, inside Vajrā, which is, again, within Su*sh*um*n*ā.

120 The Mantra "Om."

121 Shuddhabodhasvarūpā. From her is derived Jnāna by those who are pure (Shangkara).

122 The Brahmanā*d*ī is not a Nā*d*ī separate from the Chitri*n*ī, but the channel in the latter.

123 Shiva; here the Svayambhu-lingga.

124 The Parama Bindu . . . The Brahma-nā*d*ī reaches the proximity of, but not the Ādi-deva Himself.

125 That is, Chitri*n*ī, the interior of which is called the Brahma-nā*d*ī.

(lotus) fibre, and shines in the minds of the sages. She is extremely subtle; the awakener of pure knowledge; the embodiment of all Bliss, whose true nature is pure Consciousness.[126] The Brahmadvāra [127] shines in her mouth. This place is the entrance to the region sprinkled by ambrosia, and is called the Knot as also the mouth of Su*sh*um*n*a."[128]

As we see, there is no doubt that what confronts us here is a "subtle" body and a "mystical physiology." Yet there is nothing "abstract" in the passage—we have, not conceptualizations, but images expressing transmundane experiences. The texts insistently repeat that, in the uninitiate, the *nāḍīs* have become "impure," that they are "obstructed" and must be "purified" by *āsanas*, *prāṇāyāma*, and *mudrās*.[129] The *iḍā* and the *piṅgalā* convey the two "breaths," but also all the subtle energy of the body; they are never simply "vessels" or "ducts," physiological organs. According to the *Sammohana-tantra*,[130] *iḍā* is the Śakti and *piṅgalā* is the Puruṣa. Other texts tell us that *lalanā* (=*iḍā*) and *rasanā* (=*piṅgalā*) respectively convey the semen and the ovum.[131] But semen is of the essence of Śiva and the moon, and blood (generally assimilated to the "*rajas* of women") is of the essence of the Śakti and the sun.[132] In the commentary on Kāṇhupāda's *Dohākoṣa*, it is said that the moon is born of the *semen virile* and the sun of the ovum.[133] Moreover, the commonest names for *iḍā* and *piṅgalā* in both the Hindu and Buddhist tantras are "sun" and "moon." The *Sammohana-tantra* says that the *nāḍī* on the left is the "moon" because of its gentle nature, and the *nāḍī* on the right is the "sun" because its nature is strong. The *Haṭhayogapradīpikā* compares

126 Shuddha-bodha-svabhāvā. 127 Door of Brahman.

128 *Ṣaṭcakranirūpaṇa*, 1–3; tr. Arthur Avalon (Sir John Woodroffe), *The Serpent Power*, pp. 4–12.

129 Cf., for example, *Haṭhayogapradīpikā*, I, 58.

130 Cited in the *Ṣaṭcakranirūpaṇa*.

131 *Sādhanamālā*, *Hevajra-tantra*, and *Herukta-tantra*, cited by Dasgupta, *Introduction to Tantric Buddhism*, p. 119.

132 *Gorakṣasiddhāntasaṃgraha*, cited by Dasgupta, p. 172, n. 4.

133 Dasgupta, p. 172, n. 5.

them to day and night, and we shall soon see the importance of this temporal symbolism. But we must not forget that *iḍā* and *piṅgalā* convey the *prāṇa* and the *apāna;* now, the former is Rāhu (the Asura who swallows the moon) and the *apāna* is the "fire of time" (*Kālāgni*).[134] This in itself gives us one of the keys to their symbolism; by using the principal "breaths" and the principal "subtle channels," one can destroy time.

In the Buddhist tantras *suṣumṇā* is replaced by *avadhūtī,* and this "nerve" is regarded as the road to *nirvāṇa.* The *Sādhanamālā* says: [135] "*Lalanā* [=*iḍā*] is of the nature of *prajñā* [Gnosis] and *rasanā* [=*piṅgalā*] is of the nature of *upāya* [means]: the *avadhūtī* remains in the middle as the seat of the *mahāsukha* [the Great Bliss]." The commentaries on the *Dohākoṣa* explain the term *avadhūtī* as "that which, through its effulgent nature, destroys all sins." [136]

Now, the texts constantly return to this theme: hold to the middle way; the left and the right are snares! "Cut off the two wings called the sun and the moon!" [137] "By destroying : : : the *lalanā* and the *rasanā* on both sides . . ." [138] "When the *candra* and the *sūrya* are rubbed and mixed up together, merit and demerit immediately disappear." [139] One gains the Great Bliss "by keeping close to the (middle) way and pressing [i.e., keeping under control] the right and the left (ways)." [140] "The right and the left are the pitfalls." [141]

For the moment, let us note two aspects of this symbolism: (1) the emphasis is put on the two principal breaths, *prāṇa* and *apāna,* assimilated to the sun and the moon; what is involved, then, is a cosmicization of the human body; (2) but all of the *sādhaka's* efforts are directed toward unifying the "moon" and the "sun," and to do

134 MS. commentary on Kāṇhupāda's *Dohākoṣa,* cited by Dasgupta, p. 173, n. 1.

135 Ed. Bhattacharyya, II, 448.

136 Cited by Dasgupta, p. 107.

137 Guṇḍarī, *Caryāpada,* 4.

138 Kāṇhupāda, *Dohākoṣa,* 3.

139 Saraha.

140 *Caryā,* 8, Kambalapāda.

141 *Caryā,* 32, Sarahapāda. All these texts quoted, with many others, by P. C. Bagchi, *Studies in the Tantras,* pp. 61 ff.

so he takes the "middle way." We shall soon see how polyvalent and complex is the symbolism of this sun-moon union. But let us first conclude our analysis of the subtle body by describing the *cakras*.

The Cakras

According to Hindu tradition, there are seven important *cakras*, which some authorities refer to the six plexuses and the *sutura frontalis*.[142]

(1) The *mūlādhāra* (*mūla* = root) is situated at the base of the spinal column, between the anal orifice and the genital organs (sacrococcygeal plexus). It has the form of a red lotus with four petals, on which are inscribed in gold the letters *v*, *ṣ*, *ś*, and *s*. In the middle of the lotus is a yellow square, emblem of the element earth (*pṛthivī*); at the center of the square is a triangle with its apex downward, symbol of the *yoni*, and called Kāmarūpa; at the center of the triangle is the *svayambhū-liṅga* (the *liṅga* existing by itself), its head as brilliant as a jewel. Coiled eight times (like a serpent) around it, as brilliant as lightning, sleeps Kuṇḍalinī, blocking the opening of the *liṅga* with her mouth (or her head). In this way Kuṇḍalinī obstructs the *brahmadvāra* (the "door of Brahman")[143] and access to the *suṣumṇā*. The *mūlādhāra cakra* is related to the cohesive power of matter, to inertia, the birth of sound, the sense of smell, the *apāna* breath, the gods Indra, Brahmā, Ḍākinī, Śakti, etc.

(2) The *svādhiṣṭhāna cakra*, also called *jalamaṇḍala* (because its *tattva* is *jala* = water) and *meḍhrādhāra* (*meḍhra* = penis), is situated at the base of the male genital organ (sacral plexus). Lotus with six vermilion petals inscribed with the letters, *b*, *bh*, *m*, *r*, *l*. In the middle of the lotus, a white half-moon, mystically related to Varuṇa. In the middle of the moon, a *bīja-mantra*, at the center of

142 For a fuller description, the reader should consult the most authoritative treatise on the doctrine of the *cakras*, the *Ṣaṭcakranirūpaṇa*, tr. Arthur Avalon. See also Note VI, 9.

143 See above, p. 239.

which is Viṣṇu flanked by the goddess Cākinī.[144] The *svādhiṣṭhāna cakra* is related to the element water, the color white, the *prāṇa* breath, the sense of taste, the hand, etc.

(3) The *maṇipūra* (*maṇi* = jewels; *pūra* = city) or *nābhiṣṭhāna* (*nābhi* = umbilicus), situated in the lumbar region at the level of the navel (epigastric plexus). Blue lotus with ten petals and the letters *ḍ, ḍh, ṇ, t, th, d, dh, n, p, ph*. In the middle of the lotus, a red triangle and on the triangle the god Mahārudra, seated on a bull, with Lākinī Śakti (blue in color) beside him. This *cakra* is related to the element fire, the sun, *rajas* (menstrual fluid), the *samāna* breath, the sense of sight, etc.

(4) The *anāhata* (*anāhahata śabd* is the sound produced without contact between two objects; i.e., a mystical sound); region of the heart, seat of the *prāṇa* and of the *jīvātman*. Color, red. Lotus with twelve golden petals (letters *k, kḥ, g, gḥ,* etc.). In the middle, two interlaced triangles forming a Solomon's seal, in the center of which is another golden triangle enclosing a shining *liṅga*. Above the two triangles is Īśvara with the Kākinī Śakti (red in color). The *anāhata cakra* is related to the element air, the sense of touch, the phallus, the motor force, the blood system, etc.

(5) The *viśuddha cakra* (the *cakra* of purity); region of the throat (laryngeal and pharyngeal plexus, at the junction of the spinal column and the medulla oblongata), seat of the *udāna* breath and of the *bindu*. Lotus with sixteen petals of smoky purple (letters *a, ā, i, u, ū,* etc.). Within the lotus a blue area, in the center of which is a white circle containing an elephant. On the elephant rests the *bīja-mantra h* (*Haṃg*), supporting Sadāśiva, half silver, half golden, for the god is represented under his androgynous aspect (*ardhanārīśvara*). Seated on a bull, he holds in his many hands a multitude of objects and emblems proper to him (*vajra*, trident, bell, etc.). One half of his body constitutes the Sadā Gāurī, with ten arms and five faces (with three eyes each). The *viśuddha cakra* is related to the color white, the ether (*ākāśa*), sound, the skin, etc.

144 According to *Śiva Saṃhitā*, V, 99, Rākinī.

(6) The *ājñā* (= order, command) *cakra*, situated between the eyebrows (cavernous plexus). White lotus with two petals bearing the letters *h* and *kṣ*. Seat of the cognitive faculties: *buddhi*, *ahaṃkāra*, *manas*, and the *indryas* (= the senses) in their "subtle" modality. In the lotus is a white triangle, apex downward (symbol of the *yoni*); in the middle of the triangle a white *liṅga*, called *itara* (the "other"). Here is the seat of Paramaśiva. The *bīja-mantra* is *OṂ*. The tutelary goddess is Hākinī; she has six faces and six arms and is seated on a white lotus.

(7) The *sahasrāra cakra:* at the top of the head, represented under the form of a thousand-petaled lotus (*sahasrā* = thousand), head down. Also called *brahmasthāna*, *brāhmarandhra*, *nirvāṇa cakra*, etc. The petals bear all the possible articulations of the Sanskrit alphabet, which has fifty letters (50 × 20). In the middle of the lotus is the full moon, enclosing a triangle. It is here that the final union (*unmanī*) of Śiva and Śakti, the final goal of tantric *sādhana*, is realized, and here the *kuṇḍalinī* ends its journey after traversing the six *cakras*. We should note that the *sahasrāra* no longer belongs to the plane of the body, that it already designates the plane of transcendence—and this explains why writers usually speak of the doctrine of the "six" *cakras*.

There are other *cakras*, of less importance. Thus, between the *mūlādhāra* and the *svādhiṣṭhāna* is the *yoniṣṭhāna;* this is the meeting place of Śiva and Śakti, a place of bliss, also called (like the *mūlādhāra*) *kāmarūpa*. It is the source of desire and, on the carnal level, an anticipation of the union Śiva-Śakti, which is accomplished in the *sahasrāra*. Near the *ājñā cakra* are the *manas cakra* and the *soma cakra*, related to the intellective functions and to certain yogic experiences. Near the *ājñā cakra* again is the *kārana-rūpa*, seat of the seven "causal forms," which are held to produce and constitute the "subtle" and the "physical" bodies. Finally, other texts refer to a number of *ādhāras* (= supports, receptacles), situated between the *cakras* or identified with them.[145]

The Buddhist tantras speak of only four *cakras*, situated respec-

145 See Note VI, 9.

tively in the umbilical, cardiac, and laryngeal regions and the cerebral plexus; this last *cakra*, the most important, is called *uṣṇīṣa-kamala* (lotus of the head) and corresponds to the *sahasrāra* of the Hindus. The three lower *cakras* are the sites of the three *kāyas* (bodies): *nirmāṇa-kāya* in the umbilical *cakra*, *dharma-kāya* in the *cakra* of the heart, *sambhoga-kāya* in the *cakra* of the throat. But there are anomalies and contradictions in regard to the number and locations of these *cakras*.[146] As in the Hindu traditions, the *cakras* are associated with *mudrās* and goddesses: Locanā, Māmakī, Pāṇḍarā, and Tārā.[147] In connection with the four *cakras*, the *Hevajra-tantra* gives a long list of quaternities: four *tattvas*, four *aṇgas*, four moments, four noble truths (*ārya-sattva*), etc.[148]

Viewed in projection, the *cakras* constitute a *maṇḍala* whose center is marked by the *brāhmarandhra*. It is in this "center" that the rupture of plane occurs, that the paradoxical act of transcendence—passing beyond *saṃsāra*, "emerging from time"—is accomplished. The symbolism of the *maṇḍala* is also a constituent element of Indian temples and sacred edifices in general: viewed in projection, a temple is a *maṇḍala*. We may, then, say that any ritual ambulation is equivalent to an approach to the center and that entrance into a temple repeats the initiatory entrance into a *maṇḍala* or the passage of the *kuṇḍalinī* through the *cakras*. Then again, the body is transformed both into a microcosm (with Mount Meru as center) and into a pantheon, each region and each "subtle" organ having its tutelary divinity, its *mantra*, its mystical letter, etc. Not only does the disciple identify himself with the cosmos; he also rediscovers the genesis and destruction of the universe in his own body. As we shall see, tantric *sādhana* comprises two stages: (1) cosmicization of the human being and (2) transcendence of the cosmos—that is, its destruction through the unification of opposites ("sun"—"moon," etc.). The pre-eminent sign of this transcendence is found in the final act of the *kuṇḍalinī's*

146 See Dasgupta, *Introduction to Tantric Buddhism*, pp. 163 ff.

147 *Śrī-samputa*, cited in Dasgupta, p. 165.

148 Dasgupta, pp. 166–67.

ascent—its union with Śiva, at the summit of the skull, in the *sahasrāra*.[149]

Kuṇḍalinī *

Some aspects of the *kuṇḍalinī* have already been mentioned; it is described at once under the form of a snake, of a goddess, and of an "energy." The *Haṭhayogapradīpikā* (III, 9) presents it in the following terms: "Kuṭilāṅgī ('crooked bodied'), Kuṇḍalinī, Bhujangī ('a she-serpent'), Śakti, Īśvarī, Kuṇḍalī, Arundhatī—all these words are synonymous. As a door is opened with a key, so the Yogī opens the door of *mukti* (deliverance) by opening Kuṇḍalinī by means of Haṭha Yoga."[150] When the sleeping goddess is awakened through the grace of the *guru*, all the *cakras* are quickly traversed.[151] Identified with Śabdabrahman, with *OṂ*, Kuṇḍalinī possesses all the attributes of all gods and all goddesses.[152] Under the form of a snake,[153] it dwells in the midpoint of the body (*dehamadhyayā*) of all creatures.[154] Under the form of Paraśakti, *kuṇḍalinī* manifests itself at the base of the trunk (*ādhāra*);[155] under the form of Paradevatā, it dwells in the middle of the knot at the center of the *ādhāra*, whence the *nāḍīs* issue.[156] Kuṇḍalinī moves in the *suṣumṇā* by the force aroused in the inner sense (*manas*) by the *prāṇa*, is "drawn upward through the *suṣumṇā* as a needle draws a thread."[157] Kuṇḍalinī is awakened by *āsanas* and *kumbhakas*; "then the Prāṇa becomes absorbed in Śūnya" (the Void).[158]

149 However, we must not forget that many tantric schools do not employ the symbolism of *kuṇḍalinī* to express the union of opposites. See below, p. 249.

150 Tr. Pañcham Sinh, cited in Bernard, p. 43. Cf. *Gorakṣa Śataka*, 51.

151 *Śiva Saṃhitā*, IV, 12–14; *Haṭhayogapradīpikā*, III, 1 ff.

152 *Śāradātilaka-tantra*, I, 14; I, 55; XXV, 6 ff.

153 Ibid., I, 54.

154 Ibid., I, 14.

155 Ibid., I, 53.

156 Ibid., XXVI, 34.

157 *Gorakṣa Śataka*, 49; tr. Briggs, p. 294.

158 *Haṭhayogapradīpikā*, IV, 10; tr. Pañcham Sinh, cited in Bernard, p. 45.

The awakening of the *kuṇḍalinī* arouses an intense heat, and its progress through the *cakras* is manifested by the lower part of the body becoming as inert and cold as a corpse, while the part through which the *kuṇḍalinī* passes is burning hot.[159] The Buddhist tantras even more strongly emphasize the fiery nature of the *kuṇḍalinī*. According to the Buddhists, the Śakti (also called Caṇḍālī, Ḍombī, Yoginī, Nairāmani, etc.) lies sleeping in the *nirmāṇa-kaya* (umbilical region); the adept wakes her by producing the *bodhicitta* in that region, and her awakening is revealed by the sensation of a "great fire." The *Hevajra-tantra* says that "the Caṇḍālī burns in the navel," and that when everything is burned, the moon (situated in the forehead) lets fall drops of nectar. A poem of Guñjarīpāda's presents the phenomenon in veiled terms: "The lotus and the thunder meet together in the middle and through their union Caṇḍālī is ablaze; that blazing fire is in contact with the house of the Ḍombī—I take the moon and pour water. Neither scorching heat nor smoke is found, but it enters the sky through the peak of Mount Meru." [160] We shall return to the signification of this symbolic vocabulary. But let us now note the following fact: according to the Buddhists, the secret force lies asleep in the umbilical region; through yogic practice, it is kindled and, like a fire, reaches the two higher *cakras* (*dharma* and *sambhoga*), enters them, reaches the *uṣṇīṣa-kamala* (corresponding to the *sahasrāra* of the Hindus), and, having "burned" everything in its path, returns to the *nirmāṇa-kaya*.[161] Other texts explain that this heat is obtained by the "transmutation" of sexual energy.[162]

The relations between the *kuṇḍalinī* (or the Caṇḍālī) and fire, the production of inner fire by the ascent of the *kuṇḍalinī* through the *cakras*, are facts requiring emphasis at this point. The reader will remember that, according to some myths, the goddess Śakti

159 Avalon, *The Serpent Power*, p. 242.

160 Cited in Dasgupta, *Obscure Religious Cults*, pp. 116 ff.

161 *Śrī-sampu-tikā*, MS. cited by Dasgupta, pp. 118–19.

162 Lama Kazi Dawa-Samdup and W. Y. Evans-Wentz, *Le Yoga tibétain et les doctrines secrètes* (French tr. of *Tibetan Yoga*), pp. 316 ff., 322 ff. See below, pp. 330 ff.

was created by the fiery energies of all the gods.[163] Then, too, it is well known that the production of "inner heat" is a very old "magical" technique, which reached its fullest development in shamanism.[164] We may note here and now that tantrism adheres to this universal magical tradition, although the spiritual content of its principal experience—the "fire" kindled by the ascent of the *kuṇḍalinī*—is on quite another plane than that of magic or shamanism. In any case, we shall have occasion, again in connection with the production of "inner heat," to examine the symbiosis tantrism-shamanism attested in certain Himālayan practices.

It is impossible to set about waking the *kuṇḍalinī* without the spiritual preparation implied by all the disciplines we have just discussed. But its actual awakening and its journey through the *cakras* are brought about by a technique whose essential element is arresting respiration (*kumbhaka*) by a special bodily position (*āsana, mudrā*). One of the most frequently used methods of arresting the breath is that prescribed by the *khecarīmudrā:* obstructing the cavum by turning the tongue back and inserting the tip of it into the throat.[165] The abundant salival secretion thus produced is interpreted as celestial ambrosia (*amṛta*) and the flesh of the tongue itself as the "flesh of the cow" that the yogin "eats."[166] This symbolical interpretation of a "physiological situation" is not without interest; it is an attempt to express the fact that the yogin already participates in "transcendence": he transgresses the strictest of Hindu prohibitions (eating cow flesh)—that is, he is no longer conditioned, is no longer in the world; hence he tastes the celestial ambrosia.

This is but one aspect of the *khecarīmudrā;* we shall see that the obstruction of the cavum by the tongue and the arrest of breathing that follows are accompanied by a sexual practice. Before presenting it, we shall add that the awakening of the *kuṇḍalinī*

163 See above, p. 203. 164 See below, p. 330.

165 To succeed, the frenum of the tongue must be cut beforehand. See Bernard's personal experience, pp. 37 ff.

166 *Haṭhayogapradīpikā*, III, 47–49.

brought about in this way is only the beginning of the exercise; the yogin further endeavors both to keep the *kuṇḍalinī* in the median "duct" (*suṣumṇā*) and to make it rise through the *cakras* to the top of the head. Now, according to the tantric authors themselves, this effort is rarely successful. We quote the following enigmatic passage from the *Tārākhaṇḍa* (it also occurs in the *Tantrasāra*): "Drinking, drinking, again drinking, drinking fall down upon earth; and getting up and again drinking, there is no re-birth." [167] This is an experience realized during total arrest of respiration. The commentary interprets: "During the first stage of Shaṭchakra Sâdhana [=penetration of the *cakras*], the Sâdhaka [disciple] cannot suppress his breath for a sufficiently long time at a stretch to enable him to practice concentration and meditation in each centre of Power [*cakra*]. He cannot therefore, detain Kuṇḍalinî within the Sushumnâ longer than his power of Kumbhaka [arresting respiration] permits. He must, consequently, come down upon earth—that is the Mûlâdhâra Chakra—which is the center of the element, earth, after having drunk of the heavenly ambrosia [which can be understood in various ways, and especially as the copious salivation provoked by obstruction of the cavum]. The Sâdhaka must practice this again and again, and by constant practice the cause of re-birth . . . is removed." [168]

To hasten the ascent of the *kuṇḍalinī*, some tantric schools combined corporal positions (*mudrā*) with sexual practices. The underlying idea was the necessity of achieving simultaneous "immobility" of breath, thought, and semen. The *Gorakṣa Saṃhitā* (61–71) states that during the *khecarīmudrā* the *bindu* (=sperm) "does not fall" even if one is embraced by a woman. And, "while the *bindu* remains in the body, there is no fear of Death. Even if the *bindu* has reached the fire (is ejaculated) it straightway returns, arrested . . . by the *yonimudrā*." [169] The *Haṭhayogapradīpikā* (III, 82) recommends the *vajrolīmudrā* for the

167 Avalon, *The Principles of Tantra*, II, cviii.
168 Ibid.
169 Tr. Briggs, *Gorakhnāth*, p. 298.

same purpose. Milk and an "obedient woman" are required. The yogin "should draw back up again with the *meḍhra* (the *bindu* discharged in *maithuna*)," [170] and the same act of reabsorption must also be performed by the woman. "Having drawn up his own discharged *bindu* [the Yogi] can preserve (it). . . . By the loss of *bindu* (comes) death, from its retention, life." [171] All these texts insist upon the interdependence between the breath, psychomental experience, and the *semen virile*. "So long as the air (breath) moves, *bindu* moves; (and) it becomes stationary (when the air) ceases to move. The Yogī should, therefore, control the air and obtain immovability. As long as *prāṇa* remains in the body, life (*jīva*) does not depart." [172]

We see, then, that the *bindu* is dependent upon the breath and is in some sort homologized to it; for the departure of the one as of the other is equivalent to death. The *bindu* is also homologized to the *citta*,[173] and thus there is finally homology of the three planes on which either "movement" or "immobility" are exercised: *prāṇa, bindu, citta*. As the *kuṇḍalinī* is weakened by a violent stoppage—whether of respiration or of seminal emission—it is important to know the structure and ramifications of the homology among the three planes. The more so as the texts do not always make it clear to which plane of reference they apply.

"Intentional Language" *

Tantric texts are often composed in an "intentional language" (*sandhā-bhāṣā*), a secret, dark, ambiguous language in which a state of consciousness is expressed by an erotic term and the vocabulary of mythology or cosmology is charged with Haṭha-yogic or sexual meanings. In the *Saddharmapuṇḍarīka* the expres-

170 Ibid., p. 333.

171 Ibid., p. 334.

172 *Gorakṣa Saṃhitā*, 90–91; tr. Briggs, p. 302.

173 In *Gorakṣa Saṃhitā*, 90, the Benares MS. reads *cittam* instead of *bindur* (cf. Briggs, p. 302), as does *Haṭhayogapradīpikā*, II, 2: "When the breath moves, the mind moves also; when the breath ceases to move, the mind becomes motionless." Cf. also ibid., IV, 21.

sions *sandhā-bhāṣita, sandhā-bhāṣya, sandhā-vacana* occur several times. Burnouf translated them as "enigmatic language," Kern as "mystery," and Max Müller as "hidden sayings." In 1916 Haraprasād Shāstri proposed "twilight language," language of "light and darkness" (*ālo-ā-dhāri*). But it was Vidhushekar Shāstri [174] who first showed that the term is based on a shortened form of the word *sandhāya*, which can be translated as "aiming at," "having in view," "intending," "with regard to," etc.[175] Hence there is no reference to the idea of a "twilight language." "It is quite possible that scribes not knowing the true significance of *sandhāya* or its shortened form *sandhā* changed it into *sandhyā* (=crepuscular), with which they were very familiar." [176] The *Hevajra-tantra* calls *sandhā-bhāṣā* the "great doctrine" (*mahāsamaya*) of the yogins, "the great language" (*mahābhāṣam*), and proclaims it "full of the meaning of the doctrines" (*samaya-saṇketa vistaraṃ*). The value of the term thus seems to be well established: "secret," "hidden." [177]

Ritual enigmas and riddles were in use from Vedic times; [178] in their particular way, they revealed the secrets of the universe. But in tantrism we find a whole system of elaborately worked-out ciphers, which the incommunicability of yogico-tantric experiences does not suffice to explain; to signify these kinds of experiences, symbols, *mantras*, and mystical letters had long been employed. The *sandhā-bhāṣā* pursues a different end—it seeks to conceal the doctrine from the noninitiate, but chiefly to project the yogin into the "paradoxical situation" indispensable to his training. The semantic polyvalence of words finally substitutes ambiguity for the usual system of reference inherent in every ordinary language. And this destruction of language contributes, in its way too, toward "breaking" the profane universe and replacing it by a universe of convertible and integrable planes. In general, symbolism

174 In his essay, "Sandhābhāṣā," *Indian Historical Quarterly*, IV, 2 (1928), 287–96.

175 Ibid., p. 289.

176 Ibid., p. 296.

177 See also Note VI, 10, with bibliography and summary of progress.

178 *Ṛg-Veda*, I, 164; I, 152, 3; VIII, 90, 14; X, 55, 5, etc.; *Atharva Veda*, VII, 1; XI, 8, 10.

brings about a universal "porousness," "opening" beings and things to transobjective meanings. But in tantrism "intentional language" becomes a mental exercise, forms an integral part of *sādhana.* The disciple must constantly experience the mysterious process of homologization and convergence that is at the root of cosmic manifestation, for he himself has now become a microcosm and, by "awakening" them, he must become conscious of all the forces that, on various planes, periodically create and absorb the universes. It is not only in order to hide the Great Secret from the noninitiate that he is asked to understand *bodhicitta* at once as "thought of awakening" and *semen virile;* through language itself (that is, by the creation of a new and paradoxical speech replacing the destroyed profane language) the yogin must enter the plane on which semen can be transformed into thought, and vice versa.

This process of destroying and reinventing language can be observed in the tantric poets, especially in the Buddhist Siddhacaryās, authors of "ciphered" songs, *caryās.* A poem by Kukkurīpāda reads: "When the *two* (teats) are milked (or when the tortoise is milked), it cannot be preserved in the pot; the tamarind of the tree is eaten by the crocodile. The front is near the house . . . The earring . . . is stolen away in the middle of the night. The father-in-law falls asleep, the daughter-in-law awakes —the thief has stolen away the earring, where can it be searched? Even in the day-time, the daughter-in-law shrieks in fear of the crow—where does she go at night? Such a *caryā* is sung by Kukkurī-pāda, and it has entered into the heart of only one among scores." [179]

According to the commentaries, the meaning seems to be this: the *two* are the two "veins," *iḍā* and *piṅgalā;* the liquid that is "milked" is the *bodhicitta* (N.B., which can be understood in several senses), and the "pot" (*pīta* = *pīṭha*) is the *maṇipūra* (the *cakra* of the umbilical region). The "tree" (*rukha* = *vṛkṣa*) signifies the body, and the "tamarind" the *semen virile* in its form of *bodhicitta,* the "crocodile" that "eats" it being yogic arrest of

179 Tr. Dasgupta, *Obscure Religious Cults,* pp. 480 f.

respiration (*kumbhaka*). The "house" is the seat of bliss; the "ear-ring" signifies the principle of defilement, the "thief" symbolizes *sahajānanda* (the bliss of the *sahaja*, which we shall discuss later); "midnight" is the state of complete absorption in supreme happiness. The "father-in-law" (*śvaśura*) is the breath; "day" signifies the active state (*pravṛtti*) of the mind, and "night" its state of repose (*nivṛtti*), etc.[180]

We find ourselves in a universe of analogies, homologies, and double meanings. In this "intentional language" any erotic phenomenon can express a Haṭha-yogic exercise or a stage of meditation, just as any symbol, any "state of holiness," can be given an erotic meaning. We arrive at the result that a tantric text can be read with a number of keys: liturgical, yogic, tantric, etc. The commentaries especially stress the two last. To read a text with the "yogic key" is to decipher the various stages of meditation to which it refers. The tantric meaning is usually erotic, but it is difficult to decide whether the reference is to a concrete act or to a sexual symbolism. More precisely, it is a delicate problem to distinguish between the "concrete" and the "symbolic," tantric *sādhana* having as its goal precisely the transubstantiation of every "concrete" experience, the transformation of physiology into liturgy.

Several stereotyped terms of Mahāyāna Buddhism are invested in tantrism with an added erotic meaning: *padma* (lotus) is interpreted as *bhaga* (womb); *vajra* (lit., "thunderbolt") signifies *liṇga* (= *membrum virile*). Thus it can be said that Buddha (*vajrasattva*) rests in the mysterious *bhaga* of the Bhagavatīs.[181] M. Shahidullah has reconstructed several series of equivalents, after the *Dohākoṣas;* P. C. Bagchi has studied the symbolism of certain technical vocabularies in the *Caryās;* but the interpretation of

180 Dasgupta, pp. 480 ff. It is remarkable that this enigmatic style has been continuously employed in modern Indian literature, from the *Caryāpādas* to our day; see ibid.

181 La Vallée Poussin, *Bouddhisme: Études et matériaux*, p. 134. For the equivalence *vajra* = *liṇga* in the *Haṭhayogapradīpikā*, cf. the index to Walter's edn., s.v. *vajrakandara.*

ciphered texts in "intentional" and allegorical language is still far from being completed.

We give a few examples, drawn chiefly from the *Dohākoṣas*:

vajra (thunderbolt) = *liṅga* = *śūnya* (emptiness).

ravi, sūrya (sun) = *rajas* of women (menses) = *piṅgalā* = right nostril = *upāya* (means).

śaśin, candra (moon) = *śukra* (*semen virile*) = *iḍā* = left nostril = *prajñā* (perfect wisdom).

lalanā (woman) = *iḍā* = *abhāva* (nonbeing) = *candra* = *apāna* = *nāda* = *prakṛti* (nature) = *tamas* (one of the three *guṇas*) = *gaṅgā* (the Ganges) = *svara* (vowels) = *nirvāṇa*, etc.

rasanā (tongue) = *piṅgalā* = *prāṇa* = *rajas* (one of the *guṇas*) = *puruṣa* = *vyañjana* (consonants) = *kāli* = *yamunā* (the river Yamunā) = *bhāva* (being), etc.

avadhūti = female ascetic = *suṣumṇā* = *prajñā* = *nairātma*, etc.

bodhicitta = the thought of awakening = *śukra* (*semen virile*).

taruṇī = girl = *mahāmudrā*.

gṛhiṇī = wife = *mahāmudrā* = *divyamudrā*, *jñānamudrā*.

samarasa = identity of enjoyment = coitus = arrest of breath = immobility of thought = arrest of semen.

Kāṇha [182] writes: "The Woman and the Tongue are immobilized on either side of the Sun and the Moon." The first meaning is Haṭha yogic—arrest of the two breaths (*prāṇa* and *apāna*) in the *iḍā* and the *piṅgalā*, followed by immobilization of the activity of these two "subtle veins." But there is a second meaning: the Woman is knowledge (*prajñā*) and the Tongue effort, means of action (*upāya*)—both Gnosis and the effort expended toward realization must be arrested, and this "immobilization" can be obtained only through Yoga (arrest of breath). But in this context "arrest of breath" is to be understood as accompanying arrest of

182 Shahidullah incorrectly describes him as a "nihilist"; cf. *Les Chants mystiques de Kāṇha et de Saraha*, p. 14: "Kāṇha and Saraha are nihilists. As with the Mādhyamika philosophers, nothing exists, neither *bhava* nor *nirvāṇa*, neither *bhāva* (being) nor *abhāva* (nonbeing). Truth is the Innate (*sahaja*), that is to say, emptiness." In fact, Kāṇha rejects the "thought of duality," the pairs of opposites, conditions—and seeks the unconditioned (*sahaja*).

seminal emission. Kāṇha expresses this in his sibylline style: "The Motionless embraces the Thought of Illumination" (so Shahidullah translates it; it can also be rendered "thought of awakening") "despite the dust that ornaments it. One sees the lotus seed, pure by nature, in one's own body." The Sanskrit commentary explains: if in *maithuna* (coitus) the *śukra* (sperm) remains unemitted, thought too remains motionless. In effect, the "dust" (*rajas*) is the "*rajas* of women" (both menses and genital secretions); during *maithuna*, the yogin provokes his partner's emission, at the same time immobilizing his *śukra*, with the twofold result that he both arrests his thought and becomes able to absorb the "lotus seed" (=the *rajas*).

We find here, then, the three "retentions" or "immobilities" referred to in Haṭha-yogic texts: arrest of breath, of semen, and of thought.[183] The deeper meaning of this "immobility" is not easy to penetrate. Before studying it, we may usefully consider the ritual function of sexuality in ancient India and in the yogico-tantric techniques.

Mystical Erotism

Maithuna was known from Vedic times, but it remained for tantrism to transform it into an instrument of salvation. In pretantric India, we must distinguish two possible ritual values of sexual union—both of which, we may note, are archaic in structure and of unquestionable antiquity: (1) conjugal union as a hierogamy; (2) orgiastic sexual union, to the end either of procuring universal fecundity (rain, harvests, flocks, women, etc.) or of creating a "magical defense." We shall not dwell upon the marital act transformed into a hierogamy: "I am the heaven; thou, the earth," says the husband to the wife.[184] The union is a ceremony, comprising many preliminary purifications, symbolical homologi-

183 See above, p. 248.

184 *Bṛhadāraṇyaka Upaniṣad*, VI, 4, 20; tr. Hume, *Thirteen Principal Upanishads*, p. 171.

zations, and prayers—just as in the performance of the Vedic ritual. The woman is first transfigured; she becomes the consecrated place where the sacrifice is performed: "Her lap is a sacrificial altar; her hairs, the sacrificial grass; her skin, the soma-press. The two lips of the vulva are the fire in the middle [of the vulva].[185] Verily, indeed, as great as is the world of him who sacrifices with the Vājapeya ('Strength-libation') sacrifice, so great is the world of him who practices sexual intercourse, knowing this." [186] Let us note a fact that is of importance. From the *Bṛhadāraṇyaka Upaniṣad* on, the belief becomes prevalent that the fruit of "works"—the result of a Vedic sacrifice—can be obtained by a ritually consummated marital union. The identification of the sacrificial fire with the female sexual organ is confirmed by the magical charm cast on the wife's lover: "You have made a libation in my fire," etc.[187] A ritual detail of the union, when it is wished that the woman shall not conceive, suggests certain obscure ideas concerning the reabsorption of semen: "He should first exhale, then inhale, and say: 'With power, with semen, I reclaim the semen from you!' Thus she comes to be without seed." [188] Hence the Haṭha-yogic technique may have existed, at least in the form of a "magical spell," from the period of the Upaniṣads. In any case, the preceding text connects the aspiration of semen with a respiratory act and a magical formula.

Conception takes place in the name of the gods:

> Let Vishṇu make the womb prepared!
> Let Tvashṭṛi shape the various forms!
>
> Prajāpati, let him pour in!
> Let Dhātṛi place the germ for thee!

185 Senart comments that the text appears to be corrupt. But no other translation is possible. Moreover, we have here a very old belief, according to which fire originates from the vagina; cf. Eliade, *Shamanism*, p. 363, n. 78.

186 *Bṛhadāraṇyaka Upaniṣad*, VI, 4, 3; tr. Hume, p. 168.

187 Ibid., VI, 4, 12; tr. Hume, p. 170.

188 Ibid., VI, 4, 10; tr. Hume, p. 169.

O Sinīvālī, give the germ;
O give the germ, thou broad-tressed dame!
Let the Twin Gods implace thy germ—
The Aśvins, crowned with lotus-wreaths! [189]

An adequate comprehension of such behavior will suffice to show us that here sexuality was no longer a psychophysiological situation, that it was valorized as ritual—whereafter the way was open to the tantric innovations. If the sexual plane is sanctified and homologized to the planes of ritual and myth, the same symbolism also operates in the opposite direction—the ritual is explained in sexual terms. "If, in the course of a recitation, the priest separates the first two quarters of a verse and brings the other two close together, this is because the woman separates her thighs and the man presses them during pairing; the priest thus represents pairing, so that the sacrifice will give a numerous progeny (*Ait. Brāhmaṇa*, X, 3, 2–4). The hotar's inaudible recitation is an emission of semen; the adhvaryu, when the hotar addresses the sacrificial summons to him, goes down on all fours and turns away his face; this is because quadrupeds turn their backs to emit semen (id., X, 6, 1–6). Then the adhvaryu rises and faces the hotar; this is because bipeds face each other to emit semen." [190]

We have seen [191] that, during the *mahāvrata*, a *puṃścalī* copulated ritually with a *brahmacārin* or a *māgadha* in the place consecrated for the sacrifice.[192] Probably this was at once a rite of "defense" and of "prosperity," as in the great horse sacrifice, the *aśvamedha*, in which the sacrificer's wife, the *mahiṣī*, pantomimed copulation with the sacrificial animal; at the end of the ceremony, the four wives were given over to the four great priests.[193] The ceremonial

189 *Bṛhadāraṇyaka Upaniṣad*, VI, 4, 21; tr. Hume, p. 172.

190 Lévi, *La Doctrine du sacrifice*, p. 107.

191 Above, p. 104.

192 See also *Āpastamba Śrauta Sūtra*, XXI, 17, 18; *Kāṭhaka Saṃhitā*, XXXIV, 5; *Taittirīya Saṃhitā*, VII, 5, 9, etc.

193 Cf. the texts in Paul Émile Dumont, *L'Aśvamedha*, pp. 260 ff. For the sexual elements in the agricultural fertility ceremonies, cf. J. J. Meyer, *Trilogie altindischer Mächte und Feste der Vegetation.*

union between the *brahmacārin* (lit., "chaste young man") and the *puṃścalī* (lit., "prostitute") may well express a desire to effect the *coincidentia oppositorum*, the reintegration of polarities, for we find the same motif in the mythologies and the iconographic symbolism of many archaic cults. However this may be, both in the *aśvamedha* and the *mahāvrata*, sexual rites still preserve their cosmological valence (the *aśvamedha* is a repetition of the cosmogony). It is when the deeper meaning of the "conjunction of opposites" begins to be lost from view that the sexual rite is renounced; *tad etad purāṇam utsannaṃ na kāryam*, says the *Śāṇkhāyana Śrauta Sūtra* (XVII, 6, 2), "this is an old custom; let it be done no longer." Louis de la Vallée Poussin saw in this injunction "the protest of the Dakṣiṇācāras against 'left-hand' ceremonies," [194] but this is unlikely, for sexual symbolism was far from being an innovation brought in by the *vāmacāras*. We have cited passages from the Brāhmaṇas and the Upaniṣads above; we may add one from the *Chāndogya Upaniṣad* (II, 13, 1–2), in which sexual union is transposed and valorized as liturgical chant (*sāman*), in particular the *vāmadevya* (the melody accompanying the pressing of the noonday *soma*):

One summons—that is a Hiṅkāra.
He makes request—that is a Prastāva.
Together with the woman he lies down—that is an Udgītha.
He lies upon the woman—that is a Pratihāra.
He comes to the end—that is a Nidhana.
He comes to the finish—that is a Nidhana.

This is the Vāmadevya Sāman as woven upon copulation.

He who knows thus this Vāmadevya Sāman as woven upon copulation comes to copulation, procreates himself from every copulation. . . . One should never abstain from any woman. That is his rule.[195]

Now, it is difficult to see how such a text could belong to the ideology of the "left hand"—what is primary here is the transmu-

194 *Bouddhisme: Études et matériaux*, p. 136.
195 Tr. Hume, p. 196.

tation of sexual union into liturgical chant (with all the religious consequences that ensue!). As we said, this transmutation of a psychophysiological activity into a sacrament is characteristic of every archaic spirituality. "Decadence" begins with the disappearance of the symbolical meaning of bodily activities; this is why the "old customs" are finally abandoned. But the symbolism of the conjunction of opposites continues to play an important role in Brāhmanic thought. That sexual union was felt as a "conjunction of opposites" is further proved by the fact that some texts replace the term *maithuna* by the term *saṃhitā*, "union"; this latter term is used to express the binary grouping of syllables, meters, melodies, etc., but also to express union with the gods and with Brahman.[196] Now, as we shall soon see, the conjunction of opposites constitutes the metaphysical constant of all tantric rituals and meditations.

The Buddhist texts also speak of *maithuna* (Pāli *methuna*),[197] and Buddha mentions certain ascetics who regard sensuality as one of the ways to gain *nirvāṇa*.[198] "We must bear in mind," writes L. de la Vallée Poussin,[199] "that several sects allowed monks to enjoy any 'unguarded' woman (that is, not married, not engaged, etc.). . . . The episode of the former donkey driver (or bird catcher) Ariṭṭha, who, though a monk, claimed that love was no obstacle to the holy life; that of the monk Magandika, who offered the Buddha his daughter Anupamā, the 'Incomparable,' should be noted (*Culla*, VI, 32; etc.)." We have too little data to be in a position to decipher the deeper meaning of all these customs. We must bear in mind that, from prehistoric times, India has known countless rites implying sexuality, and in the most various cultural contexts. Some of these rites, attested in the strata of "popular"

196 Cf. *Aitareya Araṇyaka*, III, 1, 6; *Śāṅkhāyana Araṇyaka*, VII, 14, etc. For the philosophical basis of the conjunction of opposing principles, see A. K. Coomaraswamy, *Spiritual Authority and Temporal Power in the Indian Theory of Government*.

197 Cf. *methuno dhammo*, *Kathāvatthu*, XXIII, 1–2.

198 Cf. *Dīgha-nikāya*, I, 36.

199 *Nirvāṇa*, p. 18 n.

magic, will demand our attention later. But it is highly probable that they are not related to the tantric technique of *maithuna.*

Maithuna

Every naked woman incarnates *prakṛti.*[200] Hence she is to be looked upon with the same adoration and the same detachment that one exercises in pondering the unfathomable secret of nature, its limitless capacity to create. The ritual nudity of the *yoginī* has an intrinsic mystical value: if, in the presence of the naked woman, one does not find in one's inmost being the same terrifying emotion that one feels before the revelation of the cosmic mystery, there is no rite, there is only a secular act, with all the familiar consequences (strengthening of the karmic chain, etc.). The second stage consists in the transformation of the woman-*prakṛti* into an incarnation of the Śakti; the partner in the rite becomes a goddess, as the yogin must incarnate the god. The tantric iconography of divine couples (in Tibetan: *yab-yam,* "father-mother"), of the innumerable "forms" of Buddha embraced by their Śaktis, constitutes the exemplary model of *maithuna.* We should note the immobility of the god; all the activity is on the side of the Śakti. (In the yogic context, the static *puruṣa* contemplates the creative activity of *prakṛti.*) Now, as we have seen before in the case of Haṭha Yoga, in tantrism immobility simultaneously realized on the three planes of "movement"—thought, respiration, seminal emission—constitutes the supreme goal of *sādhana.* Here again, there is imitation of a divine model—the Buddha, or Śiva, pure Spirit, motionless and serene amid the cosmic play.

Maithuna serves, in the first place, to make respiration rhythmical and to aid concentration; it is, then, a substitute for *prāṇāyāma* and *dhāraṇā,* or rather their "support." The *yoginī* is a girl whom the *guru* has instructed and whose body has been consecrated

200 Cf. Horace Hayman Wilson, *Sketch of the Religious Sects of the Hindus,* p. 156.

(*adhiṣṭhita*) by *nyāsas*. Sexual union is transformed into a ritual through which the human couple becomes a divine couple. "Prepared for the performance of the rite (*maithuna*) by the meditation and the ceremonies that make it possible and fruitful, he (i.e., the yogin) considers the *yoginī*, his companion and mistress, under the name of some Bhagavatī, as the substitute and the very essence of Tārā, sole source of joy and rest. The mistress synthesizes the entire nature of woman, she is mother, sister, wife, daughter; in her voice, demanding love, the officiant recognizes the voices of the Bhagavatīs supplicating Vajradhara, Vajrasattva. Such, for both the Śaiva and Bauddha tantric schools, is the way of salvation, of *bodhi*." [201] Moreover, the woman chosen for the *maithuna* rite is not always the common woman of orgies. The *Pañcakrama* presents a traditional ritual: "The *mudrā*, wife of the yogin, chosen according to established rules, offered and consecrated by the *guru*, must be young, beautiful, and learned: with her, the disciple will perform the ceremony, scrupulously observing the *śikṣās*: for if no salvation is possible without love (*strīvyatirekeṇa*), bodily union does not suffice to bring salvation. The practice of the Pāramitās, the goal of *kriyā*, must not be separated from it; let the *sādhaka* love the *mudrā* according to the rites: *nātikāmayet striyam*." [202]

Prāṇāyāma and *dhāraṇā* represent only means by which, during *maithuna*, the disciple achieves "immobility" and suppression of thought, the "supreme great happiness" (*paramamahāsukha*) of the *Dohākoṣas;* this is *samarasa* (Shahidullah translates it "identity of enjoyment"; but it is rather a "unity of emotion," or, more precisely, the paradoxical, inexpressible experience of the discovery of Unity). "Physiologically," *samarasa* is obtained, during *maithuna*, when the *śukra* and the *rajas* remain motionless.[203] But, as Shahidullah observes, "in accordance with the mystical language of the *Dohākoṣas*, we may explain *maithuna*, union of lotus (=*padma*) and thunder (=*vajra*), as realization of the state of emptiness (*vajra*=*śūnya*) in the plexus of the cerebral nerves (=*padma*). We may

201 La Vallée Poussin, *Bouddhisme: Études et matériaux*, p. 135.

202 Ibid., p. 141.

203 Shahidullah, p. 15.

also understand 'girl' as emptiness. In the *Caryās* (Bauddha Gāna), *nairātmya*, state of nonego, or *śūnya*, 'emptiness,' is described as a girl of low caste or a courtesan." [204] According to the *Pañcakrama*, studied by La Vallée Poussin, *maithuna* can be understood under the aspects both of a concrete act and an interiorized ritual made up of *mudrās* (=*yoginī*)—that is, of gestures, bodily postures, and strongly visualized images. "For monks, *maithuna* is an essential act of initiation (*saṃpradāya*). At the order of their *guru*, they disobey the laws of chastity, which they are thenceforth to observe. Such, it appears to me, is the doctrine of the *Pañcakrama* (III, 40). . . . He who does not actually practice *maithuna*, if he has

204 The role played by girls of low caste and courtesans in the tantric "orgies" (*cakra*, the tantric wheel) is well known. The more depraved and debauched the woman, the more fit she is for the rite. *Ḍombī* ("the washerwoman"; but, in the secret language, signifying *nairātmya*) is the favorite of all the tantric writers (cf. Kāṇha's *Caryās*, in Shahidullah, pp. 111 ff.). "O *ḍombī*! thou art all besoiled . . . Some call thee ugly. But the wise clasp thee to their bosoms. . . . O *ḍombī*! no woman is more dissolute than thou!" (Shahidullah, p. 120 n.). In the legends of the eighty-four *mahāsiddhas* (magicians), translated from the Tibetan by A. Grünwedel ("Die Geschichten der vier undachtzig Zauberer," *Baessler-Archiv*, V [1916], 137–228), we frequently find the motif of the low-caste girl, full of wisdom and possessing magical powers, who marries a king (pp. 147–48), who can make gold (pp. 221–22), etc. This exaltation of low-caste women has several causes. First, it is a part of the "popular" reaction against the orthodox systems, which also represents a counteroffensive of the autochthonous elements against the ideology of castes and the hierarchies introduced by the Indo-Āryan society. But this is only one aspect of the problem, and the least important. It is the symbolism of the "washerwoman" and the "courtesan" that is of chief significance, and we must reckon with the fact that, in accordance with the tantric doctrines of the identity of opposites, the "noblest and most precious" is hidden precisely in the "basest and most common." (The alchemists of the West did exactly the same when they affirmed that the *materia prima*, identical with the *lapis philosophorum*, was present everywhere and under the basest form, *vili figura*.) The authors of the *Caryās* saw the *ḍombī* as the representative of "emptiness"—that is, of the unqualified and unformulable *Grund*, for only the "washerwoman" was free from every qualification and attribute, social, religious, ethical, etc. For the role of woman as spiritual guide in tantrism, see W. Koppers, "Probleme der indischen Religionsgeschichte," *Anthropos*, XXV–XXVI (1940–41), 798 ff.

practiced it once in his life, at the time of his initiation, obtains the supreme *samāpatti* by virtue of Yoga. . . . *Maithuna* is not actually practiced (*saṃvṛtyā = lokavyavahārataḥ*): it is replaced by exercises of an inner nature, by acts in which the *mudrā* (*yoginī*) is an intellectual form, a symbolic gesticulation, an impression or a curious operation of physiology." [205]

The texts frequently emphasize this idea that *maithuna* is above all an integration of the principles; "the true sexual union is the union of the Paraśakti [*kuṇḍalinī*] with Ātman; other unions represent only carnal relations with women." [206] The *Kālīvilāsa-tantra* (X–XI) gives the ritual, but stipulates that it is only to be performed with an initiated wife (*parastrī*). A commentator adds that the ceremony called *pañcatattva* (the five *makāras*—that is, the five terms beginning with the letter *m: matsya*, fish; *māṃsa*, meat; *madya*, intoxicating drink; *mudrā*, and *maithuna*) is performed in its literal meaning only by the low castes (*śūdra*). The same text elsewhere says (V) that this ritual is designed for the *kali-yuga*—that is, it is adapted to the present cosmico-historical stage, in which the Spirit is hidden, "fallen" into a carnal condition. But the author knows very well that the *pañcatattva* is interpreted literally, especially in magical circles and in the less orthodox regions, and he quotes the *Nigama-tantra-sāra:* "In Gaura and other countries, one can obtain *siddhis* through the *paśubhāva*" (the *pañcatattva* practiced physically).

We have already noted that the tantrics are divided into two classes: the *samayins*, who believe in the identity of Śiva and Śakti and attempt to awaken the *kuṇḍalinī* by spiritual exercises, and the *kaulās*, who venerate the Kaulinī (= *kuṇḍalinī*) and employ concrete rituals. This distinction is no doubt valid, but it is not always easy to be perfectly sure how far a ritual is to be understood literally: we have seen [207] in what sense "drunkenness" carried to the point of "falling to the ground" was to be interpreted. Now, coarse and brutal language is often used as a trap for the noninitiate. A cele-

205 La Vallée Poussin, *Bouddhisme: Études et matériaux*, pp. 142–43.
206 *Kulārṇava-tantra*, V, 111–12. 207 See above, p. 248.

brated text, the *Śaktisaṅgama-tantra*, devoted almost entirely to the *ṣaṭcakrabheda* (= "penetration of the six *cakras*"), employs an extremely "concrete" vocabulary [208] to describe spiritual exercises.[209] The ambiguity of the erotic vocabulary of tantric literature cannot be too strongly emphasized. The ascent of the Caṇḍālī through the yogin's body is often compared with the dance of the "washerwoman" (*ḍomḅī*). "With the *ḍomḅī* in [his] neck" (i.e., in the *sambhogakāya* near the neck), the yogin "passes the night in great bliss." [210]

Nevertheless, *maithuna* is also practiced as a concrete ritual. By the fact that the act is no longer profane but a rite, that the partners are no longer human beings but "detached" like gods, sexual union no longer participates in the cosmic plane. The tantric texts frequently repeat the saying, "By the same acts that cause some men to burn in hell for thousands of years, the yogin gains his eternal salvation" (*karmaṇāyena vai sattvāh kalpakotiśatānyapi, pacyante narake ghore tena yogī vimucyate*).[211] This, as we know, is the foundation stone of the Yoga expounded by Kṛṣṇa in the *Bhagavad Gītā:* (XVIII, 17): "He who has no feeling of egoism, and whose mind is not tainted, even though he kills (all) these people, kills not, is not fettered (by the action)." [212] And the *Bṛhadāraṇyaka Upaniṣad* (V, 14, 8) had already said: "One who knows this, although he commits very much evil, consumes it all and becomes clean and pure, ageless and immortal." [213]

Buddha himself, if we are to believe the mythology of the tantric cycle, had set the example; it was by practicing *maithuna* that he

208 To such a point that the editor of the text, Benoytosh Bhattacharyya, has taken the precaution of substituting *X's* for the sexual terms; cf. *Śaktisaṅgama-tantra*, I: *Kālīkhaṇḍa*; II: *Tārākhaṇḍa*.

209 See ibid., II, 126–31, on the five *makāras;* according to Bhattacharyya, the terms are not to be taken as "fish," "meat," *maithuna*, etc., but as technical terms referring to meditations.

210 See the texts quoted in Dasgupta, *Obscure Religious Cults*, pp. 120 ff.

211 Indrabhuti, *Jñānasiddhi*, 15; ed. Bhattacharyya, *Two Vajrayāna Works*, p. 32. See further texts in Note VI, 11.

212 Tr. Telang, p. 123.

213 Tr. Hume, p. 157.

had succeeded in conquering Māra, and the same technique had made him omniscient and the master of magical powers.[214] Practices "in the Chinese fashion" (*cīnācāra*) are recommended in many Buddhist tantras. *Mahācīnā-kramā-cāra*, also entitled *Cīnācāra-sāra-tantra*, tells how the sage Vasiṣṭha, son of Brahmā, goes to find Viṣṇu, under the aspect of the Buddha, to ask him about the rites of the goddess Tārā. "He enters the great country of China and sees the Buddha surrounded by a thousand mistresses in erotic ecstasy. The sage's surprise verges on indignation. 'These are practices contrary to the Vedas!' he cries. A voice from space corrects him: 'If,' says the voice, 'thou wouldst gain my favor, it is with these practices in the Chinese fashion that thou must worship me!' He approaches the Buddha and receives from his lips this unexpected lesson: 'Women are the gods, women are life, women are adornment. Be ever among women in thought!' "[215] According to a legend of Chinese tantrism, a woman of Yen-chu gave herself to every young man; after her death it was discovered that she was the "Bodhisattva of chained bones" (that is, the bones of her skeleton were linked together like chains).[216]

This entire aspect goes beyond *maithuna*, properly speaking, and is part of the great movement of devotion to the "Divine Woman" that, from the seventh to eighth century, dominates all India. We have seen the predominance of Śakti in the economy of salvation and the importance of woman in spiritual disciplines. With Viṣṇuism in its Kṛṣṇaist form, love (*prema*) is called upon to assume the leading role. It is chiefly an adulterous love, love of *parakīyā rati*, "another's wife"; in the famous Bengalese Courts of Love disputes were arranged between the Viṣṇuist adherents of the *parakīyā* and

214 É. Senart, *Essai sur la légende du Buddha*, pp. 303–08.

215 S. Lévi, *Le Népal*, I, 346–47. See also id., "Notes chinoises sur l'Inde," *Bulletin de l'École française d'Extrême-Orient*, V (1905), 253–305. Cf. Sir John Woodroffe, *Shakti and Shākta*, pp. 179 ff.

216 Chou Yi-liang, "Tantrism in China" (*Harvard Journal of Asiatic Studies*, VIII [1945], 241–332), pp. 327–28. But this praise of carnal love can be explained by the importance accorded (especially in Taoist circles) to sexual techniques as a means of prolonging life; cf. Note VI, 12.

the champions of conjugal love, *svakīyā*—and the latter were always the losers. The exemplary love remained that which bound Rādhā to Kṛṣṇa—a secret, illegitimate, "antisocial" love, symbolizing the rupture that every genuine religious experience imposes. (It should be noted that, from the Hindu point of view, the conjugal symbolism of Christian mysticism, in which Christ plays the part of the Bridegroom, does not sufficiently emphasize such an abandonment of all social and moral values as mystical love implies.)

Rādhā is conceived as the infinite love that constitutes the very essence of Kṛṣṇa.[217] Woman participates in the nature of Rādhā and man in the nature of Kṛṣṇa; hence the "truth" concerning the loves of Kṛṣṇa and Rādhā can be known only in the body itself, and this knowledge on the plane of "corporeality" has a universal metaphysical validity. The *Ratna-sāra* proclaims that he who realizes the "truth of the body" (*bhāṇḍa*) can then attain to the "truth of the universe" (*brahmāṇḍa*).[218] But, as in all the other tantric and mystical schools, when man and woman are mentioned, it is not the "ordinary man" (*sāmānya mānuṣ*), the "man of passions" (*rāger mānuṣ*), who is meant, but the essential, archetypal man, man "unborn" (*ayoni mānuṣ*), "unconditioned" (*sahaja mānuṣ*), "eternal" (*nityer mānuṣ*); similarly, it is not with an "ordinary woman" (*sāmānya rati*) that one can discover the essence of Rādhā, but with the "extraordinary woman" (*viśeṣa rati*).[219] The "meeting" between man and woman takes place in Vrindaban, the mythical scene of the loves of Kṛṣṇa and Rādhā; their union is a "play" (*līlā*)—that is, it is freed from the weight of the cosmos, is pure spontaneity. Besides, all the mythologies and techniques of the conjunction of opposites are homologizable; Śiva-Śakti, Buddha-Śakti, Kṛṣṇa-Rādhā can be translated into any "union" (*iḍā* and *piṅgalā*, *kuṇḍalinī* and Śiva, *prajñā* and *upāya*, "breath" and "thought," etc.). Every conjunction of opposites produces a rupture of plane and ends in the rediscovery of the primordial spontaneity. Often a mythological schema is at once interiorized and

217 See the texts quoted by Dasgupta, *Obscure Religious Cults*, pp. 142 ff.

218 Ibid., p. 165.

219 Ibid., p. 162.

"incarnated" by the employment of the tantric theory of the *cakras*. In a Viṣṇuist poem, the *Brahma Saṃhitā*, the *sahasrāra cakra* is assimilated to Gokula, the abode of Kṛṣṇa. And a nineteenth-century Viṣṇuist poet, Kamalā-Kānta, in his *Sādhaka-rañjana*, compares Rādhā with *kuṇḍalinī* and describes her running to her secret tryst with Kṛṣṇa as the ascent of the *kuṇḍalinī* to unite with Śiva in the *sahasrāra*.[220]

More than one of the Buddhist or Viṣṇuist mystical schools continued to employ the yogico-tantric *maithuna* even when "devotional love" evidently played the essential role. The profound mystical movement known as Sahajīyā, which continues tantrism, and which, like tantrism, is as Buddhist as it is Hindu, still accords their old priority to erotic techniques.[221] But, as in tantrism and Haṭha Yoga, sexual union is understood as a means of obtaining "supreme bliss" (*mahāsukha*), and it must never end in seminal emission. *Maithuna* makes its appearance as the consummation of a long and difficult apprenticeship. The neophyte must acquire perfect control of his senses, and, to this end, he must approach the "devout woman" (*nāyīkā*) by stages and transform her into a goddess through an interiorized iconographic dramaturgy. Thus, for the first four months, he should wait upon her like a servant, sleep in the same room with her, then at her feet. During the next four months, while continuing to wait upon her as before, he sleeps in the same bed, on the left side. During a third four months, he will sleep on the right side, then they will sleep embracing, etc. The goal of all these preliminaries is "autonomization" of sensual pleasure—regarded as the sole human experience capable of bringing about the nirvāṇic bliss—and control of the senses—that is, arrest of semen.

In the *Nāyīkā-sādhana-ṭīkā* ("Commentaries on Spiritual Discipline in Company with Woman"), the ceremonial is described in detail. It comprises eight parts, beginning with *sādhana*, mystical concentration with the help of liturgical formulas; then follow

220 Dasgupta, pp. 150 ff.

221 See Note VI, 13.

smaraṇa ("recollection," "penetration into consciousness"); *āropa* [222] ("attribution of qualities to the object"), in which flowers are ceremonially offered to the *nāyīkā* (who is beginning to be transformed into a goddess); *manana* ("remembering the woman's beauty when she is absent"), which is already an interiorization of the ritual. In the fifth stage, *dhyāna* ("mystical meditation") the woman sits on the yogin's left and is embraced "in such wise that the spirit is inspired." [223] In the *pūjā* (the "cult," properly speaking), the place where the *nāyīkā* is seated receives worship, offerings are made, and the *nāyīkā* is bathed as if she were the statue of a goddess. During this time, the yogin mentally repeats formulas. His concentration reaches its maximum when he carries the *nāyīkā* in his arms and lays her on the bed, repeating the formula: *Hlīng klīng kandarpa svāhā*. The union that takes place is between two "gods." The erotic play is realized on a transphysiological plane, for it never comes to an end. During the *maithuna*, the yogin and his *nāyīkā* embody a "divine condition," in the sense that they not only experience bliss but are also able to contemplate the ultimate reality directly.

The "Conjunction of Opposites"

We must not forget that *maithuna* is never allowed to terminate in an emission of semen: *bodhicittam notsṛjet*, "the semen must not be emitted," the texts repeat. [224] Otherwise the yogin falls under the

222 *Āropa* plays an important role in Sahajīyā. It designates the first movement toward transcendence: ceasing to see the human being in its physical, biological, and psychological aspects and viewing it instead in an ontological perspective; cf. texts in Dasgupta, *Obscure Religious Cults*, pp. 158 ff.

223 "The woman must not be touched for the sake of bodily pleasure, but for the perfecting of the spirit," the *Ānandabhairava* specifies; quoted by M. M. Bose, *The Post-Caitanya Sahajiā Cult of Bengal*, pp. 77–78.

224 Cf., for example, *Guṇavratanirdeśa*, cited in *Subhāṣitasaṃgraha*, ed. C. Bendall, *Muséon*, n.s., IV-V, 44: *bhage liṅgaṃ pratiṣṭhāpya bodhicittam na cotsṛjet*. Taoism, too, knows similar techniques, though in a cruder form; cf. H. Maspéro, "Les Procédés de 'Nourrir le principe vital,' " pp. 383 ff. But

law of time and death, like any common libertine.[225] In these practices, "sensual pleasure" plays the part of a "vehicle," for it produces the maximum tension that abolishes normal consciousness and inaugurates the nirvāṇic state, *samarasa*, the paradoxical experience of Unity. As we have seen earlier, *samarasa* is obtained by the "immobilization" of breath, thought, and semen. Kāṇha's *Dohākoṣas* constantly revert to this theme: the breath "does not descend and does not rise; doing neither, it remains motionless." [226] "He who has immobilized the king of his spirit through identity of enjoyment [*samarasa*] in the state of the Innate [*sahaja*], instantly becomes a magician; he fears not old age and death." [227] "If one fixes a strong lock on the entrance door of breath, if in that terrible darkness one makes the spirit a lamp, if the jewel of the *jina* touches the supreme heaven above, Kāṇha says, one accomplishes *nirvāṇa* while still enjoying existence." [228]

It is in "identity of enjoyment," in the inexpressible experience of Unity (*samarasa*), that one reaches the state of *sahaja*, of nonconditioned existence, of pure spontaneity. All these terms are, of course, difficult to translate. Each of them attempts to express the paradoxical state of absolute nonduality (*advaya*) that issues in *mahāsukha*, the "Great Bliss." Like the *brahman* of the Upaniṣads and Vedānta, and the *nirvāṇa* of the Mahāyānists, the state of *sahaja* is indefinable; it cannot be known dialectically, it can only be apprehended through actual experience.[229] "The whole world,"

---

the aim of these techniques was not to obtain a paradoxical nirvāṇic state, but to economize the "vital principle" and prolong youth and life. These Taoist erotic rituals sometimes assumed the proportions of a collective orgy (Maspéro, pp. 402 ff.); they were probably vestiges of ancient seasonal festivals. But the spiritual horizon peculiar to *maithuna* is entirely different from that of the archaic orgies, whose sole purpose was to ensure universal fertility. See Note VI, 12.

225 Cf. Kāṇha, *Dohākoṣa*, 14; *Haṭhayogapradīpikā*, III, 88, etc.

226 *Dohākoṣa*, 13; after Shahidullah's tr.

227 Ibid., 19.

228 Ibid., 22.

229 See the texts from the *Dohākoṣa* and tantras given by Dasgupta, pp. 91 ff.

says the *Hevajra-tantra*, "is of the nature of *sahaja*—for *sahaja* is the quintessence (*svarūpa*) of all; this quintessence is *nirvāṇa* to those who possess the perfectly pure *citta*." [230] One "realizes" the state of *sahaja* by transcending the dualities; this is why the concepts of *advaya* (nonduality) and *yuganaddha* (principle of union) have an important place in tantric metaphysics. The *Pañcakrama* discusses the concept of *yuganaddha* at length: it is a state of unity obtained by doing away with two polar and contradictory notions, *saṃsāra* (=the cosmic process) and *nivṛtti* (=absolute arrest of all process); one transcends these two notions by becoming conscious that the ultimate nature of the phenomenal world (*saṃkleśa*) is identical with that of the absolute (*vyavadāna*); hence one realizes synthesis between the notions of formal existence and of the nonformed, etc.[231]

In this dialectic of opposites we recognize the favorite theme of the Mādhyamikas and, in general, of the Mahāyānist philosophers. But the tantrist is concerned with *sādhana*; he wants to "realize" the paradox expressed in all the images and formulas concerning the union of opposites, he wants concrete, experimental knowledge of the state of nonduality. The Buddhist texts had made two pairs of opposites especially popular—*prajñā*, wisdom, and *upāya*, the means to attain it; *śūnya*, the void, and *karuṇā*, compassion. To "unify" or "transcend" them was, in sum, to attain the paradoxical position of a Bodhisattva—in his wisdom, the Bodhisattva no longer sees persons (for, metaphysically, the "person" does not exist; all that exists is an aggregation of the five *skandhas*), and yet, in his compassion, he undertakes to save persons. Tantrism multiplies the pairs of opposites (sun and moon, Śiva and Śakti, *iḍā* and *piṅgalā*, etc.) and, as we have just seen, attempts to "unify" them through techniques combining subtle physiology with meditation. This fact must be emphasized: on whatever plane it is realized, the conjunction of opposites represents a transcending of the phenomenal world, abolishment of all experience of duality.

230 Tr. Dasgupta, p. 90.
231 Unprinted text quoted by Dasgupta, p. 32, n. 1.

The images employed suggest return to a primordial state of nondifferentiation; unification of sun and moon represents "destruction of the cosmos," and hence return to the original Unity. In Haṭha Yoga, the adept works to obtain "immobility" of breath and semen; there is even supposed to be a "return of semen"—that is, a paradoxical act, impossible to execute in a "normal" physiological context dependent upon a "normal" cosmos; in other words, the "return of semen" stands, on the physiological plane, for a transcendence of the phenomenal world, entrance into freedom. This is but one application of what is termed "going against the current" (*ujāna sādhana*), or of the "regressive" process (*ulṭā*) of the Nātha Siddhas, implying a complete "inversion" of all psychophysiological processes; it is, basically, the mysterious *parāvṛtti* that is already to be found in Mahāyānic texts, which, in tantrism, also designates the "return of semen." [232] For one who realizes them, this "return," this "regression," imply destruction of the cosmos and hence "emergence from time," entrance into "immortality." In the *Gorakṣa Vijaya*, Durgā (=Śakti, Prakṛti) asks Śiva: "Why is it, my Lord, that thou art immortal, and mortal am I? Advise me the truth, O Lord, so that I also may be immortal for ages." [233] It is on this occasion that Śiva reveals the doctrine of Haṭha Yoga. Now, immortality cannot be gained except by *arresting manifestation*, and hence the process of disintegration; one must proceed "against the current" (*ujāna sādhana*) and once again find the primordial, motionless Unity, which existed before the rupture. This is what the Haṭha yogins do when they unite the "sun" and "moon." The paradoxical act takes place on several planes at once: through the union of Śakti (=*kuṇḍalinī*) with Śiva in the *sahasrāra*, the yogin brings about inversion of the cosmic process, regression to the undiscriminated state of the original Totality; "physiologically," the conjunction sun-moon is represented by the "union" of the *prāṇa* and *apāna*—that is, by a "totalization" of the breaths; in short, by their arrest; finally, sexual union,

232 See Note VI, 1.
233 For this and other texts, see Dasgupta, pp. 256 ff.

through the action of the *vajrolīmudrā*,[234] realizes the "return of semen."[235]

As we have seen, the union of "sun" and "moon" is brought about by unification of the breaths and vital energies circulating in the *iḍā* and *piṅgalā;* it takes place in the *suṣumṇā*. Now, the *Haṭha-yogapradīpikā* (IV, 16–17) says that "the *suṣumṇā* devours time." The texts dwell upon the "conquest of death" and the immortality that the yogin who "conquers time" obtains. To arrest respiration, suspend thought, immobilize the semen—these are only formulas expressing the same paradox of the abolishment of time. We have noted that every effort to transcend the cosmos is preceded by a long process of "cosmicizing" the body and the psychomental life, for it is from a perfect "cosmos" that the yogin sets out to transcend the cosmic condition. But "cosmicization," first realized through *prāṇāyāma*, already modifies the yogin's temporal experience.[236] The *Kālacakra-tantra* relates inhalation and exhalation to day and night, then to the half months, months, years, thus progressively reaching the longest cosmic cycles. This is equivalent to saying that, through his own respiratory rhythm, the yogin repeats and, as it were, relives the cosmic Great Time, the periodical creations and destructions of the universes (the cosmic "days and nights"). By arresting his breathing, by "unifying" it in the *suṣumṇā*, he transcends the phenomenal world, he passes into that nonconditioned and timeless state in which "there is neither day nor night," "neither sickness nor death"—naïve and inadequate formulas to signify "emergence from time." To transcend "day and night" means to transcend the opposites. In the language of the Nātha Siddhas, it is the reabsorption of the cosmos through inversion of all the processes of manifestation. It is the coincidence of time and eternity, of *bhāva* and *nirvāṇa;* on the purely "human" plane, it is the reintegration of the primordial androgyne, the conjunction, in one's own being, of male and female—in a word, the reconquest of the completeness that precedes all creation.

234 See above, p. 248.

235 Cf. texts in Dasgupta, pp. 274 ff.

236 Cf. Eliade, *Images and Symbols*, pp. 86 ff.

In short, this nostalgia for the primordial completeness and bliss is what animates and informs all the techniques that lead to the *coincidentia oppositorum* in one's own being. We know that the same nostalgia, with an astonishing variety of symbolisms and techniques, is found almost everywhere in the archaic world; [237] we know, too, that many aberrant ceremonies have their basis and theoretical justification in the desire to recover the "paradisal" state of primordial man. Most of the excesses, cruelties, and aberrations referred to as "tantric orgies" spring, in the last analysis, from the same traditional metaphysics, which refused to define ultimate reality otherwise than as the *coincidentia oppositorum*. Some of these excesses, certain "popular" forms connected with tantric theories and methods, will be examined in a later chapter.

But we have still to emphasize an aspect of tantric *sādhana* that is generally overlooked; we refer to the particular meaning of cosmic reabsorption. After describing the process of creation by Śiva (I, 69–77), the *Śiva Saṃhitā* describes the inverse process, in which the yogin takes part: he sees the element earth become "subtle" and dissolve in water, water dissolve in fire, fire in air, air in ether, etc., until everything is reabsorbed into the Great Brahman. Now, the yogin undertakes this spiritual exercise in order to anticipate the process of reabsorption that occurs at death. In other words, through his *sādhana*, the yogin already witnesses the reabsorption of these cosmic elements into their respective matrices, a process set in motion at the instant of death and continuing during the first stages of existence beyond the world. The *Bardo Thödol* gives some invaluable information on the subject. Viewed from this angle, tantric *sādhana* is centered on the experience of initiatory death, as we should expect, since every archaic spiritual discipline implies initiation in one form or another—that is, the experience of ritual death and resurrection. In this respect the tantrist is a "dead man in life," for he has experienced his own death in advance; he is, by the same token, "twice born," in the

237 Cf. Eliade, *Patterns in Comparative Religion*, pp. 419 ff.

initiatory sense of the term, for he has not gained this "new birth" on a purely theoretical plane, but by means of a personal experience. It is possible that many references to the yogin's "immortality," references that are especially frequent in Haṭha-yogic texts, ultimately stem from the experiences of such "dead men in life."

Yoga and Alchemy

Legends of Yogins as Alchemists

THE tantric Vajrayāna was directed to obtaining a "body of diamond," incorruptible, not subject to becoming. Haṭha Yoga strengthened the body to prepare it for the final "transmutation" and make it fit for "immortality." As we have just seen, the tantric processes took place in a subtle body, which was homologized with both the cosmos and the pantheon, a body in some sort already divinized. An important detail is that the disciple was required to contemplate the dissolution and creation of the universe and finally to experience in himself the "death" (= dissolution) and "resurrection" (= re-creation) both of the cosmos and of his own subtle body.[1] This process of dissolution and re-creation suggests the *solve et coagula* of Western alchemy. Like the alchemist, the yogin effects transformations in "substance"; and in India "substance" is the work of Prakṛti or of Śakti (or of Māyā, archetype of the magician). Hence tantric yoga inevitably opened the way to an alchemical continuation. On the one hand, by mastering the secrets of the Śakti, the yogin is able to imitate its "transformations," and the transmutation of common metals into gold is soon included among the traditional *siddhis;* on the other hand, the "diamond body" of the Vajrayānists, the *siddha-deha* of the Haṭha yogins is not unlike the "body of glory" of the Western alchemists; the adept realizes the transmutation of the flesh, constructs a divine body

1 See above, p. 272.

(*divya-deha*), a "body of wisdom" (*jñāna-deha*), a receptacle worthy of him who is "liberated in this life" (*jīvan-mukta*).

The unity between Yoga and alchemy was felt not only by the first foreign travelers to India, but also by the Indian people, who soon elaborated a whole yogico-alchemical folklore by incorporating the themes of the elixir of immortality and the transmutation of metals into the mythology of the yogin-magician. Before examining the alchemical texts proper, we may profitably cite some travelers' observations and some legends of famous alchemists; as is so often the case, myth is more eloquent than historical reality, and enables us to apprehend the deeper meaning of a historical fact better than the documents that record it.

Marco Polo, describing the *chugchi* (yogins) who "live 150 or 200 years," writes: "These people make use of a very strange beverage, for they make a potion of sulphur and quicksilver mixt together and this they drink twice every month. This, they say, gives them long life; and it is a potion they are used to take from their childhood." [2] Polo seems not to have attached much importance to the yogin-alchemists. François Bernier, on the contrary, who had observed various sects of Indian ascetics, made them the subject of several penetrating pages, which, until the beginning of the nineteenth century, remained the principal source of information concerning yogins and fakirs.[3] He did not fail to note their alchemical knowledge: "There are others, very different from these, who are strange people; they are almost constantly traveling hither and thither; they are men who scoff at everything, who take no care for anything; men possessing secrets, and who, the people say, even know how to make gold and to prepare mercury so admirably, that one or two grains taken in the morning restore the body to perfect health and so fortify the stomach that it digests very well and can hardly be satisfied." [4]

The tradition that the Indian ascetics knew the secret of obtaining

2 Sir Henry Yule, *The Book of Ser Marco Polo*, ed. Henri Cordier, II, 365 ff.

3 Cf. *Voyages de François Bernier*, II, 121–31. 4 Ibid., II, 130.

longevity through drugs is also found in the Moslem historians: "I have read in a book that certain chiefs of Turkistán sent ambassadors with letters to the kings of India on the following mission, viz.: that they, the chiefs, had been informed that in India drugs were procurable which possessed the property of prolonging human life, by the use of which the kings of India attained to a very great age . . . and the chiefs of Turkistán begged that some of this medicine might be sent to them, and also information as to the method by which the Ráís preserved their health so long." [5]

According to Emir Khosru, the Indians also obtained long life through *prāṇāyāma:* "Through their art they [the Brāhmans] can procure longevity by diminishing the daily number of their expirations of breath. A *jogí* who could restrain his breath in this way lived . . . to an age of more than three hundred and fifty years." [6] The same writer gives the following account of the yogins: "They can tell future events by the breath of their nostrils, according as the right or left orifice is more or less open. They can also inflate another's body by their own breath. In the hills on the borders of Kashmír there are many such people. . . . They can also fly like fowls in the air, however improbable it may seem. They can also, by putting antimony on their eyes, make themselves invisible at pleasure. Those only can believe all this who have seen it with their own eyes." [7] We recognize most of the yogic *siddhis,* first of all power to "fly through the air." We may note in passing that this *siddhi* was finally taken over into alchemical literature.[8]

Indian literature is full of references to yogin-alchemists. "When I was a boy," says the famous Jain ascetic Hemacandra to Devacandra, "a lump of copper, having been smeared with the juice of a

5 Tr. Sir Henry M. Elliot, *The History of India as Told by Its Own Historians,* II, 174. The legend of an Indian plant that would confer eternal life was known in Persia from the time of King Khosru (531–579); cf. J. T. Reinaud, *Mémoire géographique, historique et scientifique sur l'Inde,* p. 130. There are references to the potion of immortality in the *Jātakas* too, but this potion probably derives from the legend of ambrosia rather than from alchemy.

6 *Nuh Sipihr,* "The Nine Heavens (or Spheres)," tr. Elliot, III, 563.

7 Ibid., III, 563–64.

8 See Note VII, 1.

creeper . . . had fire applied to it under your instructions and became gold. Tell us the name of that creeper and its characteristics, and other necessary particulars connected with it."[9] But it was especially around the famous Nāgārjuna that alchemical legends crystallized. To be sure, this legendary personage, referred to by Somadeva (eleventh century) in his *Kathāsaritsāgara* and by Merutunga in his *Prabandhacintāmaṇi*, is not the same as the illustrious Mādhyamika doctor; we know that a whole tantric, alchemical, and magical literature was added to the biography of the famous philosopher. But it is important to emphasize to what an extent, in the exemplary image of Nāgārjuna (the only image that imposed itself, and has been retained by the collective memory), tantrism and magic are presented as saturated with alchemy. In the *Kathāsaritsāgara*, we read that Nāgārjuna, minister of Chirāyus, succeeded in preparing the elixir, but that Indra commanded him not to communicate the use of it to anyone.[10] Somadeva, as a good Brāhman, was determined to uphold the prestige of Indra even in comparison with so powerful a magician as Nāgārjuna. In the *Prabandhacintāmaṇi*, Nāgārjuna concocts an elixir that enables him to fly through the air.[11] According to other legends, when famine was ravaging the land, he made gold and exchanged it for grain imported from distant countries.[12] We shall later have occasion to return to Nāgārjuna. But for the present we should emphasize that belief in the ability of yogins to transmute metals is still alive in India. Russell and William Crooke encountered yogins who claimed to change copper into gold; they said they had received the power from one of their masters in the time of Sultan

9 *Prabandhacintāmaṇi*, tr. C. H. Tawney, p. 147; cf. ibid., p. 173: a monk obtains an elixir that changes everything it touches into gold. The author is the Jain monk Merutunga (fourteenth century), who also wrote a commentary on the alchemical treatise *Rasādhyāya;* cf. A. B. Keith, *A History of Sanskrit Literature*, p. 512. On the "man of gold," see *Prabandhacintāmaṇi*, p. 8; Johannes Hertel, *Indische Märchen*, p. 235. The legend of the philosophers' stone in India also occurs in the *Āīn-i-Akbarī* of Abū'l Faḍl (1551–1602), tr. H. Blochmann and H. S. Jarrett, II, 197.

10 Tr. C. H. Tawney, ed. N. M. Penzer, *The Ocean of Story*, III, 257 ff.

11 Tr. Tawney, pp. 195–96.

12 See Note VII, 2.

Altitmish (or Altamsh). Oman too tells of a *sādhu* who was an alchemist.[13] We shall see that alchemical powers crystallized especially around the eighty-four tantric *siddhas* and that, in some regions, alchemy merges with tantric yoga and magic.

Tantrism, Haṭha Yoga, and Alchemy

In his description of India, al-Bīrūnī especially emphasizes the connections of alchemy with longevity and the restoration of youth. "They have a science similar to alchemy which is quite peculiar to them. They call it *Rasâyana*, a word composed with *rasa, i.e.* gold. It means an art which is restricted to certain operations, drugs, and compound medicines, most of which are taken from plants. Its principles restore the health of those who were ill beyond hope, and give back youth to fading old age, so that people become again what they were in the age near puberty; white hair becomes black again, the keenness of the senses is restored as well as the capacity for juvenile agility, and even for cohabitation, and the life of people in this world is even extended to a long period. And why not? Have we not already mentioned on the authority of Patañjali that one of the methods leading to liberation is *Rasâyana?*" [14] And it is true that Vyāsa and Vācaspatimiśra, commenting on a *sūtra* of Patañjali's [15] that mentions simples (*auṣadhi*) as one of the means of gaining the "perfections," interpret *auṣadhi* as elixir of long life, obtained by *rasāyana*.

Some Orientalists (A. B. Keith, Lüders) and most historians of the sciences (J. Ruska, Stapleton, R. Müller, E. von Lippmann) have maintained that alchemy was introduced into India by the Arabs; they have particularly stressed the alchemical importance of

13 R. V. Russell and Rai Bahadur Hīra Lāl, *The Tribes and Castes of the Central Provinces of India*, II, 398; William Crooke, *Tribes and Castes of the North-western Provinces and Oudh*, III, 61; J. C. Oman, *The Mystics, Ascetics and Saints of India*, pp. 59 ff.

14 Tr. Edward C. Sachau, *Alberuni's India*, I, 188–89.

15 *Yoga-sūtras*, IV, 1.

mercury and its late appearance in the texts. Now, mercury is mentioned in the Bower Manuscript (fourth cent. A.D.) [16] and perhaps even in the *Arthaśāstra* (third cent. B.C.), and always in connection with alchemy.[17] In addition, a number of Buddhist texts mention alchemy long before the influence of Arabic culture. The *Avataṃsaka Sūtra*, which can be dated approximately between A.D. 150 and 350 (it was translated into Chinese by Sikṣānanda in 695–99), says: "There is a drug-juice called Hataka. One *liang* of it will turn a thousand *liangs* of bronze into pure gold." [18] The *Mahāprajñāpāramitopadeśa* (translated by Kumārajīva in 402–05) is still more explicit: "By drugs and incantations one can change bronze into gold. By skilful use of drugs silver can be changed into gold, and gold into silver." [19] These are not the only texts,[20] but we shall restrict ourselves to citing a passage from the *Mahāprajñāpāramitāśāstra*, the important treatise by Nāgārjuna translated into Chinese by Kumārajīva (A.D. 344–413, hence a good three centuries before the flowering of Arabian alchemy, which begins with Jābir ibn-Ḥayyān, *c.* A.D. 760). Among the "metamorphoses" (*nirmāṇa*), Nāgārjuna cites a long list of *siddhis* (shrinking to the size of an atom, enlarging to the point of filling space, etc.; passing through stone walls, walking on air, touching the sun and moon with one's hand), ending with the transformation "of stone into gold and gold into stone." He then adds: "There are four further kinds of *nirmāṇas* (metamorphoses): (1) in the world of desire (*kāmadhātu*) one can transform substances (*dravya*) by herbs (*oṣadhi*), precious objects, and magical artifices; (2) beings

16 Cf. A. F. R. Hoernle, ed., *The Bower Manuscript*, p. 107.

17 According to R. Müller and E. von Lippmann (*Entstehung und Ausbreitung der Alchemie*, II, 179), the term *rāsa* in the Bower Manuscript does not refer to mercury; but the problem is not yet closed. On mercury and alchemy in the *Arthaśāstra*, cf. R. V. Patvardhan, "Rasavidyā or Alchemy in Ancient India," *Proceedings and Transactions of the First Oriental Congress*, I, clv; Moriz Winternitz, *Some Problems of Indian Literature*, p. 101.

18 Tr. Arthur Waley, "References to Alchemy in Buddhist Scriptures," *Bulletin of the School of Oriental Studies*, London Institution, VI, 4 (1932), 1102.

19 Ibid.

20 See Note VII, 3.

endowed with the superknowledges (*abhijñā*) can transform substances by the force of their magical power (*ṛddhibala*); (3) the Devas, Nāgas, Asuras, etc., by the force of retribution (*vipākabala*) of their (previous) existences, can transform substances; (4) beings retributed in an existence in the material world (*rūpadhātu*) can transform substances by the force of concentration (*samādhibala*)." [21] From which we must conclude that the transmutation of metals could be accomplished not only by vegetable or mineral alchemy and magic but also by the "force of *samādhi*"—that is, by Yoga. We shall soon see that the same tradition is attested in other texts.

We may say at once that nothing proves any dependence of Indian alchemy upon Arabic culture. On the contrary, alchemical ideology and practices are found in ascetic circles—that is, precisely where, when India is later invaded by the Moslems, Islamic influence produces almost no effect. Alchemy is connected with Yoga and tantrism, which are archaic and pan-Indian traditions. We find alchemical tantras preponderantly in regions where Islam hardly penetrated, in Nepāl and in the Tamil country (where alchemists are called *sittars*—that is, *siddhas*).

It is especially in the literature and traditions of tantrism that we find the most distinct references to alchemy and the greatest number of names of alchemist-*siddhas*. The *Subhāṣitasaṃgraha* [22] gives mercury an important role; the *Sādhanamālā* [23] mentions *rasarasāyana* as the fifth *siddhi*. A work by Siddha Carpaṭi speaks of alchemical processes.[24] The *Śiva Saṃhitā* (III, 54) says that the yogin can make gold from any metal by rubbing it with his own excrement and urine; there is a similar statement in the *Yogatattva Upaniṣad* (74), in which, however, alchemy is regarded (30) as an obstacle on the road of yogic perfection. The great tantric

21 Tr. after Lamotte, *Traité*, I, 382–83.

22 Ed. Bendall, p. 40, strophe beginning *rasaghṛṣṭaṃ yathā*.

23 Ed. Bhattacharyya, I, 350; cf. introd., pp. 85–86.

24 Cf. the fragment of the *Devamanusyastotra*, in G. Tucci, "Animadversiones Indicae," *Journal of the Asiatic Society of Bengal*, XXVI (1930), 137.

treatise translated from the Tibetan by A. Grünwedel under the title "Die Geschichten der vierundachtzig Zauberer" [25] informs us concerning the alchemical practices of the *siddhas:* Karnari obtains the elixir from urine [26] and can transmute copper into silver and silver into gold; [27] Capari knows the dye by which gold can be made; [28] Guru Vyāli attempts to make gold from silver and drugs,[29] etc. Writing of another tantric master, Vāgīśvarakirti, Tāranātha said that he "conjured up quantities of the elixir of life, and distributed it to others, so that old people, 150 years old and more, became young again." [30]

All these legends and all these references to the symbiosis tantrism-alchemy leave no doubt of the soteriological function of alchemical operations. We have here no prechemistry, no science in embryo, but a spiritual technique, which, while operating on "matter," sought first of all to "perfect the spirit," to bring about deliverance and autonomy. If we set aside the folklore that proliferated around the alchemists (as around all "magicians"), we shall understand the correspondence between the alchemist working on "vulgar" metals to transmute them into "gold" and the yogin working on himself to the end of "extracting" from his dark, enslaved psychomental life the free and autonomous spirit, which shares in the same essence as gold. For, in India as elsewhere, "gold is immortality" (*amṛtam āyur hiraṇyam*).[31] Gold is the one perfect, solar metal and hence its symbolism meets the symbolism of Spirit, of spiritual freedom and autonomy. The adept hoped to prolong life indefinitely by absorbing gold. But, according to an alchemical treatise, the *Rasaratnasamuccaya,* before gold could be absorbed, it had to be purified and "fixed" with mercury.[32]

That we are not dealing with an empirical science, with a pre-

25 *Baessler-Archiv,* V (1916), 137–228.

26 Ibid., pp. 165–67.

27 Ibid., pp. 205–06.

28 Ibid., p. 202.

29 Ibid., pp. 221–22.

30 Cited in Edward Conze, *Buddhism, Its Essence and Development,* p. 179.

31 *Maitrāyaṇī Saṃhitā,* II, 2, 2; *Śatapatha Brāhmaṇa,* III, 8, 2, 27; *Aitareya Brāhmaṇa,* VII, 4, 6, etc.

32 Text cited by P. C. Rāy, *A History of Hindu Chemistry,* I, 105.

chemistry, is sufficiently clear from the chapter that Mādhava devotes to the *raseśvaradarśana* (lit., the "science of mercury") in his *Sarvadarśanasaṃgraha.*[33] For liberation depends on the "stability of the human body"; hence mercury, which strengthens and prolongs life, is also a means of liberation. A text cited in the *Sarvadarśanasaṃgraha* declares that "liberation results from knowledge, knowledge from study, and study is only possible in a healthy body." The ideal of the ascetic is to obtain "liberation in this life," to be a *jīvan-mukta. Rasa* (mercury)[34] is the quintessence of Śiva; it is also called *pārada,* because it leads to the further shore of the world. It is likewise the seed of Hara (=Śiva), and *abhra* (mica) is the ovum of the goddess (Gaurī); the substance produced by their union can make man immortal. This "glorified body" was obtained by a great number of *jīvan-muktas,* among whom the text cites Carvati, Kapila, Vyāli, Kāpāli, Kandalāyana.

Mādhava emphasizes the soteriological function of alchemy. "The mercurial system is not to be looked upon as merely eulogistic of the metal, it being immediately, through the conservation of the body, a means to the highest end, liberation."[35] And the *Rasasiddhanta,* a treatise on alchemy cited by Mādhava, says: "The liberation of the personal soul [*jīva*] is declared in the mercurial system, O subtile thinker."[36] A text from the *Rasārṇava,* and another that Mādhava does not name (*anyatrāpi*), say that the merit that accrues from seeing mercury is equal to the merit one gains by seeing and worshiping the phallic emblems at Benares or any other sacred place.

Like other tantric and Haṭha-yogic treatises, the *Rasārṇava* begins with a dialogue between Bhairava (Śiva) and the goddess: she asks him for the secret of *jīvan-mukti,* and Śiva tells her that it is seldom known, even among the gods. Deliverance after death is

33 Ānandāśrama Series ed., pp. 48–53; tr. E. B. Cowell and A. E. Gough, pp. 137–44.

34 In some tantras mercury is regarded as the generative principle and instructions are given for making a mercurial phallus dedicated to Śiva; cf. Rāy, I, introd., 79.

35 Tr. Cowell and Gough, p. 140. 36 Ibid.

worthless (stanzas 4–5). According to the same treatise, the body can be kept alive indefinitely if one learns to control the breath (*vāyu*, lit. "vital wind") and to apply mercury. Now, this suggests the yoga of the Nātha Siddhas, which attempts to master the "vital wind" and to regulate the secretion of *soma;* the technique is even named *somarasa.*[37] There is another group of ascetics, the Siddhas of the *śuddha mārga* (the "pure way"), who distinguish two kinds of "incorruptible bodies"—that of the man "liberated in life" (*jīvan-mukta*) and that of the *parā-mukta;* the former is constituted by a sort of transmutation of Māyā, is immortal, and above all processes of disintegration, but it ends by being absorbed into the "body of pure light," or "divine body," the *divya-deha* or *jñāna-deha;* this second body, being wholly spiritual (*cinmaya*), no longer belongs to matter. In tantric terminology, these two incorruptible bodies are called *baindava* and *śakta* respectively. According to some texts, the Nātha Siddhas also distinguished the *siddha-deha* from the *divya-deha.*[38]

To summarize, we may say that the physico-chemical processes of the *rasāyana* serve as the "vehicle" for psychic and spiritual operations.[39] The "elixir" obtained by alchemy corresponds to the "immortality" pursued by tantric yoga; just as the disciple works directly on his body and his psychomental life in order to transmute the flesh into a "divine body" and free the Spirit, so the alchemist works on matter to change it into "gold"—that is, to hasten its process of maturation, to "finish" it. Hence there is an occult correspondence between "matter" and man's physico-psychic body—which will not surprise us if we remember the homology man-cosmos, so important in tantrism. Once the process of interiorization had led men to expect spiritual results from rites and physiological operations, it followed logically that similar results

37 Dasgupta, *Obscure Religious Cults*, pp. 292 ff.

38 Ibid., pp. 293 ff.

39 This tradition of alchemy is said to have adherents in India even today. Cf. C. S. Nārāyaṇaswami Aiyar, "Ancient Indian Chemistry and Alchemy of the Chemico-Philosophical Siddhānta System of the Indian Mystics," *Proceedings and Transactions of the Third Oriental Conference*, pp. 597–614.

could be obtained by interiorizing operations performed on "matter"; in a certain spiritual condition, communication between the different cosmic levels became possible. The alchemist accepted and continued the archaic tradition—attested by numerous myths and "primitive" behavior patterns—that regarded "matter" not only as alive but more especially as a reservoir of sacred forces. For him, as for the "primitive" magician and the tantrist, the problem was to awaken these forces and master them. The cosmos was not opaque, inert, "objective"; to the eyes of the initiated, it revealed itself as alive, as guided by "sympathy." Minerals, metals, and precious stones were not "objects" having a particular economic value; they incarnated cosmic forces and hence participated in the sacred.

Chinese Alchemy

We find a similar situation in China. Here, too, alchemy is built up by employing the traditional cosmological principles, the myths concerning the elixir of immortality and the Blessed Immortals (*hsien*), the techniques whose threefold goal was prolongation of life, bliss, and spiritual spontaneity.[40] Gold and jade, by the fact that they participate in the cosmological principle *yang*, preserve bodies from corruption. "If there is gold and jade in the nine apertures of the corpse, it will be preserved from putrefaction," writes the alchemist Ko Hung. And T'ao Hung-king (fifth century) gives the following details: "When on opening an ancient grave the corpse looks . . . alive, then there is inside and outside of the body a large quantity of gold and jade. According to the regulations of the Han dynasty, princes and lords were buried in clothes adorned with pearls, and with boxes of jade, for the purpose of preserving the body from decay." [41]

40 See summary of progress and bibliography, Note VII, 4.

41 B. Laufer, *Jade*, p. 299, n. 1. See also J. J. M. de Groot, *The Religious System of China*, I, 269; J. Przyluski, "L'Or, son origine et ses pouvoirs magiques" (*Bulletin de l'École française d'Extrême-Orient*, XIV [1914], 1–17), p. 8.

For the same reason, vessels made of alchemical gold have a peculiar virtue: they prolong life forever. The magician Li Shao-chün says to the emperor Wu Ti of the Han dynasty: "Sacrifice to the stove (*tsao*) and you will be able to summon 'things' (i.e., spirits). Summon spirits and you will be able to change cinnabar powder into yellow gold. With this yellow gold you may make vessels to eat and drink out of. You will then increase your span of life. Having increased your span of life, you will be able to see the *hsien* of P'êng-lai that is in the midst of the sea. Then you may perform the sacrifices *fêng* and *shan*, and escape death." [42] The most celebrated of Chinese alchemists, Pao P'u Tzŭ (pseudonym of Ko Hung, 254–334),[43] says: "If with this alchemical gold you make dishes and bowls, and eat and drink out of them, you shall live long." [44] To be efficacious, gold must be "prepared." "Made" gold is better than natural gold.[45] The Chinese believed that substances found in the ground were impure and that they needed "preparation," just like foodstuffs, in order to be assimilable.[46]

> If even the herb *chü-shēng* can make one live longer,
> Why not try putting the Elixir into the mouth?
> Gold by nature does not rot or decay;
> Therefore it is of all things most precious.
> When the artist [i.e., alchemist] includes it in his diet

42 Ssŭ-ma Ch'ien, *Shih Chi* ("History"), ch. XXVII. The tr. given is by A. Waley, "Notes on Chinese Alchemy" (*Bulletin of the School of Oriental Studies*, London Institution, VI, 1 [1930], 1–24), p. 2. The passage has also been translated by Édouard Chavannes, *Les Mémoires historiques de Se-ma-Ts'ien*, vol. III, pt. 2, p. 465; by O. S. Johnson, *A Study of Chinese Alchemy*, pp. 76–77, and by H. H. Dubs, "The Beginnings of Alchemy" (*Isis*, XXXVIII [1947], 62–86), pp. 67–68.

43 Cf. Note VII, 4.

44 Tr. Waley, "Notes," p. 4.

45 Gold produced by the alchemical processes of sublimation and transmutation possessed a higher vitality, which was of help in obtaining salvation and immortality. The alchemist sought to find the gold of transcendental quality that would make possible the spiritualization of the human body. Cf. Laufer, review of O. S. Johnson, *A Study of Chinese Alchemy*, in *Isis*, XII (1929), 331.

46 Waley, p. 18.

The duration of his life becomes everlasting . . .
When the golden powder enters the five entrails,
A fog is dispelled, like rain-clouds scattered by wind . . .
Hairs that were white all turn to black;
Teeth that had fallen out grow in their former place.
The old dotard is again a lusty youth;
The decrepit crone is again a young girl.
He whose form is changed and has escaped the perils of life,
Has for his title the name of True Man.[47]

The first historical reference to alchemy is in connection with the making of gold; in 144 B.C. an imperial edict decreed public execution for anyone who should be caught counterfeiting gold.[48] According to W. H. Barnes, the earliest references to alchemy may be of the fourth or third century B.C. Dubs believes [49] that the founder of Chinese alchemy was Tsou Yen, a contemporary of Mencius (fourth century B.C.). Whether or not this view is warranted, it is important that we distinguish between the historical beginning and development of a prechemistry, on the one hand, and alchemy as a soteriological technique, on the other; the latter was intimately connected (and so remained until the eighteenth century of our era) with methods and mythologies—in large part Taoistic—that pursued a very different end from "making gold."

Gold was associated with empire: it was found at the "center" of the earth and had mystical connections with *jue* (realgar or sulphur), yellow quicksilver, and the future life (the "yellow springs"). So it is presented in a text of 122 B.C., the *Huai Nan Tzŭ*, in which we also find evidence of a belief in a hastened metamorphosis of metals.[50] This text may come from the school of

47 *Ts'an T'ung Ch'i*, ch. XXVII; tr. Waley, "Notes," p. 11; tr. Lu-Ch'iang Wu and T. L. Davis, "An Ancient Chinese Treatise on Alchemy Entitled *Ts'an T'ung Ch'i*," *Isis*, XVIII (1932), 240–41. *Ts'an T'ung Ch'i*, the title of the popular alchemical treatise by Wei Po-yang (a pseudonym in the "style" of Lao Tzŭ, fl. A.D. 120–150), means "Union of Composite Correspondences." On this treatise, see Lu-Ch'iang Wu and Davis, pp. 212–16; Johnson, *A Study of Chinese Alchemy*, p. 133.

48 Text in Dubs, "Beginnings," p. 63. 49 Ibid., p. 77.

50 Fragment tr. by Dubs, pp. 71–73.

Tsou Yen, if not from the master himself.[51] Belief in the natural metamorphosis of metals was quite old in China, and is also found in Annam, India, and the Indian Archipelago. The Tonkinese peasants say: "Black bronze is the mother of gold." Gold is naturally engendered by bronze. But if this natural transmutation is to take place, the bronze must lie in the ground for a long time. "Thus the Annamese are convinced that the gold found in mines has been slowly formed on the spot during the course of ages, and that if the ground had been opened in the beginning, bronze would have been discovered where gold is found today."[52] The alchemist only hastens the growth of metals; like his Western colleague, the Chinese alchemist contributes to the work of nature by accelerating the rhythm of time. But we must not forget that the transmutation of metals into gold also has a "spiritual" side; gold being the imperial, "perfect" metal, "liberated" from impurities, the alchemical operation implicitly pursues the "perfecting" of nature—that is, in the last analysis, its absolution and freedom. The gestation of metals in the depths of the earth obeys the same temporal rhythms that "bind" man in his carnal and fallen condition; to hasten the growth of metals by the alchemical *opus* is equivalent to absolving them from the law of time. By a like application of suitable techniques, the yogin and the tantric emancipate themselves from their temporal condition and conquer "immortality." Let us recall the Vedic adage: gold is immortality.

This explains the fact that alchemical operations are always connected with liberation from time. In China "preparing gold," obtaining the "drug of immortality," and "evoking" the Immortals are clearly interrelated: Luan Tai presented himself before the Emperor Wu and offered to perform these three miracles, but he succeeded only in "materializing" the Immortals.[53] Another celebrated figure, Liu Hsiang (79–8 B.C.), undertook to "make gold," but also failed.[54] Some centuries later, Pao P'u Tzŭ (Ko

51 Ibid., p. 74.

52 Przyluski, "L'Or," p. 3.

53 Ssŭ-ma Ch'ien, tr. Chavannes, *Mémoires*, III, 479.

54 Texts in Dubs, p. 74.

Hung) attempts to explain Liu Hsiang's ill success by saying that he did not possess the "true medicine" (the "philosophers' stone"), and that he had not been spiritually prepared (the alchemist must fast a hundred days, purify himself with perfumes, etc.). Nor, he adds, can transmutation be performed in a palace; one must live in solitude, far from the profane. Books are inadequate; what is found in books suffices only for beginners; all the rest is secret and is taught only by word of mouth, etc.[55]

The search for the elixir is connected with the search for the distant and mysterious islands where the Immortals live; to meet the Immortals is to transcend the human condition and to share in an atemporal and blissful existence. It is quite possible that many expeditions undertaken to find the "supernatural islands" resulted in geographical discoveries. Was not the Western search for Paradise or the Isles of the Blest a point of departure for the great geographical discoveries beyond the Atlantic? Yet we must not forget that, at the basis of such enterprises, there was always the myth, the primordial image, of a paradisal land, beyond time, inhabited by the "perfected," the Immortals (in other cultures we find Śvetadvīpa,[56] the Isle of the Blest, Avalon, etc.). The search for the Immortals of the faraway islands preoccupied the first emperors of the Chin dynasty (219 B.C.)[57] and the Emperor Wu of the Han dynasty (in 110 B.C.).[58] Nostalgia for a mythical land where the "drug of immortality" is to be found persists into the Middle Ages; the "supernatural islands in the midst of the Eastern Sea" are replaced by distant but not less miraculous lands—India, western Asia. The emperor T'ai Tsung (seventh century) had at his

55 See the summary given by Dubs, pp. 79–80, and the texts translated by T. L. Davis and Ch'ên Kuo-fu, "The Inner Chapters of *Pao-p'u-tzŭ*," *Proceedings of the American Academy of Arts and Sciences*, LXXIV (1940–42), 297–325. See further, on the ascetic and spiritual preliminaries for alchemical operations, the passages from Wei Po-yang's *Ts'an T'ung Ch'i*, tr. T. L. Davis and Lu-Ch'iang Wu, "Chinese Alchemy" (*The Scientific Monthly*, XXXI [1930], 225–35), pp. 230, 231, 234.

56 On which, see Note VII, 1.

57 Chavannes, II, 143, 152; III, 437.

58 Ibid., III, 499; Dubs, p. 66.

court a Brāhman named Nārāyaṇasvāmin whom Wang Hsüan-ts'e had brought from India in 648.[59] This alchemist specialized in the art of prolonging life. In 664–65, Kao Tsung sent the Buddhist monk Hsüan-chao to Kashmir to bring back an Indian magician named Lokāditya, who was said to possess the elixir of life.[60] In 1222 Genghis Khan summoned the Taoist alchemist Ch'ang Ch'un to Samarkand.[61] Asked by the Khan if he possessed the elixir of life, Ch'ang Ch'un frankly replied: "I have a means of protecting life [talismans against evil influences], but no elixir of immortality." [62]

From a certain period, authors begin to distinguish between esoteric and exoteric alchemy. Peng Hsiao (who lived from the end of the ninth century to the first half of the tenth), in his commentary on the *Ts'an T'ung Ch'i*, makes a definite distinction between exoteric alchemy, which is concerned with concrete substances, and esoteric alchemy, which employs only the "souls" of the same substances.[63] The distinction had been made long before by Hui-ssŭ (A.D. 515–577). "Esoteric" alchemy is clearly expounded in Su Tung-p'o's *Treatise on the Dragon and the Tiger*, written in A.D. 1110. The "pure," transcendental metals are identified with the various parts of the body, and alchemical processes, instead of being performed in the laboratory, take place in the body and the consciousness of the experimenter. Su Tung-p'o expresses it as follows: "The Dragon is mercury. He is the semen and the blood. He issues from the kidneys and is stored in the liver. . . . The tiger is lead. He is bread and bodily strength. He issues from the mind and the lungs bear him. . . . When the mind is moved, then the breath and strength act with it. When the kidneys are flushed, then semen and blood flow with them." [64] Just as,

59 Waley, p. 23.

60 Chavannes, *Mémoire sur les religieux éminents qui allèrent chercher la loi dans les pays d'Occident, par Yi-tsing*, p. 21.

61 Waley, *The Travels of an Alchemist*, p. 131.

62 Waley, "Notes," p. 17.

63 Ibid., p. 15.

64 Cited by Waley, "Notes," p. 15; cf. also Lu-Ch'iang Wu and T. L. Davis, "An Ancient Chinese Treatise," p. 255 (*Ts'an T'ung Ch'i*, ch. LIX).

in India, alchemy was incorporated into tantric yoga, so in China it was always closely connected with Taoist techniques. This is why rhythmic breathing—so important in Taoist circles [65]—forms part of the discipline of the alchemist. Pao P'u Tzŭ writes: "In the beginning to learn the proper use of the breath, one should inhale a breath through the nose, stop up the nose (by holding it with two fingers) and mentally count one's heart beats. When one has counted one hundred and twenty heart beats, the breath should be exhaled through the mouth. In this method of breathing, every one should make it his aim that his own ears might not hear the sound of either inhalation or exhalation. . . . With gradual practice, one should increase correspondingly the count of heart beats during which the breath is held. . . . When an old man has arrived at that stage, then he will be transformed into a young man." [66]

Alchemy as a Spiritual Technique

We shall not here enter into the problem of the "origins" of Chinese alchemy; whether they are connected with the quest for "gold," for the "drug of immortality," or [67] for artificial cinnabar, the symbolic and sacred character of the substances employed is patent. (The color red represents the vital principle, the blood; cinnabar was held to prolong life, hence its presence in burials from prehistoric times.) We must also take into consideration the symbolism and sacred character of metallurgy, a secret technique by which minerals were "ripened" and metals "purified," and which was continued by alchemy, because it hastened the "perfecting" of metals.[68] Perhaps, at a certain period a rudimentary chemistry began to develop by the side of alchemical operations, finally becoming an empirical science based solely on observation and experiment. This is possible. But we must be very careful not to

65 See above, pp. 59 ff.

66 Tr. Johnson, pp. 47–48.

67 As Waley believes, "Notes," pp. 18–19.

68 On the "secrets of metallurgy" and its connections with alchemy, see Note VII, 5.

confuse these two types of experimentations—alchemical and pre-chemical. There is no proof that the alchemists were interested in chemical phenomena. Writing of the Alexandrian alchemists, F. Sherwood Taylor says: "No one who had used sulphur, for example, could fail to remark the curious phenomena which attend its fusion and the subsequent heating of the liquid. Now while sulphur is mentioned hundreds of times there is no allusion to any of its characteristic properties except its action on metals. This is in such strong contrast to the spirit of the Greek science of classical times that we must conclude that the alchemists were not interested in natural phenomena other than those which might help them to attain their object. . . . We shall not find in alchemy any beginnings of a science. . . . At no times does the alchemist employ a scientific procedure." [69]

Even in Europe, the alchemistic ideal survived down to the eighteenth century. It was believed that man could collaborate in the work of nature. "What nature made in the beginning, we can likewise make, by returning to the procedure that she followed. What she is perhaps still making, by help of the centuries, in her subterranean solitudes, we can cause her to finish in a single instant, by aiding her and surrounding her with better circumstances. As we make bread, so we can make metals." [70]

The relations between Yoga and alchemy can be understood if we take into consideration the soteriological nature of the two techniques. Both experiment on the "soul," using the human body as a laboratory; the goal is "purification," "bringing to perfection," final transmutation. This correspondence between the two methods of experimentation—the alchemical and the mystical—is also found elsewhere. We know that the symbolism of ascetic

69 "A Survey of Greek Alchemy" (*The Journal of Hellenic Studies*, L [1930], 109–39), p. 110.

70 Jean Reynaud, *Études encyclopédiques*, IV, 487, cited by M. A. Daubrée, "La Génération des minéraux métalliques dans la pratique des mineurs du Moyen Âge, d'après le *Bergbüchlein*" (*Journal des savants* [1890], 379–92, 441–52), p. 383.

purification of the soul and the symbolism of the alchemical quest were closely connected among the earliest Ṣūfīs (in the sense of "those who possessed and experimented with the secret and mysterious procedure of transmutation," a sense that is very old)—for example, Jābir ibn-Hayyān, Sāi'ih'Alawī, and Dhū'l Nūn al-Miṣrī. As Massignon remarks, "in the realm of literature, an affinity was inescapable a priori between these two legendary dramas of human experimentation—that of science and that of mysticism; between the alchemist in search of an elixir, the potion of youth, the agent of universal transmutation, and the ascetic in search of a spirit, the minister of sanctification." [71]

In India, the tendency of Yoga to assimilate all concrete techniques could not disregard an experimentation as precise as that of alchemy. At certain moments the osmosis between these two spiritual sciences is perfect. Both oppose the purely speculative path, purely metaphysical knowledge; both work on "living matter" to the end of transmuting it—that is, of changing its ontological status; both pursue deliverance from the laws of time—seek, that is, to "decondition" life, to conquer freedom and bliss: in a word, "immortality."

71 *La Passion d'al-Hosayn-ibn-Mansour al-Hallâj, martyr mystique de l'Islam*, II, 931. On alchemy in relation to Ismailite Gnosticism, see Henry Corbin, "Le livre du Glorieux de Jâbir ibn Ḥayyân. Alchimie et archétypes," *Eranos-Jahrbuch*, XVIII (1950), 47–114.

CHAPTER EIGHT

Yoga and Aboriginal India

The Roads to Freedom

IN OUR survey of the imposing spiritual synthesis that bears the name of tantrism, we were able to distinguish elements different in their origins and their importance: on the one hand, the legacy of the Vedic cult and of Brāhmanism, the innovations of the *Bhagavad Gītā*, and the sectarian trends; on the other, the contributions of medieval Buddhism, of alchemy, and of the autochthonous spiritualities. We saw the fundamental role that yogic techniques played in tantrism: in virtue of them, planes of experience as heterogeneous as, for example, iconography, sexuality, and alchemy were homologized and integrated, until finally they became equivalent planes of a single spiritual itinerary. As in the earlier syntheses (the *Mahābhārata*, the *Bhagavad Gītā*, etc.), it was the specifically yogic disciplines that furnished the basis for the new valorizations. This process of incorporation continued, in a constantly increasing degree, even after the triumph of tantrism, the decadence of Vajrayāna Buddhism, and the Islamic invasion. We shall not undertake to trace its history, which is often extremely involved, for it touches almost every aspect of the cultural and religious life of India. (We shall mention only that the different forms of Yoga—devotional, mystical, erotic, or magical—exerted a basic influence on the birth of the vernacular literatures and, in general, on the formation of the spirit of modern India.) We propose, by a series of examples chosen from the most various milieus (folklore, popular devotion, sects, superstitions, etc.), to show the many and contradictory valorizations of Yoga on all cultural levels. This brief investigation will be pursued through increasingly eccentric and archaic strata, finally including a considerable part of the protohistory of India. Our borings will be instructive; we shall see that the yogin and the *sannyāsi* can assume countless forms, from the sorcerer and fakir who perform cures and miracles to the noblest ascetics and loftiest mystics, taking in cannibal magicians and extremist Vāmacārīs along the way.

If the yogins were confused with all these types of magico-religious behavior, it is because all Indian spiritual techniques shared in Yoga to some degree. Among the populace, the yogins have always been regarded as redoubtable magicians, gifted with superhuman powers.[1] Despite the reservations expressed by Patañjali and by other forms of Yoga in regard to the *siddhis*, the assimilation of the yogin to the magician was almost inevitable. For the uninstructed could easily confuse *liberation* and *absolute freedom*, the *jīvan-mukta* and the "immortal" magician, who had access to all experiences without being subject to their karmic effects. Texts to be cited later will give some examples of such confusions in regard to Gorakhnāth and the Nātha Siddhas. The phenomenon becomes intelligible if we consider that freedom manifests itself under countless forms, some of them antisocial—a free man no longer feels bound by the laws and prejudices of society; he takes his stand outside of all ethics and all social forms. The excesses and aberrations echoed in the legends of the Vāmacārīs, the cruelties and crimes of the Kāpālikas and the Aghorīs, are, for Indian feeling, so many proofs of a total freedom conquered from the human condition and outside of society. We must not forget that, for Indian thought, the "normal" human condition is equivalent to bondage, ignorance, and suffering; freedom, knowledge, and bliss are inaccessible so long as this "normality" is not de-

1 See Maurice Bloomfield, "On False Ascetics and Nuns in Hindu Fiction" (*Journal of the American Oriental Society*, XLIV [1924], 202–42), especially pp. 213–18.

stroyed. And the same premise is the metaphysical justification for all excesses and all aberrations, which are also effective methods of abolishing the human condition. Let us say at once that, in India, the extremists have always remained a minority, that the great spiritual movements have never encouraged these manifestations in which nihilism vied with turpitude, that the cynics, the libertines, and the adepts of the "terrible schools" have for the most part existed on the margin of Indian asceticism and mysticism. But all such literal interpretations of transcending the human condition were justified by respectable ideologies, both Hinduistic and Mahāyānic.

On the other hand, such excesses, adopted in the name of a doctrine of salvation, opened the way to almost inevitable syncretisms with rites relegated to the lower levels of spirituality and with the behavior patterns of subordinate groups; tantrism finally incorporates the major and minor magic of the people, erotic Yoga encourages the open emergence of secret orgiastic cults and of licentious maniacs, which, but for the prestige of the tantric *maithuna* and the techniques of Haṭha Yoga, would have continued their obscure existence in the margin of society and of the community's religious life. Like every Gnosticism and every mysticism that spread and triumph, tantric Yoga does not succeed in avoiding degradation as it penetrates increasingly broad and eccentric social strata. Those who cannot practice a full Yoga will content themselves with imitating certain external aspects of it, will interpret certain technical details literally. This is the risk run by every spiritual message that is assimilated and lived by masses lacking in a preliminary initiation. From the Indian point of view, this phenomenon of degradation corresponds to the movement of accelerated descent typical of the end of the cycle; during the *kali-yuga*, truth is buried in the darkness of ignorance. This is why new masters continually appear and readapt the timeless doctrine to the slender aptitudes of a fallen humanity. But we shall see, in connection with Gorakhnāth and the eighty-four Siddhas that the constantly renewed message of these new masters undergoes the erosive action of the masses (for the appearance of the masses is the characteristic note of the *kali-yuga*) and ends by being degraded and forgotten; more precisely, on a certain "popular" level, every spiritual master ends by coinciding with the archetypal image of the Great Magician, of the *jīvan-mukta,* liberated in life and possessor of all the *siddhis.*

Aghorīs, Kāpālikas

In this spiritual process, we find one point important. It is the degradation of an ideology through failure to comprehend the symbolism that forms its vehicle. We shall give an example. The role that the cemetery (*śmaśāna*), together with meditations performed while sitting on corpses, plays in a number of Indian ascetic schools is well known. The symbolism is frequently emphasized in the texts: the cemetery represents the totality of psychomental life, fed by consciousness of the "I"; the corpses symbolize the various sensory and mental activities. Seated at the center of his profane experience, the yogin "burns" the activities that feed them, just as corpses are burned in the cemetery. By meditating in a *śmaśāna* he more directly achieves the combustion of egotistic experiences; at the same time, he frees himself from fear, he evokes the terrible demons and obtains mastery over them.

Now, there is a class of Śivaist ascetics, the Aghorīs or Aghorapanthīs, who have at times interpreted this symbolism of the "cemetery" and "corpses" materially. Their name has been translated "not terrific" (*a-ghora*); the *aghorapanthī* would, then, be one who follows the path (or the cult) of Śiva under this form. The connections with tantrism are patent. These Aghorīs eat from human skulls, haunt cemeteries, and still practiced cannibalism at the end of the nineteenth century; Crooke cites the case of an Aghorī from Ujjain who, in 1887, ate a corpse from the pile at the burning ghat.[2] They eat all sorts of refuse and any kind of meat except horse meat. They justify these practices by saying that all of man's natural

2 See Note VIII, 1.

inclinations and tastes should be destroyed, that there is neither good nor evil, pleasant nor unpleasant, etc. Even as human excrement fertilizes a sterile soil, so assimilating every kind of filth makes the mind capable of any and every meditation.[3] For them, there is no distinction of castes or religions; parents are mere accidents.[4] They are divided into two branches: the *śuddhs* (the pure) and the *malins* (the dirty). As to cult, some of them profess that they worship Sītalā Devi, others Parnagīrī Devi,[5] yet others Kālī. Any Śaiva of any caste can become an Aghorī. According to Barrow, even Jainas are admitted, but not Viṣṇuists.[6] They do not worship images. Except God, they respect only their *guru.*[7] Celibacy is obligatory. They lead a life of vagabondage, and a disciple (*chela*) cannot become a *guru* until twelve years after the death of his spiritual master. Every *guru* is always accompanied by a dog. Their bodies are not buried in the recumbent position, but seated, with the legs crossed.[8]

These Aghorīs are only the successors to a much older and more widespread ascetic order, the Kāpālikas, or "wearers of skulls." The *Maitrāyaṇī Upaniṣad* (VII, 8) already mentions a *kāpālin;* an inscription from the first half of the seventh century names the god Kāpāleśvara and his ascetics.[9] The Kāpālikas venerated Śiva under his aspects of Mahākāla (the Great Destroyer) and Kāpālabhṛt (he who carries a skull). They resemble the tantric Vāmacārīs, but they carry orgiastic practices and ritual cruelty to the extreme. From the sixth century on, references become more frequent: the *Daśakumāracarita* in the sixth century; Hiuen Tsiang, who encountered them on his journey through India (630–645); Bhava-

3 H. W. Barrow, "On Aghorīs and Aghorapanthīs" (*Proceedings on the Anthropological Society of Bombay*, III [1893], 197–251), p. 222.

4 Ibid., p. 223.

5 Goddess worshiped at Pāli, near Ajmēr, and regarded as the tutelary goddess of ascetics; cf. Barrow, p. 210.

6 Ibid., p. 210.

7 Ibid., p. 233.

8 See Note VIII, 4.

9 R. G. Bhāndārkar, *Vaiṣṇavism, Śaivism and Minor Religious Systems,* p. 118. Cf. *Brahma-sūtras,* II, 2, 37.

bhūti (eighth century), who, in his play *Mālatī-Mādhava*, represents a Kāpālika named Aghoraghanta on the point of sacrificing the virgin Mālatī to the goddess Cāmuṇḍā. There is a similar episode in the *Prabodha Chandrodaya*, which was performed in 1065; the author is a *sannyāsi* named Kṛṣṇamiśra, who seems to have known the Kāpālikas well. He makes one of them say: "My necklace and ornaments are of human bones; I dwell among the ashes of the dead and eat my food in human skulls. . . . We drink liquor out of the skulls of Brāhmans; our sacred fires are fed with the brains and lungs of men mixed up with their flesh, and human victims covered with the fresh blood gushing from the dreadful wound in their throats, are the offerings by which we appease the terrible god [Mahā Bhairava]. . . . The might of our religion is such that I control Hari-Hara and the greatest and most ancient of the gods; I stop the course of the planets in the heavens; I submerge the earth in water, with its mountains and cities, and I again drink up the waters in a moment. . . . He who resembles the gods, whose crest is the lunar orb, and who with delight embraces women as beautiful as Pārvatī, feels supreme bliss."[10] In the *Prabodha Chandrodaya*, a Kāpālinī accompanies the Kāpālika; in attire like his, the heavy-breasted Kāpālinī dances with him under Bhairava's direction. There is no possible doubt about the licentious rites practiced by the Kāpālikas; "without renouncing the pleasures derived through the organs of sense, the eight great *siddhis* may be obtained."[11] Rāmānuja, who distinguishes two classes of Kāpālikas, one extremist, the other moderate, emphasizes their connections with sexual techniques.[12] He makes the Kāpālas say: "He who knows the true nature of the six mudrâs, who understands the highest mudrâ, meditating on himself as in the position called bhagâsana [i.e., visualizing himself as seated on the *pudendum muliebre*], reaches Nirvâṇa."[13]

10 Tr. Briggs, *Gorakhnāth*, p. 226.

11 Ibid.

12 *Śrībhāṣya*, II, 2, 35–38.

13 Tr. G. Thibaut, *The Vedānta Sūtra* (Sacred Books of the East, XLVIII), p. 520.

Both the European travelers to India and the *Dabistān* confuse the Kāpālikas and the Aghorīs with yogins in general. The description given by the *Dabistān* could not be more vivid: "There are some of this sect [of *yogins*], who, having mixed their excretions and filtered them through a piece of cloth, drink them and say, that such an act renders a man capable of great affairs, and they pretend to know strange things. They call the performer of this act Atília and also Akhórí." [14] Further on, the author of the *Dabistān* probably confuses the Kāpālikas with some Vāmacārī sect. For, writing of the *liṅga* and *bhaga*, he says: "In many places and among a great number of the Hindus, this worship exists: a great many follow the Agama, in which wine drinking is approved, and if, instead of a common cup, a man's skull (which they call *kapāla*) be used, the beverage is much more agreeable. They hold the killing of all animals, even of man, to be permitted and call it *bala* [daring]. At night they go to the places which they call *śmaśāṇa* [cemetery], and where the dead bodies are burnt; there they intoxicate themselves, eat the flesh of the corpses burnt, and copulate before the eyes of others with women, whom they name *śakti pūjā*." The information given by the author of the *Dabistān* is substantially correct. He says that these tantrics prefer incest to ordinary union. He knows that *lulīs* (public women) are prized and that they are called *deva kanyā*; that there are two kinds of cults, *bhadram* (pure) and *vakam* (impure), but that the second is preferred. He knows, too, that in the sexual act the woman personifies the goddess. The author had seen a Kāpālika meditating on a corpse, and in Gujarāt he came upon a certain Mahadeo who spent his nights seated on a corpse. Sterile women spent a night with the *guru*.

Muḥsin-i-Fāni very probably misunderstood his sources to some extent and confused certain sexual rites of the Kāpālikas with the orgy (the *rāsamaṇḍalī*) of the Vallabhācāryas.[15] However, there is

14 *The Dabistān; or, School of Manners*, tr. D. Shea and A. Troyer, II, 129–60. We remind the reader that the *Dabistān* was compiled by Muḥsin-i-Fāni in the seventeenth century.

15 On the latter, see Note VIII, 2.

no doubt about the orgiastic tendency of the Kāpālikas; we even have evidence of seasonal collective orgies, in which all the members of the sect participated. According to the *Kaumudīmahotsava Nāṭaka*, these festivals took place in the spring (*vasantotsava*) and autumn (*kaumudīmahotsava*) and were strongly orgiastic in character.[16] Now, those who took part in these ceremonies were not only all the Kāpālikas, but also the "materialists" and the "cynics," the Lokāyatikas—that is, those who rejected the Vedic tradition and all the values of Hinduism. Seasonal festivals and the orgies accompanying them were specific features of the archaic, pre-Indo-European cult of vegetation. It is interesting to note that some traditions make the Kāpālikas the originators of the seasonal orgies in which the Lokāyatikas also took part; here festivals of vegetation, tantric orgies, and the eccentric practices of the "materialists," cannibals, and wearers of skulls are merged in a single system. This detail shows us the direction of the future coalescence between tantric yoga and the aboriginal spiritual values.

Heine-Geldern has established a connection between the human sacrifices and skull hunts that are abundantly attested in Assam and Burma, and a matriarchal ideology that still survives in Tibet and the Himālayan regions. In India proper, some of the archaic cultural elements played their part later in the prodigious advance of tantric Śaktism (whose center was none other than Assam-Kāmarūpa). Such are the ethnological elements of the problem. But it also has a historico-religious aspect—the spiritual revalorization of prehistoric customs entailing human sacrifices and the cult of skulls. And it is this aspect which is of chief interest to us here.

The process may be imagined as follows. (1) An archaic ideology, connected with a particular lunar symbolism, implied, among other things, human sacrifice and skull hunting; populations holding these ideas were, during the historical period, settled in zones bordering on Hinduism. (2) On the level of the highest Indian spirituality, the cemetery, corpses, and skeletons were revalorized

16 Cf. D. Shāstri, "The Lokāyatikas and the Kāpālikas," *Indian Historical Quarterly*, VII (1931), 135.

and incorporated into an ascetico-mystical symbolism; to meditate seated on a corpse, to wear a skull, etc., now represented spiritual exercises that pursued a wholly different order of values from those, let us say, of the head-hunters. (3) When the two ideologies came into contact—whether in the frontier regions (Assam, Himālayas), or in the districts of inner India in which the elements of archaic culture had been best preserved—we witness phenomena of pseudomorphism and devalorization. In this light, we can understand how one or another tantric yoga becomes licentious on a certain cultural level imbued with matriarchal elements; we also understand why a particular Kāpālin forgets the yogic meaning of the "corpse" and the "skeleton" and becomes a head-hunter, thus reverting to cannibal behavior (minus the "philosophy" of cannibalism, which, as Volhard has shown, was not as aberrant as it appears to modern eyes). Above all, these reciprocal degradations and devalorizations are explained by "symbolic confusionism," by a symbolism being forgotten or inadequately comprehended. We shall have occasion to observe the same phenomenon again in other cultural contexts and in connection with other symbolisms, mythologies, or techniques incorporated into Yoga.

Gorakhnāth and the Eighty-four Siddhas *

A considerable number of yogins claim to be followers of Gorakṣanātha (Gorakhnāth) and call themselves "Gorakhnāthis" or "Kānphaṭa Yogīs"; this latter term derives from the fact that, at the initiation ceremony, the disciple's ears are split to permit the insertion of enormous earrings (*kān* = ear, *phaṭa* = split). As we saw above,[17] Haṭha Yoga also claims that its founder was Gorakhnāth, the supposed author of the school's first treatise (now lost). In any case, the connections between Gorakhnāth, the Kānphaṭas, and Haṭha Yoga are beyond question; the Kānphaṭas call themselves simply "yogīs," and their literature contains a number of Haṭha-

17 See above, p. 228.

yogic texts, among them the most famous treatises, including the *Haṭhayogapradīpikā*, the *Gheraṇḍa Saṃhitā*, the *Śiva Saṃhitā* the *Gorakṣa Śataka*, etc. But this ascetic order goes far beyond the limits of the Haṭha-yogic ideology and disciplines. In fact, we are dealing with a movement of considerable importance that seems to have been highly popular after the twelfth century of our era and that formed the point of convergence for a large number of religious, magical, and alchemical traditions and practices, most of them Śivaistic, but some of them Buddhist.

The movement originated by the historical figures who were later mythicized under the names of Gorakhnāth, Matsyendranāth, and other famous Siddhas seems to represent a fresh ground swell of the deep spirituality that reaches down to the aboriginal strata of India. Today, the Gorakhnāthis show all the symptoms of a sect in decomposition, and the origins of this process probably go back several centuries. But the mythologies and folklores that have crystallized around their masters permit us to estimate the enormous popular response these masters aroused between the collapse of Buddhism in eastern India and the dawn of modern times. These mythologies and folklores, though comparatively "recent" from a strictly chronological point of view, actually represent extremely archaic contents; they are the emergence of spiritualities long unknown, and hence unrecorded, by the "official" cultural circles—that is, by circles more or less dependent upon a *learned tradition*, whether Brāhmanic, Buddhist, Jaina, or "sectarian." The popular legends and vernacular literatures created around Gorakhnāth, the Nāthas, and the Siddhas give expression to the real spiritual longings of the superficially Hinduized masses. Now, it is noteworthy that such folkloric and literary creations were inspired precisely by tantric and alchemistic saints and masters, and especially by the supposed "inventor" of Haṭha Yoga—that is, by Siddhas who understood liberation as the conquest of immortality. We shall see the enormous importance of the motif of immortality in the folklores and literatures of the Gorakhnāthis and the Nāthas—an importance that leads us to believe that this particular motif (which continues and completes that of the *jīvan-mukta*, the "liberated while living") expresses the nostalgia of the whole Indian soul.

We know almost nothing of the historical personality of Gorakhnāth. It was very soon distorted by myth, almost deified—witness the countless myths and legends found almost everywhere in western and northern India, from Nepāl to Rājputāna, from the Punjab to Bengal, from Sind to the Deccan. His life may probably be dated between the ninth and the twelfth century, and he accomplished a new synthesis among certain Śivaist traditions (Pāśupata), tantrism, and the doctrines (unfortunately, so imperfectly known) of the Siddhas—that is, of the "perfect" yogīs. In some respects, the Gorakhnāthis continue such Śivaist sects as the Pāśupata, Lakulīśa Kālāmukha, and Kāpālika.[18] But they also practice the rites of "left-hand" tantrism,[19] and, in addition to Gorakhnāth, whom they identify with Śiva, they venerate the nine Nāthas and the eighty-four Siddhas. It is in this "milieu" of the Siddhas and the Nāthas that we must place Gorakhnāth's message (for, concerning his historical personality, nothing definite has come down to us).

We cannot here enter into the problem (still so little elucidated) of the eighty-four Siddhas.[20] We shall only note that all yogins who attained "perfection" could receive the name of *siddha*, but the fact that this term is connected with "miraculous power" (*siddhi*) indicates that what was in question was primarily a "magical perfection." The *Haṭhayogapradīpikā* (I, 5–9) contains a list of *mahāsiddhas*, beginning with Ādinātha (mystical name of Śiva) and mentioning Matsyendranāth, Gorakṣa, Kāpāla, Carpaṭi, etc. Other more or less complete lists have come down to us, but they seldom agree in respect to the names of the Siddhas. The confusion was heightened by coalescence with the traditions of the Siddhas and Siddhacaryās peculiar to Sahajīyā Buddhism. Some names—especially those of Matsyendranāth, Gorakhnāth, Nāgārjuna, Kāpāla,

18 Briggs, p. 218.

19 Daniel Wright, *History of Nepāl* (Cambridge, 1877), p. 140; Crooke, *Tribes and Castes*, III, 158 (citing F. Buchanan); Briggs, p. 172.

20 See Note VIII, 3.

Carpaṭi, etc.—occur with great frequency. We may note that, aside from Matsyendranāth and Gorakhnāth, the most important Siddhas are Nāgārjuna and the alchemists (Capari, Carpaṭi, etc.).

The number 84 corresponds to no historical reality; it is a mystical number, attested in all Indian traditions, whether Hindu, Buddhist, Ājīvika, or Jaina.[21] It probably expresses completeness, totality. Thus, the eighty-four Siddhas would represent the "totality of a revelation." As for the nine Nāthas, their number also symbolizes the integrality of a doctrine. The *Gorakṣasiddhānta-saṃgraha* cites two tantric texts clearly illustrating this symbolism: the *Soḍaśa-nitya-tantra* tells us that the nine Nāthas propagated tantrism in the different cosmic periods, and the *Tantra-mahārṇava* says that eight Nāthas reside in the eight directions and the ninth at the center.[22] In other words, the doctrine propagated by these nine masters covers the "totality" of time and space. The Nāthas—especially Matsyendranāth, Gorakhnāth, Carpaṭi, Kāpāla—also appear in the lists of the eighty-four Siddhas. Hence we see that Sahajīyā tantrism (both Hindu and Buddhist), alchemy (Nāgārjuna, Carpaṭi), Haṭha Yoga (Gorakhnāth), and the Kāpālikas here coincide: their representatives are included in the lists both of the nine Nāthas and of the eighty-four Siddhas. This may perhaps give us the key to the symbolism of the Nāthas and Siddhas—at a certain period (probably between the seventh and the eleventh century), a new "revelation" occurred, formulated by masters who no more claimed to be original than their predecessors had done (were they not "identified" with Śiva or with Vajrasattva?), but who had reinterpreted the timeless doctrines to conform to the needs of their day. One of the essential points of this new "revelation" was that it finally completed the synthesis among the elements of Vajrayāna and Śivaist tantrism, magic, alchemy,[23] and Haṭha Yoga. In a way, it was a continuation of the tantric synthesis. But a number of the

21 See some examples in Dasgupta, *Obscure Religious Cults*, pp. 234 ff.

22 Quoted by Dasgupta, p. 237.

23 The *Gorakṣa Saṃhitā*, attributed to Gorakhnāth, figures among the alchemical treatises; cf. Rāy, *History of Hindu Chemistry*, II, xcvi.

Nāthas and Siddhas put more emphasis than their predecessors had done upon the value of magic and Yoga as inestimable means for the conquest of freedom and immortality. It was especially this aspect of their message that struck the popular imagination; we still find it echoed today in folklore and the vernacular literatures. It is for this reason that the latter seem to us of great value for our inquiry.

As for the order of Kānphaṭa Yogīs, strictly speaking, we saw [24] that it adheres to the tradition of extremist Śivaism. The Kānphaṭas serve as *pūjāris* (officiants) in the temples of Bhairon, Śakti, and Śiva.[25] Many of them make pilgrimages to the Vāmacāra temple of Hinglāj, in Baluchistan, and wear a necklace of white pebbles as a souvenir.[26] In fact, the first Europeans to mention the Kānphaṭas (e.g., Buchanan) saw resemblances between them and the Vāmacārīs. Their relations with the Aghorīs are quite close; after his first initiation, the Kānphaṭa receives the name of Aughar, and occasionally an Aughar becomes an Aghorī.[27] Some Aghorīs serve in the temple of Kāmākhyā (=Durgā) in Assam. Now, this temple was famous for the human sacrifices that were performed there into the nineteenth century (they were suppressed by the English government in 1832). In 1565, 140 victims were beheaded in the course of a single sacrifice.[28]

If we bear in mind that Assam (=Kāmarūpa) was the tantric country par excellence, that important tantras exalted Durgā-Kāmākhyā and described her bloody and licentious cult,[29] that the Aghorīs were famous for their cruelties and their orgies, we shall understand how the name *yogī* sometimes came to designate the most extremist among tantrics. A detail of the human sacrifices performed in Assam is of interest for the problem under consideration. Those who volunteered were called *bhogīs*, and from the moment they announced their intention of allowing themselves to

24 Above, p. 301.
25 Briggs, p. 139.
26 Farquhar, *Outline*, p. 348.
27 Briggs, p. 71.
28 E. A. Gait, *A History of Assam*, p. 58.
29 E.g., *Yoni-tantra*, *Mahānirvāṇa-tantra*, and *Kālikā Purāṇa*.

be sacrificed they became almost sacred and everything was put at their disposition; in particular, they were allowed as many women as they wished. They were sacrificed at the annual festival of the goddess, and the *Kālikā Purāṇa* even devotes a chapter to the details of their decapitation, stipulating, however, that this ritual must not be performed by the first three castes.[30] According to the same text, the victim incarnated Śiva himself. All this reminds us of another bloody Indian sacrifice; the *meriah* of the Khonds was strangled, then cut into pieces, which were buried in the fields to promote fertility.[31] The *meriah* too incarnated the divinity. Now, it is significant that, here, in a tantric context that brings together the Aghorīs and the Kānphaṭa Yogīs, we find the same bloody sacrifice that was elsewhere performed for the sake of agricultural fertility. It is one more example of the coalescence between Śaktism and the archaic ideology of fecundity, in which sexuality and violent death coexist.

As for the theology of the Gorakhnāthis, it is extremely elementary: Śiva is their supreme god, and salvation consists in union with the divinity through Yoga.[32] It is for this reason that the Gorakhnāthis assert their mastery of the art of respiration.[33] But they are chiefly known and respected for their magical prowess: they have a considerable reputation as healers and magicians, they are supposed to be able to bring rain, they exhibit snakes.[34] The ability to tame wild beasts is also attributed to them; they are said to live in the jungle, surrounded by tigers, who sometimes serve them as mounts.[35] This motif is archaic and shamanic, for the tiger is the "master of initiation"; in central Asia, in Indonesia, and elsewhere the tiger or other wild animals appear and carry the neophyte into the jungle on their backs (symbol of the beyond).[36]

30 Cf. Briggs, pp. 167 ff.

31 Cf. Eliade, *Patterns in Comparative Religion*, p. 344 f.

32 L. P. Tessitori, "Yogīs (Kānphaṭā)," *Encyclopaedia of Religion and Ethics*, XII, 833.

33 Briggs, pp. 125 ff.

34 Ibid., pp. 127 ff., 142 ff.

35 Ibid., p. 136.

36 Cf. Eliade, *Shamanism*, pp. 72 ff., 344 ff., etc.

Gorakhnāthis may marry; [37] in the Bombay Province almost all of them are married, and one of the important books of the sect, the *Gorakhbodh*, written in Hindi, probably in the fourteenth century, permits marriage. When they die, they are not cremated but are buried in the posture of meditation. It is supposed that they continue to remain in *samādhi*, hence the name given their tombs, *samādh*.[38] Above the tomb are set symbols of the *liṅga* and *yoni*.[39] The custom of burying ascetics and yogins is quite old in India; it is a way of proclaiming that the *sannyāsi* has identified himself with Śiva, whose sign (*liṅga*) hallows the tomb and can in time transform it into a sanctuary.[40] Let us note in passing the "materialization" of *samādhi* on the level of popular spirituality; the tomb becomes a sacred place because it contains not a corpse but the body of one "liberated," in a state of permanent meditation. In connection with the same phenomenon of "materialization," characteristic of the popular mind, we may note that the *siddhis*, the yogic powers par excellence, become in the eyes of peasants "spirits" or "demons" (Siddhis), which are supposed to have received their magic directly from Gorakhnāth. In some parts of the Punjab, the Siddhis are even venerated under different names and under the form of stones.[41] Ancient local hierophanies are revalorized through the prestige of Gorakhnāth and are incorporated into the new magico-religious synthesis effected on all the cultural planes of aboriginal India.

Matsyendranāth and the Myth of "Transmission of the Doctrine"

Like all other great Indian movements, the Kānphaṭa Yogīs claim that their sect existed before the creation and that the gods Brahmā, Viṣṇu, and Śiva were Gorakhnāth's first disciples.[42] This is a way

37 Tessitori, p. 835; Briggs, p. 46.

38 Briggs, p. 41.

39 Ibid., p. 154.

40 On the custom of burying yogins, see Note VIII, 4.

41 Briggs, pp. 137 ff.

42 Ibid., p. 228.

of expressing the atemporal and eternal nature of the doctrine. The majority of the traditions, however, say that Ādināth and Matsyendranāth preceded Gorakhnāth, Matsyendra having been his immediate *guru*. It is difficult to disentangle the historical reality that may perhaps lie hidden under these traditions. The names themselves designate degrees of spirituality rather than flesh-and-blood personages. Ādināth is an incarnation of Śiva, and his name is also given to Buddha Vajrasattva; in some Buddhist tantras, Ādināth and Bhūtanāth are epithets of Vajrasattva.[43] This amounts to saying that the founder of the sect was God himself. Through Yoga, Gorakhnāth identifies himself with Śiva, and iconography and cult regard him as an incarnation of Śiva.[44] As for Matsyendranāth, he became the tutelary divinity of Nepāl, where he was identified with Avalokiteśvara.[45] The historical persons and concrete events were very soon transfigured and acquired the mythical dimensions of exemplary figures and divine gestures.

We might conclude from this that Matsyendranāth and Gorakhnāth brought a new "revelation," which they declared that they had received directly from Śiva. The myth of the "transmission of the doctrine" was well known and had often been employed in the past; it was represented by the initiatory dialogue between God and his "wife," overheard by a semidivine being who then becomes the messenger. In the case of Matsyendranāth, the story runs: Śiva was one day teaching the doctrine of Yoga to his wife Pārvatī by

43 Dasgupta, *Obscure Religious Cults*, p. 224.

44 Briggs, p. 181, and Note VIII, 3.

45 Lévi, *Le Népal*, I, 347 ff. According to Tucci ("Animadversiones Indicae," pp. 133–34), Matsyendranāth is a mystical name bestowed upon every Siddha who has reached a particular degree of spiritual perfection: *matsya*, "fish," is interpreted by the school of Kashmir to mean the "senses" (*indriya*). P. C. Bagchi (*Kaulajñāna-nirṇaya and Some Minor Texts of the School of Matsyendranātha*, pp. 6 ff.) rejects this hypothesis. According to him, the name Matsyendranāth indicates the trade of "fisherman." But still to be explained is the entire symbolism of "fish" and "fisherman," which occurs in innumerable cultural contexts and always in connection with a "revelation," or, more precisely, the passage of a doctrine from the state of oblivion or "eclipse" to the state of complete manifestation.

the seaside; Pārvatī fell asleep during the lesson. But Lokeśvara (=Avalokiteśvara) had heard everything, for he had hidden in the water in the form of a fish—whence the name he has since borne, Matsyendranāth.[46] The earliest reference in literature to Matsyendranāth occurs in the *Kaulajñāna-nirṇaya* (an eleventh-century MS. of which was used by Bagchi for his edition). The story presents some variants from the Nepālese version: Śiva (Bhairava) reveals to his wife that, his disciple Kārttikeya having thrown the *Śāstra* ("Doctrine") into the sea, a fish swallowed it.[47] Another legend relates that Śiva, implored by a woman to grant her a child, gave her a substance to eat. But the woman did not eat it and threw it on a dunghill. Matsyendranāth, who, in the shape of a fish, had overheard Śiva teaching the doctrine to Pārvatī, went to the woman twelve years later and asked her to show him the child. Learning what had happened, he sent her to search the dunghill. She found a twelve-year-old boy, who was given the name Gorakhnāth.[48] And in fact the name could be interpreted as derived either from *ghor-*, "mud," "slime," "ordure," or from *ghoṛ-*, "intense," "terrifying," applied especially to ascetic austerities. The name Gorakhnāth can also mean "lord of flocks," and in this case would suggest one of the names of Śiva.

The myth clearly states the sequence of the transmission of the doctrine: Śiva, Matsyendranāth, Gorakhnāth. The legends concerning the relationship between the last two—that of master and disciple—are equally instructive. We are told that Matsyendranāth, having gone to Ceylon, fell in love with the Queen and took up residence in her palace. Gorakhnāth followed him, found him in the palace, and "recalled him to reality" (the motif of "recall to reality" will engage our attention later). Matsyendranāth abandoned the Queen, taking with him his two sons, Pārasnāth and Nīmnāth. According to another legend, found in Nepāl, Matsyendranāth succumbed to temptation under the following circumstances. Leaving his body to be guarded by his disciple, his spirit entered

46 Wright, *History of Nepāl*, pp. 140 ff.

47 *Kaulajñāna-nirṇaya*, vv. 22 ff. 48 Lévi, I, 351–52.

the corpse of a king who had just died, and revived it. (This is the well-known yogic miracle of entering another's body; the saints sometimes employ it to experience sensual pleasure without being polluted; Śaṇkara himself is said to have done so.) After some time Gorakṣa came to the king and reminded him of his true identity.[49]

The legends of the cycle of Matsyendranāth, his two sons, and Gorakhnāth are of great interest, for they not only evince the archaic character of the initiation of the two boys but also reveal certain occult connections between the Siddhas and Jainism. We are told that Gorakhnāth one day became angry with the two boys and killed them; he washed their entrails "after the way of washer-women" and hung their skins on a tree. But at Matsyendranāth's request he later revived them.[50] This is clearly an initiatory death and resurrection. But some of the details are distinctly shamanic (washing the entrails, hanging up the skins); they are found in the initiations of Siberian, central Asian, and Australian shamans.[51] Hence we may conclude that, in addition to such aboriginal archaic elements as we have already cited (and further examples will be given later), the sect of the Gorakhnāthis had also assimilated certain shamanic initiatory ceremonies of unquestionable antiquity. The legend just cited may indicate that Gorakhnāth possessed occult wisdom unknown to his master, and that the latter asked him to initiate his two sons into it. However this may be, the real initiation was conferred by Matsyendranāth himself, for it was only after it that Nīmnāth and Pārasnāth founded the two Jain sects that are still in existence today.[52] According to the folklore of the Kānphaṭa Yogīs, the two sons were the founders of Jainism. This anachronism probably conceals certain obscure relations between the Jain ascetics and the secret doctrine of Matsyendranāth and Gorakhnāth. There are other indications pointing in the same direction; in a Jain temple near Paidhoni (Pāe Dhūnī), there is an idol of Ghorajīnāth decorated with precious stones,[53] and the

49 Briggs, p. 233.

50 Ibid., p. 72; Dasgupta, p. 244.

51 Eliade, *Shamanism*, pp. 36 ff., 45 ff., etc.

52 Briggs, p. 72

53 Ibid., p. 72, n. 1.

Nīmnāthīs and Pārasnāthīs, although they profess to be followers of Gorakhnāth, behave like the Jainas (they wear a strip of cloth over their mouths to avoid killing invisible animalcula).

Shamanistic Magic and the Quest for Immortality

The folklore that crystallized around Gorakhnāth bears witness not only to the tremendous impression that his magical powers made on the popular imagination but also to certain shamanic elements that confirm the archaism of the myths and symbols launched by the appearance of the Siddhas. The well-known story of the drought in Nepāl [54] has come down to us in several versions. Gorakhnāth, not having been received with fitting honors in the course of a visit, shut up the clouds (or the Nāgas who governed them) in a bale, sat down on it, and remained there for twelve years, lost in meditation. The King begged Avalokiteśvara (=Matsyendranāth), who was living on a mountain named Kāpōtal (near Kāmarūpa), to save the country, and the saint came to Nepāl; upon seeing his *guru* approach, Gorakhnāth got up from the bale, the clouds escaped, and rain began to fall. After this service, Matsyendranāth-Avalokiteśvara became the tutelary divinity of Nepāl. We may note in passing that this legend clearly points to a historical fact: it was from Kāmarūpa (=Assam) that "Matsyendranāth" brought tantrism, or, more precisely, the new "revelation" of the Siddhas and Nāthas, to Nepāl. Certain variants allow us to glimpse something more: Gorakhnāth is said to have shut up the clouds because he wanted to have a conversation with Matsyendranāth; the latter was lost in meditation on Kāpōtal, but Gorakhnāth knew that he would be moved to pity and would come to Nepāl to save the country from the great drought. This perhaps shows us that Gorakhnāth wanted to force his master to reveal secrets that the disciple had not yet learned.

54 Lévi, I, 352 ff.; H. A. Oldfield, *Sketches from Nipal*, II, 325 ff.; Briggs, pp. 196 ff.

Commanding rain is a power universal among shamans and magicians. Other legends make the shamanic character of the Siddha legends even clearer. Gorakhnāth one day left his body "asleep on his mat" (that is, he was in shamanic trance rather than in *samādhi*) and went down to the subterranean world of the god of snakes to obtain the magical incense that would enable him to save the life of a woman, Vāchal.[55] This is a typical shamanistic descent into hell (all the elements are present: ecstatic trance, the journey underground, and especially the purpose, saving a human life). Like the shamans, Gorakhnāth turns himself into a fly, a frog, and even into iron.[56] The *Dabistān*[57] tells of a combat with a *sannyāsi* during which Gorakhnāth turned himself into a toad—which is strangely reminiscent of combats between shamans under animal forms. He changes the water of a well into gold and then into crystal.[58] He reaches out his hand for hundreds of miles to interrupt a yogin's meditation and prevent him from destroying the land of Sind.[59] He restores many people to life. He creates men from horse dung, then burns them to ashes and revives them seven times.[60] In the Bengali poem *Gopī-candrer Pāṃcālī*, when Gorakhnāth initiated the princess Mayanāmatī, he made a banana tree grow from a seed in a few hours (this is the miracle known as the "mango trick"). At the same initiation, Gorakhnāth fed 25,000 yogins and disciples on a single grain of rice.[61]

His disciples have the same magical powers. The Nāthas fly through the air; Mayanāmatī and Hāḍī Siddha work miracles simply by uttering *mantras*. Hāḍī Siddha makes the sun and the moon his earrings,[62] Indra himself fans him, and Lakṣmī prepares his food; he touches heaven with his hand, his feet reach down to hell, the hairs of his body are like trees, etc. (We may note the macranthropic symbolism of all these feats, a symbolism indicat-

55 Briggs, p. 188.
56 Ibid., p. 187.
57 Ed. Shea and Troyer, II, 140.
58 Briggs, p. 186.
59 Ibid., p. 193.
60 Ibid., p. 190.
61 Dasgupta, p. 245.
62 But we must not forget the symbolical meaning of this expression; see above, p. 253.

ing the cosmic structure of the experience.)[63] Once Hāḍī Siddha recites a *mantra* on a broom; instantly countless brooms fall from the sky and sweep the market place. He ties twelve knots in a rag and throws it into a river, and the river immediately dries up. As he sits in the attitude of meditation in the royal park, coconuts fall before him; Hāḍī Siddha drinks their milk and eats their pulp, and the nuts return to their places in the trees. He exchanges the heads of the queens Adunā and Padunā, cuts a man in two and immediately revives him, etc. And the vernacular literatures are full of the same kinds of magical feats.[64]

Many of these miracles belong to the universal magical tradition, but some of them are definitely shamanic in structure and will occupy our attention later. For the moment, we shall emphasize the flowering of myths around the immortality conquered by Gorakhnāth and the other Nāthas and Siddhas. The Bengali poem *Gorakṣa Vijaya* presents the famous episode of Matsyendranāth's "captivity" as follows. Learning that his master is held prisoner by women in the country of Kadalī, Gorakhnāth descends into Yama's realm. On seeing him, Yama comes down from his throne, salutes him, and asks him what has brought him to the kingdom of the dead. Gorakhnāth answers him roughly, reminding him that he has no right to interfere in the affairs of the Siddhas, and threatens to ruin his kingdom; in fact, no sooner has he murmured the *mantra huṃkāra* than the city begins to shake to its foundations. Seized with panic, Yama offers to show the master the Book of Fate; Gorakhnāth searches it carefully, finds the leaf containing the destiny of his *guru*, changes it, and strikes his name from the list of the dead.[65]

We may note the shamanic character of this descent into hell to save the soul of a beloved person; similar undertakings are found in other oral literatures (central Asia, Polynesia, North America).

63 See above, p. 102.

64 Cf. Dasgupta, pp. 247 ff., citing *Gopī-candrer Gān*, *Gopī-candrer Sannyās*, etc.

65 Dasgupta, pp. 254–55.

But the story told by the *Gorakṣa Vijaya* has a further value for us. It discloses the yogic symbolism of death and immortality. Upon learning that his *guru* is the prisoner of women in Kadalī, Gorakhnāth understands that Matsyendranāth is doomed to die; this is the reason he descends into hell, reads his master's fate, and will not go until he has changed it. He then goes to Matsyendranāth, in Kadalī, presenting himself under the form of a dancing girl, and falls to dancing, at the same time singing enigmatic songs. Little by little, Matsyendranāth remembers his true identity; he understands that the "way of the flesh" leads to death, that his "oblivion" was, basically, forgetfulness of his true and immortal nature, and that the "charms of Kadalī" represent the mirages of profane life. Gorakhnāth urges him to resume the way of Yoga and to make his body "perfect" through the *kāya-sādhana*.[66] Now, we know that this "perfection," gained through alchemy and Haṭha Yoga, implied absolute mastery of body and mind, a mastery unattainable by a "prisoner of women."

The conquest of immortality is one of the favorite themes of the literature that developed around Gorakhnāth and his disciples. It is interesting to recall that the *Gorakṣa Vijaya* opens with Durgā's question to Śiva: "Why is it, my Lord, that thou art immortal, and mortal am I? Advise me the truth, O Lord, so that I also may be immortal for ages." [67] Now, it was none other than Durgā who had brought on the "oblivion" that almost cost Matsyendranāth his immortality; she had cast the spell of "forgetfulness" on him, and, as Gorakhnāth was later to explain to his master, this malediction symbolizes the eternal curse of ignorance that "nature" (=Durgā) lays upon the human being.[68]

A whole epic cycle grew up around Queen Mayanāmatī, Gorakhnāth's disciple, her husband Māṇik-candra, and her son Gopīcandra, whom Mayanāmatī endeavors to initiate in order to make him immortal. The struggle with death constitutes the central epic theme. Through her mystical gifts, Mayanā recognizes that

66 Ibid., p. 256. 67 See above, p. 270.

68 *Gorakṣa Vijaya*, cited by Dasgupta, p. 256.

her husband is doomed to die, and she offers to teach him the *mahājñāna* (the secrets of Yoga) so that he can nullify Yama's decree. But the king refuses. When Yama's messengers come to the palace to take her husband's soul, Mayanā murmurs *mantras*, magically changes herself into the goddess Kālī, and strikes and routs the messengers with her saber. One of their leaders, Godā-yama, goes to Śiva for counsel. Taking advantage of the absence of Mayanā, who had gone to the river to draw water, Godā-yama "extracts" the king's life and flies away in the shape of a bee. But Mayanāmatī, whose gift of yogic clairvoyance lets nothing escape her, pursues him down to hell. She seizes him and strikes him with an iron rod. After many episodes, Godā-yama succeeds in escaping, and Mayanā again pursues him, continually changing shape: Godā-yama hides in a heap of straw, she changes into a snake; he becomes a mouse, she a cat; he takes the form of a dove, she that of an eagle, until at last she succeeds in recovering her husband's soul. Together with widespread folklore motifs (the "magical pursuit"), these legends exploit themes that are unmistakably shamanic—the descent into hell, the theft of the soul by the demon of death, its recovery by the shaman, etc.

Other poems of the same epic cycle dwell on Mayanāmatī's initiation. Seeing her when she was still only a child, Gorakhnāth was touched by the thought that a girl so beautiful and chaste could be doomed to death like the rest of humankind, and he initiated her into Yoga, which made her immortal. After the initiation ceremony, he proclaimed: "Death himself has now given a written bond (not to extend his hands over Mayanā)"; [69] he specified that she could not die by fire, or water, or a wound from a weapon, etc. And, in fact, when later Mayanāmatī performed *satī* for her dead husband and mounted the pyre, the fire could not touch her. On another occasion, her own son Gopī-candra, egged on by one of his wives, submitted her to terrible tortures, but to no effect. We may note that all these ordeals have initiatory characteristics, and especially the characteristics of shamanic initiation.

69 Tr. Dasgupta, p. 259, n. 1.

Mayanāmatī is cast into the fire, but her dress is not even soiled by the smoke; she is tied in a sack and thrown into the river, but the goddess Gaṇgā receives her in her arms as if she were a child; she crosses a bridge made of a hair, and walks on a razor's edge; she is cooked for seven days and nights in a pot of boiling oil; she crosses every river in a boat made from the husk of a grain of wheat, etc.[70] She herself declares to her son: "By the practice of the mystic knowledge one becomes immortal (and the course of life will retard toward immortality from its natural flow toward death) just like the current of the tide-wave running backward. Through the boon granted by Gorakhnāth I am deathless; I can remain in the void for full fourteen ages—in water for full thirteen ages, in the fire for twelve years. When the creation will sink below and finally dissolve, and the earth will be not and there will remain only all-pervading water, the sun and the moon will set for ever and the whole universe will be destroyed—I shall float on for ever—I shall have no death."[71] Until this period, only the greatest gods—a Brahmā, a Nārāyaṇa—had dared so emphatically to proclaim their indestructible perenniality through the cosmic cycles. We feel how great was the thirst for immortality that found its expression in these epic poems, and we understand their extraordinary reverberations on all levels of Indian society.

Another of Gorakhnāth's disciples, Hāḍī Siddha—some of whose fakiric exploits we have already mentioned—is also known as a conqueror of death. Meeting Yama and one of his servants, he beats them for eight hours at a stretch. It is Hāḍī Siddha whom Mayanā chooses as *guru* for her son. She knows very well that, once Gopī-candra has been initiated, she will have no son, she mourns that no one in the world will then call her "mother"—but the desire to make her child immortal is stronger than maternal love, and she makes every effort to persuade him to forsake his wives and seek initiation. When Gopī-candra sets out into the

70 *Gopī-candrer Pāṃcālī, Govinda-candra-gītā, Gopī-candrer Gān,* summarized by Dasgupta, pp. 259 ff.

71 *Govinda-candra-gītā,* tr. Dasgupta, p. 260 (modified).

jungle with Hāḍī Siddha (and this isolation in the forest is a pre-eminently initiatory motif), he is unable to keep up with his master's pace and falls some way behind. Yama's messengers take advantage of this to "extract his life" (a shamanic theme) and then take refuge in hell. Returning in search of him, Hāḍī Siddha finds the young king's lifeless body; furious, he commands all the tigers in the jungle to keep watch around the corpse, descends into hell, and beats Yama and all his servants until he recovers Gopī-candra's soul.[72]

All these moving adventures in search of immortality, these dramatic descents into hell to fight Death and recover souls stolen by his messengers, these victories over the mortal and fallen condition of man, kindled the imaginations of poets and consoled the longing of the masses; here as elsewhere, these initiatory themes constituted the great literary subjects cherished by unlettered audiences. Yogic mythology and folklore finally nourished all the vernacular literatures of India. Their immense success shows us once again in what direction Indian thought valorized Yoga; it was the unrivaled means of conquering death, of gaining "miraculous powers," of enjoying absolute freedom even in this life. Despite the intrusion of magical exploits—which have always exercised a sort of fascination for the popular soul—the exemplary image of the conqueror of death, as presented in folklore and literature, corresponded precisely with that of the *jīvan-mukta*, of the man "liberated in life," the supreme goal of all yogic schools.

To be sure, the folklore and mythology that crystallized around Gorakhnāth and the other Siddhas could give but little place to the ideology and techniques that made the conquest of immortality possible. Yet the few allusions that occur, especially in the *Gorakṣa Vijaya*, are sufficiently explicit, and we understand that the method employed was that of tantrism, Haṭha Yoga, and alchemy. A short treatise, the *Yoga-vīja*, tells us that there are two kinds of bodies, the "unripe" (*apakva*) and the "ripe" (*pakva*), and that this second body is obtained through practicing Yoga (and hence is called

72 *Gopī-candrer Gān*, cited by Dasgupta, pp. 260–61.

yoga-deha, the "yoga-body").[73] Here, then, we have the alchemical theme par excellence—that of the "unripe" (imperfect) and "ripe" (perfect, "free") metals. Immortality is none other than the state of Śiva; this explains why Matsyendranāth, Gorakhnāth, and other Siddhas were "identified" with Śiva. As we have seen, the divine state is gained by him who realizes in his own body the union of the two polar principles, Śiva and Śakti. The school of the Nāthas and Siddhas employed a well-known yogico-tantric technique: *ulṭā sādhana* or *ujāna sādhana*, the process of "regression" or "going against the current"—that is, the complete reversal of human behavior, from "respiratory behavior" (replaced by *prāṇāyāma*) to "sexual behavior" (annulled by the technique of the "return of semen"). In other words, we here find once again the fundamental discipline of tantric Yoga, although the alchemistic and Haṭha-yogic themes are strongly stressed. The supreme ideal of the school is freedom, perfect health (*ajara*), and immortality (*amara*)—which is perfectly comprehensible if we bear in mind that Gorakhnāth was regarded as the "inventor" of Haṭha Yoga. Naturally, all these technical details, although documented in the literary texts, were relegated to the background; it was the *results* of Yoga that fired a "public" haunted by the mythical images of absolute freedom and immortality. Nowhere better than in these folklores and vernacular literatures do we glimpse the real function that Yoga fulfilled in the spiritual economy of all India.

Yoga and Shamanism

We have more than once found "shamanic" characteristics in the mythologies and folklores of the Siddhas. We must now define the relations between shamanism and Yoga more systematically. To begin, let us note that late Buddhism, in its Lamaistic form, perceptibly influenced the shamanisms of northern Asia and Siberia; in other words, the symbolisms, the ideology, and the techniques found in our day among Manchu, Tungus, Buriat, and other

73 Cf. the text quoted by Dasgupta, p. 253, n. 1.

shamans have been modified by Buddhist elements—in the last analysis, by Indian magic. Moreover, this is only one instance of a more general phenomenon. Indian culture, and particularly the magico-religious spirituality of India, radiated in all directions. Strong Indian influences have been identified in southeastern Asia and in Oceania. On the other hand, similar influences, especially that of aberrant, tantric magic, affected some aboriginal peoples in India itself, as, for example, the Bhaïgas and the Santals. From all this we may conclude that the tantric synthesis, while employing a large number of elements from the pre-Āryan, aboriginal spirituality, radiated very far beyond the frontiers of India, extending, by way of Tibet and Mongolia, to the extreme north of Asia and, by way of the Indian Archipelago, even into the South Seas. But this is a comparatively recent cultural phenomenon, whose beginnings coincide with the upsurge of tantrism (sixth to seventh century of our era). If we bear in mind that the tantric synthesis, especially in its "popular" elements (ritual magic, *mantrayāna*, etc.), had employed a considerable number of aboriginal elements, one conclusion is inescapable. It was a strongly *Asianized* India that carried its message so far; it was not the India of the Vedas or the Brāhmaṇas. In other words, Asia and Oceania were fertilized by the culture of an India that had already largely absorbed and assimilated its own autochthonous spiritualities.

To have said this is not, however, to have solved the problem of the relations between shamanism and Yoga; for if Indian influence (through Lamaism) modified the various shamanisms of northern Asia and the South (Malaysia, etc.), it did not create the phenomenon of shamanism itself. For there are countless shamanisms that have never been touched by Indian magico-religious elements (North and South America, Africa, Australia). To define the elements of the problem more precisely, we repeat that shamanism proper must not be confused with the mass of "magical" ideologies and practices attested almost everywhere in the world and on all cultural levels. There are very important "magical" complexes that contain no shamanic elements whatsoever: for example, agricultural magic—the rites and customs connected with the fertility of the soil and the abundance of harvests. In India, such rites and beliefs are very old and very widespread; we have already had occasion to note their coalescence with one or another form of Yoga, and we shall return to this problem. But we must emphasize that all these magico-religious complexes are in no way shamanic. Among the elements that constitute and are peculiar to shamanism, we must count as of primary importance: (1) an initiation comprising the candidate's symbolical dismemberment, death, and resurrection, which, among other things, implies his descent into hell and ascent to heaven; (2) the shaman's ability to make ecstatic journeys in his role of healer and psychopompos (he goes in search of the sick man's soul, stolen by demons, captures it, and restores it to the body; he conducts the dead man's soul to hell, etc.); (3) "mastery of fire" (the shaman touches red-hot iron, walks over burning coals, etc., without being hurt); (4) the shaman's ability to assume animal forms (he flies like the birds, etc.) and to make himself invisible.

This shamanic complex is very old; it is found, in whole or in part, among the Australians, the archaic peoples of North and South America, in the polar regions, etc. The essential and defining element of shamanism is *ecstasy*—the shaman is a specialist in the sacred, able to abandon his body and undertake cosmic journeys "in the spirit" (in trance). "Possession" by spirits, although documented in a great many shamanisms, does not seem to have been a primary and essential element. Rather, it suggests a phenomenon of degeneration; for the supreme goal of the shaman is to abandon his body and rise to heaven or descend into hell—not to let himself be "possessed" by his assisting spirits, by demons or the souls of the dead; the shaman's ideal is to master these spirits, not to let himself be "occupied" by them.[74]

74 "Possession" by a *gandharva*, and even the spiritualistic technique of communication through a medium, are already attested in the *Bṛhadāraṇyaka Upaniṣad* (III, 7, 1), but there is nothing "shamanic" here.

If we leave aside the *recent influences* (tantric and Lamaistic elements) exercised by India on the Asiatic and Siberian shamanisms, our problem is reduced to two separate questions: (1) on the one hand, we must define the Indo-European and pre-Āryan elements that, in India, can be regarded as belonging to shamanism proper; (2) having done this, we must isolate among these elements those which show certain similarities to the techniques of Yoga. We have elsewhere studied the shamanic complex in India,[75] and we shall not here repeat the data there collected, the more so as we have already had occasion, in previous chapters, to cite a number of characteristic phenomena (for example, the "magical heat" obtained through *tapas*, the rites and myths of ascent, magical flight, descents into hell).[76] We could also have cited other shamanic elements attested to in Vedic India—for example, the reconstitution of the sick man's soul by the priest or magician.[77]

We shall, then, confine our investigation to the shamanic symbolisms and practices that have a counterpart in one or another yogic technique or fakiric *siddhi*. Only after establishing this series of comparisons shall we be in a position to attack the problem of the structural connections between shamanism and Yoga. Since the most popular of fakiric miracles is the "rope trick," so called, and since it has long been considered the prototype of yogic powers, we shall make it the starting point of our investigation.

When the Buddha, after his Illumination, paid his first visit to his native city, Kapilavastu, he exhibited a number of "miraculous attainments." To convince his kinsmen of his spiritual powers and prepare them for conversion, he rose into the air, cut his body to pieces, let his limbs and his head fall to the ground, then joined them together again before the spectators' wondering eyes. Even Aśvaghoṣa describes this miracle,[78] but it is so essentially a part of the Indian magical tradition that it has become the typical prodigy of fakirism. The celebrated rope trick of the fakirs creates the

75 See *Shamanism*, pp. 403 ff.

76 See p. 106, etc.

77 See *Shamanism*, pp. 414 ff.

78 *Buddhacarita*, XIX, 12–13.

illusion of a rope that rises very high into the sky; the master makes a young disciple climb it until he is lost to sight; the fakir then throws his knife up into the air—and the young man's limbs fall to the ground one by one.

This rope trick has a long history in India, but it is also found in places as far away as China, Java, ancient Mexico, and medieval Europe. The Moroccan traveler Ibn Baṭūṭah observed it in China in the fourteenth century, Melton saw it at Batavia in the seventeenth, and Sahagun records it, in almost identical terms, in Mexico.[79] Here is Ibn Baṭūṭah's account: "He took a wooden ball, with several holes in it, through which long ropes were passed, and, laying hold of one of these, slung it into the air. It went so high that we lost sight of it altogether. There now remained only a little of the end of a thong in the conjurer's hand, and he desired one of the boys who assisted him to lay hold of it and to mount. He did so, climbing by the rope, and we lost sight of him also! The conjurer then called to him three times, but getting no answer, he snatched up a knife as if in a great rage, laid hold of the thong, and disappeared also! Bye and bye he threw down one of the boy's hands, then a foot, then the other hand, and the other foot, then the trunk and last of all the head! Then he came down himself, all puffing and panting, and with his clothes all bloody. . . . The Amir gave [him] some order . . . and our friend then took the lad's limbs, laid them together in their places, and gave a kick, when, presto! there was the boy, who got up and stood before us! All this astonished me beyond measure." Ibn Baṭūṭah then recalls how, having seen a similar performance in India, he had been similarly astonished.[80] As for Europe, numerous texts, at least from the thirteenth century on, refer to precisely similar prodigies, performed by sorcerers and magicians, who also had the power of

79 Eliade, *Shamanism*, pp. 428 ff.

80 *Voyages d'ibn Batoutah*, ed. and tr. C. F. Defrémery and B. R. Sanguinetti, IV, 291–92. (The translation given above is the one quoted in Conze, *Buddhism*, p. 174.) For bibliographies concerning these fakirs' miracles, see Note VIII, 5.

flying and making themselves invisible, like the shamans and yogins.[81]

In this "miracle" we can distinguish two separate shamanic elements: (1) the dismemberment (initiatory rite) and (2) the ascent to heaven. For the moment, let us analyze the first. We know that, during their "initiatory dreams," future shamans witness their own dismemberment by "spirits" or "demons" who play the role of masters of initiation; their heads are cut off, their bodies chopped to bits, their bones cleaned, etc.—and, after all this, the "demons" reassemble the bones and cover them with a new flesh.[82] In short, we are here dealing with ecstatic experiences whose structure is initiatory—a symbolic death is followed by renewal of the candidate's organs and his resurrection. We shall do well to recall that similar visions and experiences are also found among the Australians, the Eskimos, and the tribes of North and South America and Africa.[83] Hence we are in the presence of an initiatory technique that is extremely archaic.

Now, if the rope trick exhibits certain spectacular elements of this shamanic initiatory schema, some Indo-Tibetan rituals are still closer to it from the structural point of view. Robert Bleichsteiner thus describes the *tcheod* (*gtchod*), a Himālayan and Tibetan tantric rite that consists in offering one's own flesh to be devoured by demons: "To the sound of the drum made of human skulls and of the thighbone trumpet, the dance is begun and the spirits are

81 Cf. the examples brought together by A. Jacoby, "Zum Zerstückelung und Wiederbelebungswunder der indischen Fakire" (*Archiv für Religionswissenschaft*, XVII [1914], 455–75), pp. 466 ff. It is still difficult to decide definitely whether the rope trick of European conjurers is due to an influence from Oriental magic or if it derives from old local shamanic techniques. The fact that, on the one hand, the rope trick is attested in Mexico and that, on the other, initiatory dismemberment of the magician is also found in Australia, Indonesia, and South America inclines us to believe that in Europe we may here have a survival of local, pre-Indo-European magical techniques.

82 See the data in Eliade, *Shamanism*, pp. 35 ff., with commentary on all these symbolisms.

83 See ibid., pp. 45 ff.

invited to come and feast. The power of meditation evokes a goddess brandishing a naked sword; she springs at the head of the sacrificer, decapitates him, and cuts him to pieces; then the demons and wild beasts rush on the still-quivering fragments, eat the flesh, and drink the blood. The words uttered refer to certain *Jātakas*, which tell how the Buddha, in the course of his earlier lives, gave his own flesh to starving animals and man-eating demons." [84]

Similar initiatory rites are found elsewhere—for example, in Australia or among some North American tribes. In the case of the *tcheod*, we are in the presence of a mystical revalorization of a shamanistic initiation schema. Its "sinister" side is more apparent than real; the experience being one of death and resurrection, it is, like all experiences of its class, "terrifying." Indo-Tibetan tantrism has even more radically spiritualized the initiatory schema of "death at the hands of demons." We cite some tantric meditations whose object is to strip the body of its flesh so that the yogin can contemplate his own skeleton. He is instructed to visualize his body as a corpse and his own intellect as an angry goddess holding a knife and a skull. "Think that she severeth the head from the corpse . . . and cutteth the corpse into bits and flingeth them inside the skull as offerings to the deities." Another exercise consists in seeing himself as "a radiant white skeleton of enormous size, whence issueth flames, so great that they fill the voidness of the Universe." And a third meditation sets the yogin the task of contemplating himself as transformed into the wrathful Ḍākinī, stripping the skin from his own body. The text goes on: "Visualize thyself as . . . that thou strippest the hide from thy body, and spreadest it out so that it covereth the Third-Void Universe, and upon it heapest up all thy bones and flesh. Then, when the malignant spirits are in the midst of enjoying the feast, imagine that the Wrathful *Ḍākinī* taketh the hide and rolleth it up . . . and dasheth it down forcibly, reducing it and all its contents to a mass of

84 *L'Église jaune* (French tr. of *Die gelbe Kirche*), pp. 194–95. On the *gtchod*, see also Alexandra David-Neel, *Mystiques et magiciens du Thibet*, pp. 126 ff.

bony and fleshly pulp, upon which many mentally-produced wild beasts feed." [85]

It is probably to meditations of this type that some Indian yogins devote themselves in cemeteries.[86] Now, this is a spiritual exercise specific of Arctic shamanism. The Eskimo shamans questioned by Knud Rasmussen concerning their ability to contemplate themselves as skeletons answered rather vaguely, for the matter is a great secret. Rasmussen writes: "Though no shaman can explain to himself how and why, he can, by the power his brain derives from the supernatural, as it were by thought alone, divest his body of its flesh and blood, so that nothing remains but his bones. . . . By thus seeing himself naked, altogether freed from the perishable and transient flesh and blood, he consecrates himself, in the sacred tongue of the shamans, to his great task, through that part of his body which will longest withstand the action of the sun, wind and weather, after he is dead." [87]

This reduction of the shaman's body to a skeleton, and his ability to see himself as a skeleton, signify passing beyond the profane human condition—that is, initiation or deliverance. We know that the ritual costume of the Siberian shamans frequently attempts to imitate a skeleton.[88] Now, the same symbolism is plentifully documented in Tibet and the Himālayan regions. According to one legend, Padmasaṃbhava mounted to the roof of his house and danced a mystical dance, wearing only the "seven ornaments of bone." The role played by human skulls and thighbones in tantric and Lamaistic ceremonies is in any case well known. The skeleton dance has a particular importance in the dramatic scenarios called *tchams*, which undertake, among other things, to familiarize the spectators with the terrible images that appear in the state of *bardo*—that is, in the state intermediate between death and a new reincarnation. From this point of view, the

85 Lama Kazi Dawa-Samdup's rendering in W. Y. Evans-Wentz, *Tibetan Yoga*, pp. 311–12, 330–31.

86 See above, p. 296.

87 *Intellectual Culture of the Iglulik Eskimos*, tr. W. Worster, p. 114.

88 Eliade, *Shamanism*, pp. 158 ff.

skeleton dance must be regarded as an initiation, for it reveals certain posthumous experiences.[89]

Ascent to Heaven. Mystical Flight

As to the second "shamanic" element that we have identified in the rope trick—that is, the "ascent to heaven"—it constitutes a more complex problem. For the rite of ascent by way of the sacrificial post (*yūpa*) exists in Vedic India and apart from any shamanic complex; it is a rite by which "rupture of plane" is realized. Nevertheless, there are striking structural resemblances between the Indian ritual and the ascent of the shamanic tree. We know that the latter symbolizes the cosmic tree. Now, the sacrificial post (*yūpa*) is also assimilated to the cosmic tree.[90] The shamanic tree has seven, nine, or sixteen steps, each symbolizing a heaven, and climbing it is equivalent to ascending the cosmic tree or pillar. And the Indian sacrificer also ascends to heaven along the *yūpa* assimilated to the cosmic post.[91] The same symbolism occurs in the legends of the birth of the Buddha; he is no sooner born than he takes seven steps and touches the summit of the world,[92] just as the Altaic shaman climbs the seven or nine notches in the ritual birch to reach the highest heaven.[93] Needless to say, this old cosmological schema of the shamanic and Vedic ascent to heaven is here enriched by the millennial contribution of Indian metaphysical speculation. It is no longer the "world of the gods" and Vedic "immortality" that are the Buddha's goal: it is transcending the human condition.

The conception of the seven heavens, to which the *Majjhima-nikāya* alludes, goes back to Brāhmanism, and probably represents the influence of Babylonian cosmology—which also (though indirectly) left its mark on Altaic and Siberian cosmological conceptions. But Buddhism also knows a cosmological schema with

89 *Shamanism*, pp. 434 ff.

90 *Ṛg-Veda*, III, 8, 3; *Śatapatha Brāhmaṇa*, III, 6, 4, 13; III, 7, 1, 14, etc.

91 *Taittirīya Saṃhitā*, VI, 6, 4, 2, etc.

92 *Majjhima-nikāya*, III, 123.

93 Cf. Eliade, *Shamanism*, pp. 259 ff., 403 ff.

nine heavens, though they have been profoundly "interiorized," for the first eight heavens correspond to the several stages of meditation and the ninth symbolizes *nirvāṇa.* Each of these heavens contains the projection of a divinity of the Buddhist pantheon, who at the same time represents a particular degree of yogic meditation.[94] Now, we know that among the Altaians the seven or nine heavens are inhabited by various divine figures whom the shaman encounters during his ascent and with whom he converses; in the ninth heaven he finds himself in the presence of the Supreme Being, Bai Ülgän. Of course, in Buddhism it is no longer a question of a symbolic ascent into the heavens, but of degrees of meditation and, at the same time, of "steps" toward final liberation.

The Brāhmanic sacrificer mounts to heaven by ritually climbing a ladder; the Buddha transcends the cosmos by symbolically traversing the seven heavens; the Buddhist yogin, through meditation, realizes an ascent whose nature is completely spiritual. Typologically, all these acts share the same structure: each on its own plane indicates a particular way of transcending the profane world and attaining to the world of the gods, or Being, or the Absolute. The one great difference between them and the shamanic experience of ascent to heaven lies in the intensity of the latter; as we have already said, the shamanic experience includes ecstasy and trance. But let us recall the *muni* of the *Ṛg-Veda* who, "in the intoxication of ecstasy," mounted the "chariot of the winds," etc.[95] In other words, Vedic India also had its ecstatics, whose experience was comparable to the shamanic ecstasy. However—and this must be said at once—the difference between the yogic method of meditation and the technique that results in "shamanic" ecstasy is too great to permit us to consolidate them under any form. We shall return to these differences at the end of our comparative study.

The symbolism of the ecstatic ascent to heaven is a subspecies of the universally disseminated symbolism of magical flight, which,

94 Cf. W. Ruben, "Schamanismus im alten Indien" (*Acta Orientalia,* XVII [1939], 164–205), p. 169; Eliade, *Shamanism,* p. 406.

95 See above, p. 102.

though documented in all shamanisms and in all primitive magics, goes beyond the sphere of shamanism, strictly speaking. We need not here repeat the documentation and commentaries that we have presented elsewhere.[96] But the idea that saints, yogins, and magicians can fly is to be found everywhere in India. For rising into the air, flying like a bird, traversing immense distances in a flash, and vanishing are among the magical powers that Buddhism and Hinduism confer on arhats and magicians. The miraculous lake, Anavatapta, could be reached only by those who possessed the supernatural power of flight; Buddha and the Buddhist saints journeyed there in the twinkling of an eye, just as, in Hindu legends, the *ṛṣis* soared through the air to the divine and mysterious northern land named Śvetadvīpa. These are, of course, "pure lands," located in a mystical space that is at once paradisal and of the nature of an "inner space" accessible only to the initiate. Anavatapta, Śvetadvīpa, or the other Buddhist paradises are only so many modalities of being, attainable by virtue of Yoga, of asceticism, or of contemplation. But we must emphasize the identity between the expression given to such experiences and the archaic symbolism of ascent and flight, so prevalent in shamanism.

Buddhist texts speak of four magical powers of translation (*gamana*), the first being ability to fly like a bird.[97] In his list of *siddhis* obtainable by yogins, Patañjali cites the power to fly through the air (*laghiman*).[98] It is always by the "power of yoga" that, in the *Mahābhārata*, the sage Nārada soars into the air and reaches the summit of Mount Meru (the "center of the world"); from there, far away in the Ocean of Milk, he sees Śvetadvīpa.[99] For "with such a [yogic] body, the yogin goes where he will." [100] But another tradition recorded in the *Mahābhārata* already makes a distinction between true mystical ascent—which cannot be said to

96 *Shamanism*, pp. 407 ff., pp. 477 ff.

97 Cf. *Visuddhimagga*, ed. C. A. F. Rhys Davids, p. 396. On *gamana*, see Sigurd Lindquist, *Siddhi und Abhiññā*, pp. 58 ff.

98 *Yoga-sūtras*, III, 45; cf. *Gheraṇḍa Saṃhitā*, III, 78. On similar traditions in the epic, cf. Hopkins, "Yoga-Technique," pp. 337, 361.

99 *Mahābhārata*, XII, 335, 2 ff.

100 Ibid., XII, 317, 6.

be always "concrete"—and magical flight, which is only an illusion: "We too can fly to the heavens and manifest ourselves under various forms, but through illusion" (*māyayā*).[101]

We see in what direction Yoga and the other Indian techniques of meditation elaborated the ecstatic experiences and magical prowesses that belonged to an immemorial spiritual heritage. However this may be, the secret of magical flight is also known to Indian alchemy. And the same miracle is so common among the Buddhist arhats that *arahant* yielded the Singhalese verb *rahatve*, "to disappear," "to pass instantaneously from one point to another." [102] The Ḍākinīs, fairy sorceresses who play an important role in some tantric schools, are called in Mongolian "they who walk through the air," and in Tibetan "they who go to heaven." [103] Magical flight and ascending to heaven by the help of a ladder or a rope are also frequent motifs in Tibet, where they are not necessarily borrowed from India, the more so since they are documented in the Bon-po traditions or in traditions deriving from them. In addition, the same motifs play a considerable role in the magical beliefs and folklores of the Lolos, the Mossos, and the Chinese; and they also occur almost everywhere in the primitive world.

Ascent to heaven and magical flight carry an extremely complex symbolism relating especially to the human soul and intelligence. "Flight" sometimes stands for intelligence, comprehension of hidden things or of metaphysical truths. "Intelligence [*manas*] is the swiftest of birds," says the *Ṛg-Veda* (VI, 9, 5). And the *Pañcaviṃśa Brāhmaṇa* (XIV, 1, 13) declares: "He who understands has wings." We know that among many peoples the soul is conceived of as a bird. Magical flight assumes the value of an "escape from the body"—that is, it translates ecstasy, the liberation of the soul, into plastic terms. But while the majority of human beings are changed into birds only at the moment of death, when they forsake

101 Ibid., V, 160, 55 ff.

102 A. M. Hocart, "Flying Through the Air" (*Indian Antiquary*, LII [1923], 80–82), p. 80.

103 Cf. P. J. van Durme, "Notes sur le Lamaïsme" (*Mélanges chinois et bouddhiques*, I [1932], 263–319), p. 374, n. 2.

their bodies and fly into the air, shamans, sorcerers, and ecstatics of all kinds realize "emergence from the body" in this world and as often as they wish. This myth of the bird-soul contains in germ a whole metaphysics of man's spiritual autonomy and freedom.

We shall cite one more well-known folkloric miracle, the "mango trick." The yogin puts a mango seed into the ground, and presently the tree comes up before the astonished eyes of the audience. According to a Buddhist tradition recorded in the commentary on the *Dhammapada*,[104] the Buddha performed the very same miracle in the garden of King Pasenadi: Gaṇḍa, the king's gardener, gives Buddha a mango fruit, and the Enlightened One tells him to bury the seed; he then washes his hands over the hole in which it has been put, and in a few moments a mango tree fifty cubits high springs up, bearing flowers and fruit at once. Now, similar exploits are attested in North American shamanic circles; the Pueblos, for example, believe that their shamans can make a grain of wheat sprout and grow under the spectator's eyes.[105]

"Magical Heat." "Inner Light"

Let us pass on to another group of shamanic techniques, the "mastery of fire" and "magical heat." Shamans and sorcerers are everywhere reputed to be masters of fire. They swallow burning coals, they touch red-hot iron, they walk on flames. During their séances, the Siberian shamans "heat themselves" to such a point that they strike their bodies with knives and are not hurt, run themselves through with swords, swallow embers, etc. Now, many yogin-fakirs exhibit similar feats. The likeness between yogins and shamans is still more patent in the case of "magical heat." One of the initiatory ordeals peculiar to shamanism involves precisely the ability to resist extreme cold. Thus, among the Manchus, nine holes are cut in the winter ice; the candidate for shamanship must dive into the first hole, swim under the ice, and come out by the

104 *Dhammapada-aṭṭhakathā*, III, 199.
105 Cf. Eliade, *Shamanism*, p. 315, n. 74.

second, and so on successively to the ninth hole.[106] The Labrador Eskimos have a similar initiatory ordeal: a candidate remained for five days and nights in the frozen ocean, and, having proved that he had not even been made wet, was immediately given the title of *angákkok*.[107]

Now, certain Indo-Tibetan initiatory ordeals consist precisely in judging a candidate's degree of preparation by his ability to dry a large number of wet sheets applied, one after the other, to his naked body during a snowy winter night. In Tibetan, this "psychic heat" is called *gtūm-mö* (pronounced *toumo*). "Sheets are dipped in the icy water. Each man wraps himself in one of them and must dry it on his body. As soon as the sheet has become dry, it is again dipped in the water and placed on the novice's body to be dried as before. The operation goes on in that way until daybreak. Then he who has dried the largest number of sheets is acknowledged the winner of the competition." [108]

Gtūm-mö is a yogico-tantric exercise well known to the ascetic tradition of India. We have already referred to the intense heat aroused by the awakening of the *kuṇḍalinī*.[109] The texts say that psychic heat is obtained both by holding the breath and by transmutation of the sexual energy,[110] and the experience is always accompanied by luminous phenomena (an important detail, to which we shall have to return). The technique of "producing inner heat" is not a tantric innovation. The *Majjhima-nikāya* (I, 244) speaks of the "heat" obtained by holding the breath, and other Buddhist texts [111] say that the Buddha is "burning." The Buddha is "burning" because he practices asceticism, *tapas*—and we have seen [112] that in India *tapas* is documented from Vedic times, but that the ideology and practices of "magical sweating" and of creation through autothermy were known from the Indo-European period

106 Ibid., pp. 112 f. 107 Ibid., pp. 59–60, n. 84.

108 Alexandra David-Neel, *With Mystics and Magicians in Tibet*, pp. 227 f.

109 See above, p. 246.

110 Cf. Lama K. D. Samdup and Evans-Wentz, *Tibetan Yoga*, pp. 156 ff., 187 ff., 196 ff.

111 *Dhammapada*, 387, for example. 112 Above, p. 106.

on; indeed, they belong to an archaic cultural stage, being attested both in primitive cosmologies and in many shamanisms.

There is every reason to believe that the experience of "inner heat" was known to mystics and magicians from the earliest times. Many primitive tribes conceive of magico-religious power as "burning" and express it by terms meaning "heat," "burn," "very hot," etc. This, by the way, is the reason why magicians and sorcerers drink salted or pungently spiced water and eat highly aromatic plants—they hope thus to increase their "inner heat." In modern India the Mohammedans believe that a man in communication with God becomes "burning." Anyone who performs miracles is termed "boiling." By extension, all kinds of persons or acts involving a magico-religious power are held to be "burning." [113]

As we should expect, the *sacred power* experienced under the form of extreme heat is not obtained only through shamanic or mystical techniques. We have already mentioned [114] some terms from the Indo-European martial vocabulary (*furor*, *ferg*, etc.) that express precisely this "extreme heat" and "rage" that characterize the bodily reception of a sacred force. Like the shaman, the young hero "heats" himself during his initiatory combat. This "rage" and this "heat" are not "profane" or "natural"; they are the syndrome of the appropriation of a sacrality. "Mastery of fire" and "inner heat" are always connected with reaching a particular ecstatic state or, on other cultural levels, with reaching an unconditioned state, a state of perfect spiritual freedom. "Mastery of fire"—insensibility to heat and hence the "magical heat" that renders both extreme cold and the temperature of burning coals tolerable—is a magico-mystical virtue that, accompanied by other no less extraordinary feats (ascent, magical flight, etc.), tangibly indicates that the shaman has transcended the human condition and already participates in the condition of the "spirits."

Obviously, the primary experience of magico-religious *power* expressed in the "rage" of martial initiations or in the "heat" of magicians, shamans, or yogins could be transformed, differentiated,

113 Cf. Eliade, *Shamanism*, pp. 474 ff. 114 Above, p. 107.

refined by a later effort toward integration and "sublimation." The Indian word *kratu*, which began by meaning the "energy of the ardent warrior, especially Indra," then "victorious force," "heroic strength and ardor," "courage," "delight in battle," and, by extension, "power" and "majesty" in general, finally came to mean "the force proper to the pious man, which makes him capable of obeying the prescriptions of the *ṛta* and attaining happiness." [115]

It remains clear, however, that the "rage" and the "heat" engendered by a violent and excessive increase in *power* are feared by the majority of mankind; this kind of power, in its "crude" state, is chiefly of interest to magicians and warriors; those who seek confidence and equilibrium in religion resist magical "heat" and "fire." The term *śānti*, which in Sanskrit designates tranquillity, peace of soul, absence of passion, relief from suffering, is derived from the root *śam*, which originally had the meaning of extinguishing the "fire," the anger, the fever—in short, the "heat"—engendered by demoniac powers.[116] The Indian of Vedic times felt the danger of magic; he resisted the temptation to excessive power,[117] just as, later, the yogin must overcome the temptation of the "miraculous powers" (*siddhi*).

We have already observed that, in yogico-tantric exercises, "inner heat" is accompanied by luminous phenomena.[118] In another direction, luminous mystical experiences are attested from the time of the Upaniṣads, in which the "inner light" (*antar jyotiḥ*)

115 Kasten Rönnow, "Ved. *kratu-*, eine wortgeschichtliche Untersuchung," *Le Monde orientale*, XXVI (1932), 1–90. Cf. G. Dumézil, *Naissance d'archanges*, pp. 145 ff. In the Gāthās "the meaning of *khratu* corresponds especially to this later moral, properly religious meaning of the Vedic *kratu: khratu* is the religious effort of the pious man, what could be called man's pious courage in the fight against evil that represents the believer's whole life" (Dumézil, p. 145).

116 Cf. D. J. Hoens, *Śānti*, especially pp. 177 ff.

117 In this behavior we sense man's ambivalent reaction to the sacred: on the one hand, he feels drawn by magico-religious *power*; on the other, he feels repelled. On the meaning of this ambivalence, see Eliade, *Patterns in Comparative Religion*, pp. 14 ff., 460 ff.

118 Above, p. 107. Cf. Evans-Wentz, *Tibetan Yoga*, pp. 223 ff.

defines the very essence of the *ātman;* [119] in some Buddhist techniques of meditation, mystical light of various colors indicates the success of the operation.[120] We shall not dwell upon the immense place accorded to the inner light in the mysticisms and theologies of Christianity and Islam; nor is there room here for a study in comparative mysticism; our investigation is restricted to the realm of shamanism. We shall only add that, in India, luminous epiphanies extend beyond the boundaries of yogic experience—witness Arjuna's ecstatic ascent of the Mountain of Śiva, an ascent that comes to its end in a supernatural light.[121]

But the inner light constitutes the decisive experience of Eskimo shamanism. We can even say that obtaining it is equivalent to an initiatory ordeal. For the candidate obtains this "illumination"—*qaumaneq*—after long hours of meditation and in perfect solitude. According to the shamans whom Rasmussen questioned,[122] the *qaumaneq* consists "of a mysterious light which the shaman suddenly feels in his body, inside his head, within the brain, an inexplicable searchlight, a luminous fire, which enables him to see in the dark, both literally and metaphorically speaking, for he can now, even with closed eyes, see through darkness and perceive things and coming events which are hidden from others; thus they look into the future and into the secrets of others." When the candidate experiences this "illumination" for the first time, "it is as if the house in which he is suddenly rises; he sees far ahead of him, through mountains, exactly as if the earth were one great plain, and his eyes could reach to the end of the earth. Nothing is hidden from him any longer."

Similarities and Differences

What conclusions can we draw from a closer examination of these comparative observations? To begin, let us eliminate the elements that do not directly concern yogic ideology and yogic techniques.

119 *Bṛhadāraṇyaka Upaniṣad*, I, 3, 28.
120 See above, p. 195.
121 *Mahābhārata*, VII, 80 ff.
122 *Iglulik Eskimos*, pp. 112–13.

We shall set aside the series of correspondences dependent upon cosmological systems and the symbolism of ascent, both of which are attested in shamanism as well as in India (the *yūpa*, the Buddha's Seven Steps, etc.); these are merely structural parallels that do not entail an approximation between shamanism and Yoga. Only two aspects of the symbolism of ascent will engage our attention—the rope trick and magical or ecstatic flight. In this connection two observations are called for: (1) the rope trick, although one of the typical fakirs' miracles, is not a constituent part of any yogic technique; it can be put in the list of *siddhis*—that is, among the countless "marvelous powers" of the Indian magical tradition; (2) as to ecstatic flight, it was known from Vedic times,[123] but it, too, was never a part of Yoga, properly speaking. On the philosophical level, the power to displace oneself at will and to "fly" symbolized the *autonomy of the spirit;* on the magical level, "flight" was one of the *siddhis* and could be obtained at will through either Yoga, or alchemy, or sorcery.[124] On the other hand, as we remarked before, "magical flight" does not belong solely to the realm of shamanism, although it is one of its characteristic elements; "flight" is an integral part of the oldest magical tradition.

The mango trick is likewise to be put among the *siddhis.* Distinctly shamanic in structure, this miracle had a curious destiny in India. On the one hand, it became the typical fakirs' miracle; on the other, it was employed by philosophers (among others, by Śaṇkara) as a striking image to explain the process of cosmic illusion. Other yogic *siddhis* are also attested in magical and shamanic traditions—for example, "entering another's body," or the reanimation of corpses. Morphologically, this *siddhi* falls among the "magical powers" rather than among shamanic feats.

On the other hand, there is a *siddhi* that is peculiar to Yoga and that does not form part of the universal magical tradition, for it

123 See above, p. 102.

124 In non-Āryan India, "flight" is the specific attribute of sorcerers and sorceresses; cf. W. Koppers, "Probleme der indischen Religionsgeschichte" (*Anthropos*, XXV [1940–41], 761–814), pp. 768 (Santal), 783 (Orissa), etc.

presupposes a long spiritual preparation. It is the ability to remember previous incarnations. This "power" is documented among North American shamans; they remember their former lives, and some of them even claim to have witnessed the beginning of the world.[125] Here we touch upon a problem of considerable complexity, which goes beyond the scope of this study—the problem of the universally disseminated belief in the pre-existence of the human soul; certain privileged persons—mystics, shamans, etc.—are able to transform this "belief" into a *personal experience.* Comparison with India is unavoidable—here, too, only yogins and the Awakened are able to remember their pre-existences; other men accept the doctrine of transmigration as a part of the traditional ideology. But neither classic Yoga nor Buddhism attributes a decisive importance to knowledge of former lives; in other words, the possession of this *siddhi* does not, by itself, solve the problem of liberation. We are here probably confronted with an aboriginal mythology and mystical technique connected with the belief in the pre-existence of the soul—a mythology and technique that both Yoga and Buddhism assimilated and revalorized from the earliest times.

Equally suggestive are the similarities between the initiatory "dismemberment" of the shamans and certain yogico-tantric meditations that imply either the yogin's dismemberment by "demons," or his contemplation of his own skeleton, or, finally, the magico-religious intervention of skulls and corpses. Spiritual exercises of this type are not attested in the tradition of classic Yoga; they were assimilated during the vogue of tantrism, though they were probably known much earlier, not only in India (the Kāpālikas, the Aghorīs, etc.), but also in the Himālayan regions and in Tibet (where Bon-po still preserved a distinctly shamanistic structure). Hence we have to do with a revalorization, in yogic terms, of an aboriginal shamanic technique; similar processes are attested all through the course of the great tantric synthesis.

125 Cf. Ake Hultkrantz, *Conceptions of the Soul Among North American Indians*, pp. 412 ff.

On the plane of mystical technique in the strict sense, the most striking similarity between shamanism and Yoga is represented by the production of "inner heat." We have shown that this is a universally disseminated technique that is not always the prerogative of ascetics and magicians; "inner heat" was also aroused by martial initiations. We have further observed that this technique is connected with the "mastery of fire," a feat of fakirdom that must be regarded as the most archaic and most generally disseminated element of the magical tradition. We may conclude that from its earliest beginnings Yoga knew the production of inner heat by retention of breath. For *tapas* is already attested in the Vedic period, and respiratory discipline was practiced by the mysterious ecstatics known as *vrātyas.* It is difficult to fix the "origin" of *prāṇāyāma;* but it is permissible to suppose that rhythmically regulated breathing was the result of certain "mystical experiments" directed toward increasing inner heat.[126]

126 J. Filliozat believes ("Les Origines d'une technique mystique indienne," *Revue philosophique,* CXXXVI [1946], 208–20) that he can connect the origins of Yoga with "a scholarly doctrine"—that of the *prāṇa* as an essential element of life. "It is clear that, seeing in the respiratory breath the common motor of psychism and of life, the Indians sought to obtain effects both spiritual and psychic by acting upon it. . . . The mere existence of the theory does not, however, account for all the details of the procedures. But it was enough that it produced the idea of having recourse to it. Experiment did the rest. The physiological results obtained in the course of attempts, and their repercussions on the psychic state, decided the choice and guided the improvement of the practical means. At least the existence of the theory explains why the attempts were made" (Filliozat, pp. 217–18). The hypothesis is tempting; but one hesitates to make the origins of a mystical technique depend upon experiments attempted in view of a philosophical theory. The contrary process seems to us more plausible: mystical experimentation first, the elaborated theory of the breaths afterward. As Dr. Filliozat reminds us (p. 217), the breaths were already assimilated to the cosmic winds in the Vedic period. It is probably in an experience "cosmic" in structure that we must seek the beginnings of *prāṇāyāma,* but such experiences were mystical in nature, they were not undertaken in consequence of a scientific theory. The polyvalence of Yoga, its increasing success in an India that became more and more Asianized, perhaps show us in what direction to look for its "origins." But let us make it clear that the alternative is not between a "scholarly"

As for ritual intoxication by hemp, opium, and other narcotics, it is a practice abundantly attested in the shamanic world as well as among some yogins. We know that Patañjali himself puts simples (*auṣadhi*), together with *samādhi*, among the means of obtaining the *siddhis*.[127] "Simples" can mean either ecstasy-inducing narcotics or the "herbs" from which the elixir of longevity was extracted.[128] In any case, hemp and similar drugs produce *ecstasy* and not the yogic *samādhi*; these "mystical means" properly belong to the phenomenology of ecstasy (of which we have had an example in the behavior of the Ṛg-Vedic *muni*),[129] and they were only reluctantly admitted into the sphere of classic Yoga. Yet the fact that Patañjali himself refers to the magico-ecstatic virtues of simples is both significant and pregnant with consequences; it proves the pressure exercised by the ecstatics, their will to substitute their methods for the disciplines of classic Yoga. And in fact a certain number of Śāktas and members of other ecstatic and orgiastic movements used, and still use, opium and hashish.[130] The majority of these ecstatics are in more or less direct dependence upon Śiva—in other words, belong to an aboriginal cultural stratum.

In the sphere of shamanism, strictly speaking, intoxication by drugs (hemp, mushrooms, tobacco, etc.) seems not to have formed part of the original practice. For, on the one hand, shamanic myths and folklore record a decadence among the shamans of the present day, who have become unable to obtain ecstasy in the fashion of the "great shamans of long ago"; on the other, it has been observed that where shamanism is in decomposition and the trance is simulated, there is also overindulgence in intoxicants and drugs. In the sphere of shamanism itself, however, we must distinguish be-

---

and a "popular" origin, but between the former and a pre-Āryan spiritual tradition, represented by peoples culturally superior to the Indo-Europeans of Vedic times. The problem of Mohenjo-daro remains open (see below, pp. 353 ff.).

127 *Yoga-sūtras*, IV, 1.

128 See above, p. 275.

129 See above, p. 102.

130 Cf. Ernst Arbman, *Rudra*, pp. 300 ff.; Lindquist, *Die Methoden des Yoga*, pp. 194 ff.

tween this (probably recent) phenomenon of intoxication for the purpose of "forcing" trance, and the ritual consumption of "burning" substances for the purpose of increasing "inner heat." Aboriginal India, then, may have known a number of immemorial traditions regarding the means for obtaining "magical heat," ecstasy, or "divine possession," and all these traditions may more than once have sought to be accepted into, or even to replace, the yogic disciplines. We find a proof of this in the fact that a considerable number of "yogins" and "fakirs," while adhering to some particular yogic school and practicing certain exercises (*prāṇāyāma*, etc.), at the same time continue many ecstatic and orgiastic traditions.

If we now attempt to draw some general conclusions from this brief comparative examination, we must begin by distinguishing three spiritual positions: (1) the *ecstasy* peculiar to shamanism; (2) *deliverance* through *samādhi*, which is proper to classic Yoga; (3) *jīvan-mukti*, which, almost indistinguishable from "immortality in the body," is a form peculiar to tantric and alchemistic Yoga, of particular appeal to the "popular" imagination, whose longings it satisfies. After what we have just said, there is no need to dwell upon the structural differences between shamanic ecstasy and yogic enstasis. As a developed spiritual technique (we are not discussing its possible "origins"), Yoga cannot possibly be confused with shamanism or classed among the techniques of ecstasy. The goal of classic Yoga remains perfect *autonomy*, enstasis, while shamanism is characterized by its desperate effort to attain the "condition of a spirit," to accomplish ecstatic flight. Nevertheless, there is a definite point where Yoga and shamanism meet. They meet in "emergence from time" and the abolition of history. The shaman's ecstasy recovers the primordial freedom and bliss of the ages in which, according to the myths, man could ascend to heaven physically and converse with the gods.[131] For its part, Yoga results in the nonconditioned state of *samādhi* or of *sahaja*, in the perfect

131 See Eliade, *Shamanism*, passim, and "Nostalgia for Paradise in the Primitive Traditions," in *Myths, Dreams and Mysteries*, pp. 59–72.

spontaneity of the *jīvan-mukta,* the man "liberated in this life." From one point of view, we may say that the *jīvan-mukta* has abolished time and history; his spontaneity in some sort resembles the paradisal existence of the primordial man evoked by the myths. This is as much as to say that the yogin, no less than the shaman, attempts to do away with historical time and to return to a situation that is nonconditioned (hence paradoxical, impossible to imagine). But while the shaman can obtain this spontaneity only through his ecstasy (when he can "fly") and only for as long as his ecstasy lasts, the true yogin, he who has gained *samādhi* and become a *jīvan-mukta,* enjoys this nonconditioned situation continuously—that is, he has succeeded in definitively abolishing time and history.

This structural difference between the shaman and the yogin is seen particularly in classic Yoga. But we have noted that, alongside the classic form of Yoga, others crystallized very early, using other approaches (for example, *bhakti*) and pursuing other ends (for example, obtaining a "divine body"). It is because of this proliferation of new yogic forms and this process of coalescence with other mystical techniques that we find ourselves before a third "spiritual position"—that which affirms the possibility of prolonging life indefinitely in an "incorruptible body," created by Haṭha Yoga and alchemy in concert. Neither classic Yoga nor, in general, any other leading form of Indian thought pursued immortality. To indefinitely prolonged existence, India preferred liberation and freedom. And yet, as we have just seen,[132] at a particular moment Yoga came to represent for the Indian mind not only the ideal instrument of liberation but also the "secret" that would conquer death. There is but one explanation for this. For part of India, and perhaps for the greater part, Yoga was identified not only with the way of sanctity and liberation but also with magic, particularly with the magical means of vanquishing death. In other words, the mythology of the *jīvan-mukta* satisfied not only the thirst for freedom but also the longing for immortality.

132 Above, p. 317.

In short, we observe a continuous process of osmosis and coalescence, which, in the end, radically changed certain fundamental aspects of classic Yoga. Although the latter is neither magic nor shamanism, many magical marvels are accepted among the *siddhis* and a number of shamanic techniques are successfully homologized with yogic exercises. From all this we can divine the pressure exerted by the immemorial magico-religious substratum that preceded the constitution of Yoga in the strict sense, a pressure that, from a particular moment on, succeeded in sending to the surface, and incorporating into Yoga, certain elements of the extremely ancient, aboriginal spirituality. It may even be that Yoga received and preserved the contribution of long-vanished civilizations, such as that of Mohenjo-daro. For, as we shall soon see, popular Hinduism displays numerous aspects that are to be found in the protohistorical religions and cultures of India. Before reviewing these aspects, let us consider the process of coalescence between certain "popular" yogas and aboriginal spiritualities. Such an examination will prove highly instructive. It will show us, in flesh and blood as it were, the many and various erosions, degradations, and transformations that, though they took place in the margin of official Hinduism, yet at the same time prepared and anticipated the final syntheses.

Coalescence and Degradation: Yoga and Popular Religions

The survival of Buddhism many centuries after the Moslem invasion and after the Brāhmanic offensive for reconversion is further proof of its success among the popular strata. In some provinces, especially in Orissa and Bengal, the Buddhist cult and dogmas continued to find adherents even after the triumph of Brāhmanism.[133] It was, of course, a popular religion, which had very little connection with the original Buddhist message. Yet the survival of "crypto-Buddhism" (as N. N. Vasu terms it) [134] is nevertheless

133 See Note VIII, 6.

134 *Modern Buddhism and Its Followers in Orissa.*

significant. It is because it became a ritual religion and a mystical devotion (*bhakti*)—that is, because it satisfied the need for worship and devotion characteristic of the aboriginal populations—that this "decadent" Buddhism was able to maintain itself against the combined offensive of Islam and Brāhmanism. On the plane of dogma, it had arrived at a synthesis between the Vajrayāna and Brāhmanism.[135] Yoga plays almost no part. But that tantric excesses had free rein under the cloak of Buddhism, we can divine from the names given to Buddhist places of worship—for example, "seat of the prostitute." [136]

The cult of Dharma has survived to our day, for its Hinduization was still in process at the beginning of this century. In a temple of Dharma, Haraprasād Shāstri had seen the priest dividing the offerings into two parts; when asked the reason, the priest had replied: "He is Dharma and Śiva at the same time and hence the division." The *mantra* employed was: "Salute be to Śiva, who is Dharma-rāja." A few years later, Shāstri visited the temple again and observed that the priest had set a symbolic representation of the female organ of generation (*gaurī-paṭṭa*) under the statue of Dharma, as if to Hinduize it completely.[137]

This Hinduization was not without its dangers. Very often it was the occasion for restoring archaic religious behavior that had long since run its course in Brāhmanic society. We shall cite an example. From the Middle Ages on, we have testimony to an autumnal ceremony, the Śabarotsava, which was held in honor of Durgā and which still survives in Bengal. The participants daubed their bodies with mud and covered them with leaves and flowers, like the Śabaras, an autochthonous people of southern India, of Australoid origin, from whom, too, the ceremony derives its name. Two verses of the *Kālikā Purāṇa* (LXI, 21–22) prove that the Śabarotsava included licentious ritual songs, erotic mimicry, and probably orgies. In addition, another Bengalese Purāṇa of the

135 Cf. the cult of Dharma in western Bengal.

136 K. R. Subramanian, *Buddhist Remains in Āndhra*, p. 30.

137 Dasgupta, *Obscure Religious Cults*, p. 321, n. 2.

seventeenth century, the *Bṛhaddharma Purāṇa* (III, 6, 81–83), says that on the occasion of this agricultural festival the names of the organs of generation must be uttered only before persons who have been initiated into the cult of Śakti, adding, however, that Śakti delights in hearing obscene words.[138]

This episode is highly instructive. We see how a Hindu vegetation festival (itself of aboriginal origin and structure, but long since Hinduized), in its effort to assimilate eccentric sacralities at all costs, adopts and validates the religious behavior of an archaic people. The Śabarotsava is a typical example of the processes by which the aboriginal religions were incorporated into the cult of the Great Goddess of fertility and vegetation, Durgā-Śakti.

As we have already seen, Durgā-Śakti plays a preponderant role in tantrism and in all forms of Śāktism. We must stress the fact that the assimilation and coalescence of aboriginal cults was effected especially on the lowest levels of religion and magic, among what are termed the popular strata. It is here that we find, for example, yogic and Śaktic complexes incorporated into the mythologies and rituals of vegetation. Certain fairies, moreover, bear the name *yoginī*, as if to emphasize the origin of their magical power, obtained through Yoga. The tantric texts describe them thus: "The *Kula Yoginīs* always dwell in all these *kula* trees. No one should sleep under the *kula* trees nor injure them." [139] They are at once nymphs and sorceresses; like the Great Goddess Durgā, whom the vast troop of them serve, but of whom they are sometimes epiphanies, the Yoginīs, the Ḍākinīs, and the Lāmās are kindly and at the same time terrible. Some texts emphasize their beauty and grace. According to the *Abhidānottara-tantra*,[140] the Yoginīs—of whom there are three classes: Kulajā, Brāhmī, Rudrā—are fairies white as lotus blossoms, with pink eyes; they are fond of white and

138 D. C. Sirkar, "The Śākta Pīṭhas" (*Journal of the Royal Asiatic Society of Bengal*, XIV, 1 [1948], 1–108), pp. 105–06.

139 *Śaktānandatāraṅgiṇī*, cited by R. Chanda, *The Indo-Āryan Races*, p. 135.

140 Text analyzed by Rājendralāla Mitra, *The Sanskrit Buddhist Literature of Nepāl*, pp. 2 ff.

perfumed attire and are devoted to the adoration of Sugata. The Ḍākinīs are red-skinned and exude the fragrance of lotus; they have gentle faces, red eyes and nails, and they like to decorate their dwellings with pictures of lotus blossoms. In the country around Mt. Girnar,[141] three kinds of Yoginīs are known: Pul-(flower), Lāl-(red), and Keśur-(hair). They are invoked when epidemics, especially cholera, afflict the region.

Fairies, she-devils, sorceresses—all these companions or local epiphanies of Durgā represent minor deities of both vegetation and destiny (they bring death or wealth), at the same time incarnating the forces of shamanic magic and of Yoga. At Udyāna, the Yoginīs were imagined under the form of tiger-women, feeding on human flesh and able to transform themselves into birds when they had to cross a river.[142] Tibetan paintings show the Ḍākinīs under their terrible aspect, with an eye in the forehead, naked save for a green scarf, or wearing "a red loincloth and carrying on their backs a corpse whose arms are knotted like a scarf around the divinity's throat."[143] Whatever be the origin of these terrible demigoddesses, they were soon incorporated into tantrism; we find them, for example, represented in the *cakras*, together with other divinities. Some of them are Tibetan in origin; the Lāmās have even kept their Tibetan name (*lhamo*, "she-devil"). This group of facts illustrates the coalescence of popular Himālayan cults with Buddhist tantrism.[144]

According to the *Rasaratnācara*, an alchemical treatise attributed to Nāgārjuna, the latter acquired the secrets of alchemy after twelve years of asceticism spent in adoration of the goddess Yak-

141 Cf. G. Oppert, *On the Original Inhabitants of Bharatavarṣa or India*, p. 571 n.

142 A. Grünwedel, "Der Weg nach Śambhala," *Abhandlungen d. könig. Bayerischen Akademie d. Wissenschaften*, Phil. u. hist. Klasse, XXIX, 3 Abh. (1915), 28 (17a). It is unnecessary to point out the shamanic structure of this mythology of sorceresses.

143 R. Linossier, "Les Peintures tibétaines de la collection Loo" (*Mélanges Linossier*, I, 1–97), p. 55.

144 See also Note VIII, 7.

ṣinī, who protects the *Ficus religiosa.*[145] The Yakṣas and the Yakṣinīs make up the great class of local divinities into which the Hindus finally incorporated all minor religious forms, most of them aboriginal. The term *yakṣa* appears for the first time in the *Jaiminīya Brāhmaṇa* (III, 203, 272), where it means "a wondrous thing," but the ordinary meaning of "spirit," "genius" becomes prevalent only with the *Gṛhya-sūtras.*[146] In the *Mahābhārata,* the Yakṣas are already fairly well known, and a late passage in the same epic says that men of a "sāttvic" temperament worship the gods (*devas*), those of "rājasic" temperament venerate the *yakṣas* and *rakṣasas,* and those of "tāmasic" temperament the *pretas* (phantoms) and *bhūtas* (spirits of the dead, generally evil spirits). This represents the first attempt at assimilation and classification by a Hinduism confronted with this crowd of geniuses and demons from the aboriginal religions. Comparatively few Yakṣas have names, but Coomaraswamy [147] regards it as highly probable that the goddess Sītalā, Olābībī (goddess of cholera), the Seven Mothers (partly connected with Kubera, "king" of the Yakṣas), the sixty-four Yoginīs and Ḍākinīs, some forms of Devī, almost all the divinities of southern India, and even the great Durgā were originally Yakṣas—that is, we may add, were regarded as such in Brāhmanic circles. In any case, the Yakṣas and the Yakṣinīs represent the type-form of aboriginal religious devotion; this is why both Hinduism and Buddhism were forced to absorb them. (Hāritī, Mother-of-demons, originally a goddess of smallpox, became a very important Yakṣinī in Buddhism.)

Altars for the worship of Yakṣas can be raised almost anywhere. The essential element is the stone tablet or altar (*veyaḍḍi, mañco*) placed under the sacred tree.[148] The alliance between tree and altar denotes an extremely old cultural type; Buddhism incorporated it into the cult of *caityas.* This term sometimes designated the hierophanic tree, without the altar; and sometimes the *caitya* was a

145 Rāy, *History of Hindu Chemistry,* II, 7.
146 Coomaraswamy, *Yakṣas,* I, 5. 147 Ibid., I, 9–10.
148 Ibid., I, 17.

construction close to a tree. The cult of *caityas* passed to Tibet (the *mc'od rten*), where it assumed a very marked funerary character; many such *caityas* were erected to preserve the ashes of Lamas.[149]

The Yakṣa cult was devotional in structure—that is, it was a part of the great popular current of *bhakti*. For, as Coomaraswamy observes,[150] Viṣṇu and Śiva were not the only gods to crystallize the popular *bhakti* around their cults; all the other religious movements, including Buddhism, did the same. The latter took over the iconographic motif of "woman and tree," of pre-Āryan origin and deeply rooted in vegetation cults. In addition, the Yakṣas were regarded as protectors of *stūpas* and were represented in the same attitudes of devotion toward the Buddha as men. This cult of Yakṣas and Yakṣinīs was also assimilated by Jainism, for we find them represented as guardians of Jain temples. All this proves the vigor of the aboriginal religious sentiment; every religious form elaborated above the popular stratum—Buddhism, Jainism, Brāhmanism—had finally to reckon with the cult (*pūjā*) and the mystical devotion (*bhakti*) that constituted the very structure of the religious experience of pre-Āryan India.

Another example will still more clearly show the coalescence among the Great Goddess (Durgā), fertility cults, and popular yoga. We refer to the *pīṭhas* or places of pilgrimage in honor of the Great Goddess (whatever her name—Devī, Śakti, Durgā, Kālī, etc.). The tantras and the Purāṇas speak of four *pīṭhas*, one of them, as we should expect, being Kāmarūpa. Since each *pīṭha* represented the actual presence of the Great Goddess, the quaternary symbolism expresses the victory of the cult of Śakti in all India (the *pīṭhas* were distributed among the four cardinal points). But soon the number of *pīṭhas* began to increase and to show variations; we have lists of seven, eight, forty-two, fifty, and even 108 *pīṭhas* (there is here a relation with the 108 names of the Goddess). A myth whose origin is Brāhmanic and Vedic, but which crystallizes,

149 Cf. G. Tucci, *"Mc'od rten" e "Ts'a-ts'a" nel Tibet indiano ed occidentale*, p. 24.

150 *Yakṣas*, I, 27 f.

in the sense that interests us, only in the *Mahābhārata* (XII, 282–83), explains the multiplicity of *pīṭhas:* Satī, wife of Śiva, dies or kills herself because she has been mistreated by her father, Prajāpati. The tantras and Purāṇas developed the myth: Śiva wanders through the world, dancing and carrying his wife's corpse on his shoulder. To put an end to Śiva's madness, the gods decide to reduce Satī's body to fragments. The operation is described in two variants: according to the first,[151] Brahmā, Viṣṇu, and Śani enter the body by Yoga and divide it into small pieces; the places where the fragments fall become *pīṭhas.* According to the other version, Viṣṇu pursues Śiva and divides Satī's body with his arrows.[152]

The myth of the dismemberment of the Goddess, though not incorporated into Indian texts until comparatively late, is extremely archaic; in different forms, it is found in southeastern Asia, Oceania, and North and South America, always in connection with the myth of the divinity's self-immolation in order to create edible species of plants.[153] The symbolism of dismemberment also occurs, though in different contexts, in lunar mythologies and in shamanism. In the case of the *pīṭhas,* we have an aboriginal fertility myth incorporated into tantrism; for, as we must not forget, the *pīṭhas* were the outstanding places of pilgrimage for tantrics and Śāktas. Now—and we consider this fact important—the *pīṭhas,* regarded as members of the Great Goddess, were at the same time aniconic altars, which had acquired their rank as holy places from the fact that ascetics and yogins had meditated and obtained *siddhis* there. In other words, the sanctity of the *pīṭhas* was similar to that of the *samādhs* where yogins were buried. Consequently, a *pīṭha* could equally well be a place containing a member of the Goddess (especially the *yoni*) or a place where an ascetic had gained his "yogic

151 *Devībhāgavata,* VII, 30; *Kālikā Purāṇa,* XVIII, etc.

152 Sirkar, "Śākta Pīṭhas," pp. 5 ff.

153 Cf. A. W. Macdonald, "À propos de Prajāpati," *Journal asiatique,* CCXL (1952), 323–38; Eliade, "La Terre-Mère et les hiérogamies cosmiques," *Eranos-Jahrbuch,* XXII (1953), 57–95.

perfection" (*siddha pīṭha*). *The Sarvānandataraṅgiṇī* calls Mehāra (in the Tippera district) a *pīṭha-sthala*, because Sarvānanda conquered his tantric *siddhis* there.[154] Here we have an illuminating example of the many complex coalescences and syntheses brought about and encouraged by yogic tantrism. An archaic myth is incorporated both into Yoga and into the popular devotion to the Great Goddess of fertility. The place consecrated by the yogic conquest of deliverance later becomes sacred because it is reputed to contain a member of the Great Goddess. Durgā, as Śakti and wife of Śiva, becomes the goddess of yogins and ascetics, at the same time remaining, for the rest of the population, the Great Goddess of vegetation and fertility.

The Dravidian Heritage, Muṇḍa, Proto-Muṇḍa

We shall not here dwell on the linguistic and cultural influences exercised upon the Indo-Āryans by the Dravidian peoples.[155] We shall only point out that the essential mark of Hinduism, the devotional cult, *pūjā*, is a Dravidian contribution. The term *pūjā* itself may be of Dravidian origin (Gundert and Kittel have referred it to a Dravidian root, Tamil *pūśu-*, Kanarese *pūru-*, "to smear," "anoint," "dye"). As for mystical devotion, *bhakti*, it is certainly aboriginal in structure, either Dravidian or pre-Dravidian; in any case, *bhakti* played a considerable role in Hinduism, purifying it from magical excesses and ritualistic scholasticism. *Bhakti* was addressed either to God or to the Great Goddess or one of the countless Grāmadevatās who represented her. The Grāmadevatās are of particular interest to us, since their cult includes elements that are extremely archaic. The entire religious life of southern India is concentrated around these local divinities, manifestations of the Great Goddess. Now, it is precisely this type of cult that has everywhere imposed itself in popular Hinduism; in devotion to the Grāmadevatās, India has rediscovered its proper religious voca-

154 Sirkar, p. 3, n. 1.

155 See some brief particulars in Note VIII, 8.

tion. Among the names of the Great Goddess as she is manifested in these "village divinities," we shall note Ellammā, Māriyamma, Piḍārī, Ambikā (from a Dravidian root, *amma*, "mother"). Their icons are everywhere simple stone images of the female organ of generation (*yoni*). But the Dravidian Great Goddess does not show the sanguinary and orgiastic characteristics of Kālī-Durgā. Traces of a primordial and androgynous Great God (Kadaval) still subsist, but his role in the cult is of little importance. Among the names of the Dravidian Great God, we shall note that of Yogī, probably introduced after his coalescence with Śiva.

The cult sites of the Grāmadevatās are almost always in the vicinity of trees. Incorporated among so many other elements of archaic culture, to which we shall presently return, this detail might denote an ancient, preagricultural stratum of the religion of vegetation. For example, the Austroasiatic peoples of the South Seas habitually call countries and ethnic groups by names borrowed from the vegetable kingdom. Now, Jean Przyluski has shown that the Sanskrit word *udumbara*, which designates both the *Ficus glomerata* and a section of the Punjab with its inhabitants, attests the existence of Austroasiatic populations in the northern Punjab. This proves that the pre-Dravidian populations, speaking Muṇḍa languages, also influenced the culture and religion of the Indo-Āryans. We shall return to this problem. For the moment, let us note the survival of other elements from the archaic, pre-Dravidian religion in the cult of the Grāmadevatās. For one of the favorite images of the Grāmadevatās is the pot, and sometimes a pot even incarnates the Goddess.[156] At the yearly festival of the Goddess, a decorated pot is carried around the village in procession.[157] On the occasion of the ceremony of expiation, the entire populace gathers outside the village and a pot (*karagam*), representing the angry Goddess, is solemnly carried to the center of the village, where it

156 H. Whitehead, *The Village Gods of South India*, pp. 37 ff., 55, 64, 98, etc. The pot-goddess is named Kumbāttāḷ in Tamil, Kumbhamātā in Sanskrit, and Garigadevara in Kanarese (Oppert, *Original Inhabitants*, pp. 274 ff.).

157 Oppert, pp. 461 ff.; Whitehead, p. 38, etc.

remains for three days; at the end of that time it is carried out of the village again and broken to pieces.[158]

Now, the symbolism and cultural function of the pot were assimilated by Hinduism. Some post-Vedic ceremonies already included the "pot dance," which was performed by girls and whose magical meaning of fertility is obvious.[159] But in this example the sexual symbolism of the pot outweighs its aquatic, marine symbolism, which is the older. A passage from the *Śrīlalitāsahasranāmastotram*[160] says that the supreme Goddess may be venerated under any form, even that of a pot. According to a tradition preserved in the South, the sage Agastya was born, together with Vasiṣṭa, in a pot of water, from the union of Mitra and Varuṇa with the apsaras Urvaśī.[161] Agastya is also called *pītābhdi*, "drinker of the ocean." Another legend tells that Brahmā performed a sacrifice to explain Sanskrit and Tamil, and that it was by virtue of the magical power generated by this sacrifice that Agastya was born in a pot; the sage later married the daughter of the Ocean.[162] We here have an example of the well-known phenomenon of myths and religions from outside the Indo-European sphere being translated into Brāhmanic language.

But sometimes the symbolism of water resists all mythological and scholastic reinterpretations and ends by forcing its way even into the sacred texts. The *Devyupaniṣad* relates that the gods, having asked the Great Goddess (Devī) who she was and whence she came, received the answer, "The place of my birth is in the water within the sea: he who knows this, obtains the dwelling of Devī" (*mama yonir apsvnataḥ samudre ya evam veda sa devīpadamāpnoti*). The Goddess is the principle and origin of the gods and the universe. "It was I who, in the beginning, created the father of this world" (*aham suve pitaram asya mūrdhan*).[163] In other words, the

158 Oppert, p. 463.

159 Coomaraswamy, *Yakṣas*, II, 46.

160 Quoted by Oppert, p. 418.

161 Whence his names Kumbhasaṃbhava (born of Kumbhamātā, the pot-goddess), Kumbhayoni, and Ghaṭodbhava (Oppert, p. 24, n. 25).

162 Oppert, pp. 67–68, n. 61.

163 Text in Oppert, pp. 425–26.

sacred force incarnated by the Goddess resides in the waters; the ocean is conceived as the great reservoir or sacrality, whence gods, saints, and heroes draw their powers and their marvels. This religious conception is characteristic of the maritime civilizations of the Southeast. Jean Przyluski has analyzed a number of Austro-asiatic myths and legends all of which contain a common characteristic—the hero owes his glorious position of king or saint to the fact that he was born of an aquatic animal. In Annam, the first mythical king bore the name *long quān*, "the dragon king." In Indonesia, the kings of San-fo-ts'i were called *long tsin*, "spirit, sperm of a *nāga*." The kings of Chotā Nāgpur were likewise descended from a *nāga* named Puṇḍarīka, who was reported to have a foul-smelling breath. Now, this detail suggests the "princess with the fishy smell" who, in Indonesian myths and legends, lay with a Brāhman and founded a dynasty. The "princess with the fishy smell" was a *nāgī*, a female aquatic spirit; she symbolized both the primordial sacrality concentrated in the ocean and the earliest aboriginal cultural forms. Her union with the representatives of an opposing spiritual principle signified the founding of a new civilization, the beginning of a new history. According to a Palaung legend, the *nāgī* Thusandi loved the prince Thuriya, son of the Sun. From their union three sons were born; the first became emperor of China, the second, king of the Palaungs, the third king in Pagan. According to the *Sedjarat Malayou*, King Souran descended to the bottom of the ocean in a glass box, was well received by the inhabitants, and married the king's daughter; from their marriage three sons were born, the first of whom became king of Palembang.[164]

We shall not dwell on the symbolism of the "union of opposites" —the *nāgī* (the formless, the virtual, the dark) and the sun, etc. To enter into it would take us too far from our subject.[165] We shall only remark the enormous importance of *nāgas* and serpents in the

164 Cf. Przyluski, "La Princesse à l'odeur de poisson et la Nāgī dans les traditions de l'Asie orientale," *Études asiatiques*, II (1925), 265–84.

165 Cf. Eliade, *Patterns*, pp. 209 ff., 419 ff.

aboriginal mythologies and cults that found their way into Hinduism. Like the aquatic *nāgī*, the *nāga* symbolizes darkness, the preformal, the primordial sacred force, here no longer concentrated in the bottom of the ocean but in the depths of the earth. In India *nāgas* and snakes represent the genii of places, the aboriginal sacrality.[166] Now, *nāgas* are always connected with magic, yoga, the occult sciences; and the folklore that developed around Nāgārjuna shows us how living was the belief that snakes preserve a timeless "hidden doctrine," which they transmit through mysterious initiations.

The elements of marine symbolism and culture attested among the Dravidians and the Muṇḍa populations are due to Micro-Polynesian migrations, which, beginning in prehistory, continued into historical times. James Hornell has demonstrated a strong Polynesian influence on the pre-Dravidian population of the south coast of India. H. C. Das-Gupta has brought out striking similarities between some Indian and Sumatran games. Populations speaking Muṇḍa (or Kolarian) languages, belonging to the Austroasiatic linguistic group, made important contributions to Indian culture. The *Ṛg-Veda* itself has been shown to contain an Austroasiatic myth: Indra shoots an arrow that passes through a mountain and kills the boar guarding a treasure (a dish of rice) on the farther side of it. The words for the bow (*drumbhūlī*), the arrow (*bunda*), the dish of rice (*odaná*), and the name of the boar (Emuṣá) are of Muṇḍa origin.[167] The names of the betel (*tāmbula*), the betel nut (*guvāka*), the coconut (*nārikela*), the banana (*kadala*), etc. are Austroasiatic. The vigesimal numeration peculiar to Bengal and some parts of northern India are of Austroasiatic origin. The cultivation of rice on terraces, on hills, and in fields is also an Austroasiatic contribution. The word *liṅga*, so important

166 See Note VIII, 9.

167 F. B. J. Kuiper, "An Austro-Asiatic Myth in the *Rig-Veda*," *Mededelingen der koninklijke Nederlandse Academie van Wetenschappen*, XIII, 7 (1950), 163–82. According to the same author, forty per cent of the vocabulary of the Indo-Āryan dialects of the North are borrowed from Muṇḍa, either directly or through Sanskrit and Prakrit.

in Hinduism, related to the word *lāṅgula* (Skr. "plow"), is derived from an Austroasiatic root *lak*, meaning both spade and the male generative organ.[168]

We have cited these few facts to show how deeply the roots of Hinduism reach back in time. Austroasiatic symbols, cults, elements of civilization, and terminology, some pre-Dravidian, others Dravidian, have vigorously nourished, enriched, and modified the society of India as well as its culture and spirituality. It is the Indian soil itself that made the most important contribution to the final synthesis of Hinduism. Especially on the plane of religion, India proves to be pre-eminently conservative; almost nothing of its immemorial heritage has been lost. We shall reach a better understanding of this fact if we examine the relations between the protohistorical civilizations of the Indus and contemporary Hinduism.

Harappā, Mohenjo-daro *

The excavations undertaken in the Punjab some thirty years ago by Sir John Marshall and his collaborators, and continued by E. Mackay, Vats, and Wheeler, have brought to light a civilization whose high point may be placed between 2500 and 2000 B.C.[169] It has been principally the two citadel-cities, Mohenjo-daro on the Indus and Harappā on the Ravi, an affluent of the Indus, which have revealed the essentials of this protohistorical civilization. What is most striking at first is its uniformity and its stagnation—intensive search has brought to light no change, no innovation, in the thousand years of the history of the Harappā civilization. The two citadel-cities were probably the capitals of the "empire." Their cultural uniformity and continuity are explicable only on the hypothesis of a regime based upon some kind of religious authority. The variety of anthropological types shows an ethnic synthesis already well advanced. The proto-Australoids seem to represent the most numerous and most "primitive" elements, the aborigines;

168 See Note VIII, 10. 169 See Note VIII, 11.

the "Mediterranean" type is probably of Occidental origin and can be regarded as the conveyor of agricultural civilization (for the type is found associated with agriculture throughout the Western world); [170] finally, two other anthropological types have been identified—the Mongoloid and the Alpine.[171]

The plan of the city of Mohenjo-daro shows the importance of a Great Bath that is strangely reminiscent of the "baths" of Hindu temples in our day. The pictographic script, displayed on a large number of seals, has not yet been deciphered; so far, it has only given rise to some fantastic hypotheses. The art, like the entire Harappā culture, is conservative and already "Indian"; one feels a definite foreshadowing of the later artistic style.[172]

But it is especially the religion of the Harappā civilization that is of interest to us. According to Sir John Marshall, it is so characteristically Indian that it can hardly be distinguished from Hinduism.[173] Side by side with the cult of the Great Goddess, and that of a god who can be considered the prototype of Śiva, we find animal worship,[174] phallism,[175] the cult of trees,[176] and of water [177]—in other words, all the elements that will later enter into the great Hinduistic synthesis. The cult of the Mother Goddess was particularly prevalent; innumerable figurines have been found, some of them representing almost naked goddesses.[178] The latest types resemble Kālī-Durgā, of whom they were probably the model. No Āryan people has raised a female divinity to the supreme rank that she held in the civilization of Mohenjo-daro and that Kālī holds in Hinduism today.

But the most important fact for our investigation is the discov-

170 Stuart Piggott, *Prehistoric India*, p. 146.

171 See the description in Sir John Marshall, *Mohenjo-Daro and the Indus Civilization*, II, 599–648; and, I, 42, the premature attempt to relate these four ethnic types with the Mūṇḍā and Dravidian linguistic families.

172 Piggott, p. 187.

173 *Mohenjo-Daro*, I, vii.

174 Ibid., I, 67.

175 Ibid., I, 58 ff.

176 Ibid., pl. XII, fig. 18.

177 Ibid., I, 75.

178 One of the names of the Great Goddess of Hinduism is Aparṇā, "she who is without her garment of leaves"—that is, who is naked.

ery, at Mohenjo-daro, of an iconographic type that may be considered the earliest plastic representation of a yogin. Here the Great God himself, in whom the prototype of Śiva has been identified, is represented in the specifically yogic posture.[179] Sir John Marshall describes the figure as follows: [180] "The God, who is three-faced, is seated on a low Indian throne in a typical attitude of *Yoga*, with legs bent double beneath him, heel to heel, and toes turned downwards. . . . Over his breast is a triangular pectoral or perhaps a series of necklaces or torques. . . . The phallus (*ūrdhvameḍhra*) [is] seemingly exposed, but it is possible that what appears to be the phallus is in reality the end of the waistband. Crowning his head is a pair of horns meeting in a tall head-dress. To either side of the god are four animals, an elephant and a tiger on his proper right, a rhinoceros and a buffalo on his left. Beneath the throne are two deer standing with heads regardant and horns turned to the center." One of the most recent writers to express an opinion on the question, Stuart Piggott, writes: "There can be little doubt that we have here the prototype of the great god Shiva as Lord of the Beasts and Prince of Yogis; he may have been conceived as four-faced, and with his four animals looks to the four quarters of the earth. This would indeed recall the symbolical elephant, lion, horse, and bull on the Mauryan column of the third century B.C. at Sarnath. The deer by the god's throne make another significant link with later religion, and with Sarnath, for, similarly placed, they are the inevitable accompaniment of Buddha in representations of the Deer Park Sermon." [181]

Representations of other divinities in the *āsana* posture have been found on the seals, too. Finally, a second statue was excavated that in all probability is that of a yogin.[182] Sir John Marshall describes it as follows: [183] "It represents someone seemingly in the pose of a yogī, and it is for this reason that the eyelids are more than half closed and the eyes looking downward to the tip of the nose. . . .

179 Marshall, pl. XII, fig. 17.
180 Ibid., I, 52.
181 *Prehistoric India*, p. 202.
182 Marshall, pl. XCVIII.
183 I, 44, 54.

Probably it is the statue of a priest or may be of a king-priest, since it lacks the horns which would naturally be expected if it were a figure of the deity himself. That it possessed a religious or quasi-religious character is suggested by the distinctive trefoil patterning of its robe—a motif which in Sumer is reserved for objects of a sacral nature." [184]

These facts can hardly be belittled, and their bearing is immense. Between the protohistorical civilization of the Indus and modern Hinduism there is no solution of continuity. The Great Goddess and the genetic God (Śiva), the cult of vegetation (the pipal tree, so characteristic of Hinduism) and phallism, the holy man in the *āsana* position, perhaps practicing *ekāgratā*—then as now, they are in the very foreground. "The links between the Harappā religion and contemporary Hinduism are of course of immense interest, providing as they do some explanation of those many features that cannot be derived from the Aryan traditions brought into India after, or concurrently with, the fall of the Harappā civilization. The old faiths die hard: it is even possible that early historic Hindu society owed more to Harappā than it did to the Sanskrit-speaking invaders." [185]

Moreover, many of the cultural elements identified at Harappā and Mohenjo-daro are to be found in India today. Thus, for example, the Harappān two-wheeled cart is the same as that used today in Sind, the boats resemble those seen today on the Indus, the technique of pottery seems to be identical with that which can be observed today in Sind villages, and the like is true of architecture, nasal ornaments, the method of applying kohl, the ivory comb, etc.[186] The use of the turban, unknown in the Vedic texts, attested from the Brāhmaṇas on, was popular in Harappā.[187] There

184 Ernest Mackay (*Early Indus Civilization*, ed. Dorothy Mackay, p. 53) is more cautious: "But this may not be so, for very much the same kind of eye has been noticed in very early clay figures from Kish and Ur."

185 Piggott, p. 203.

186 V. Gordon Childe, *New Light on the Most Ancient East*, pp. 210, 222, etc.

187 Piggott, p. 269.

can be disagreement over the details, but it is difficult to doubt the Indian character of the civilization of Mohenjo-daro, whatever its origins may have been. Quite possibly the authors of the civilization borrowed some religious forms from the aboriginal population.[188] We have seen the importance of the proto-Australoid element, which probably composed the lower stratum of society. That element survives to this day in the autochthonous tribes of southern India.[189] It doubtless entered into the Harappān synthesis, as it will later enter into the Hinduist syntheses.

About 2000 B.C., the Indus civilization was in a state of defense; not long afterward, a part of Harappā was burned by invaders coming down from the Northwest. These "barbarians" were not yet the Indo-Europeans, but their invasion was doubtless related to the general movement in the West, in which the Indo-Europeans were involved.[190] Some centuries afterward, these latter put a brutal end to all that remained of the Indus civilization. Not long ago it was still believed that, in their invasion of India, the Indo-Āryans had encountered nothing but aboriginal tribes, culturally in the ethnographic stage. These were the Dasyus, whose "forts," attacked and destroyed by the Indra of the *Ṛg-Veda*, were thought to be only humble earthworks. But Wheeler has shown that the famous hymn in the *Ṛg-Veda* (I, 53), praising Indra in his conquest of the "forts" of the Dasyus, applies to the solid defenses of the citadel of Harappā or Mohenjo-daro.[191] Whence we may conclude that, in their descent into central India, the Indo-Āryans encountered not only aboriginal tribes but also the last survivors of the Indus civilization, to which they gave the deathblow. On the cultural plane, the Harappāns were definitely superior to the Indo-Europeans; their urban and industrial civilization could not be compared with the Indo-European "barbarism." But the Harappāns were not warlike (we may even suppose them to have been a sort of industrial and mercantile theocracy); ill-prepared for an attack by a young and aggressive people, they were defeated and annihilated.

188 Mackay, p. 75.
189 Childe, p. 208.
190 Piggott, p. 255.
191 Ibid., p. 263.

Yet the destruction of the Indus culture could not be final. The collapse of an urban civilization is not equivalent to the simple extinction of its culture, but merely to that culture's regression to rural, larval, "popular" forms. (This phenomenon was amply demonstrated in Europe during and after the great barbarian invasions.) But before very long the Āryanization of the Punjab launched the great movement of synthesis that was one day to become Hinduism. The considerable number of "Harappān" elements found in Hinduism can be explained only by a contact, begun quite early, between the Indo-European conquerors and the representatives of the Indus culture. These representatives were not necessarily the authors of the Indus culture or their direct descendants; they might be tributaries, by dissemination, of certain Harappān cultural forms, which they had preserved in eccentric regions, spared by the first waves of Āryanization. This would explain the following apparently strange fact: the cult of the Great Goddess and of Śiva, phallism and tree worship, asceticism and Yoga, etc., appear for the first time in India as the religious expression of a high urban civilization, that of the Indus—whereas, in medieval and modern India, these religious elements are characteristic of "popular" cultures. To be sure, from the Harappān period on, there was certainly a synthesis between the spirituality of the Australoid aborigines and that of the "masters," the authors of the urban civilization. But we must presume that it was not only this synthesis that was preserved, but also the specific and almost exclusive contribution of the "masters" (a contribution related especially to their theocratic conceptions). Otherwise it would be impossible to explain the considerable importance assumed by the Brāhmans after the Vedic period. Very probably all these Harappān religious conceptions (which strongly contrast with those of the Indo-Europeans) were preserved, with inevitable regressions, among the "popular" strata, in the margin of the society and civilization of the new Āryan-speaking masters. Very probably it is from there that they welled up, in successive waves, during the later synthesis that ended in the formation of Hinduism.

Conclusions

NOW that we have reached the end of our study, some observations of a general nature remain to be made. Our intention is neither to summarize the general lines of our exposition nor to restate the results arrived at in the several chapters. Rather, we consider it important to draw attention to a number of facts. The first is this: Yoga constitutes a characteristic dimension of the Indian mind, to such a point that wherever Indian religion and culture have made their way, we also find a more or less pure form of Yoga.[1] In India, Yoga was adopted and valorized by all religious movements, whether Hinduist or "heretical." The various Christian or syncretistic Yogas of modern India constitute another proof that Indian religious experience finds the yogic methods of "meditation" and "concentration" a necessity. For, as we have seen, Yoga ended by absorbing and incorporating all kinds of spiritual and mystical techniques, from the most elementary to the most complex. The generic name of yogins designates not only saints and mystics but also magicians, orgiastics, common fakirs, and sorcerers. And each of these types of magico-religious behavior corresponds to a particular form of Yoga.

To become what it has been for many centuries—that is, a pan-Indian corpus of spiritual techniques—Yoga had to meet all the deepest needs of the Indian soul. We have seen how it met them.

1 See Note IX, 1.

From the beginning, Yoga marked the reaction against metaphysical speculation and the excesses of a fossilized ritualism; it represented the same *tendency toward the concrete*, toward personal experience, that we find again in the popular devotion expressed in *pūjā* and *bhakti*. We always find some form of Yoga whenever the goal is *experience of the sacred* or the attainment of a perfect *self-mastery*, which is itself the first step toward magical mastery of the world. It is a fact of considerable significance that the noblest mystical experiences, as well as the most daring magical desires, are realized through yogic technique, or, more precisely, that Yoga can equally well adapt itself to either path. Several hypotheses could account for this. The first would invoke the two spiritual traditions that, after numerous tensions and at the end of a long synthetic effort, ended by forming Hinduism—the religious tradition of the Āryan-speaking Indo-Europeans and the tradition of the aborigines (the latter, as we have seen, a complex tradition, including Dravidian, Muṇḍa, proto-Muṇḍa, and Harappān elements). The Indo-Europeans contributed a patriarchal social structure, a pastoral economy, and the cult of the gods of the sky and the atmosphere—in a word, the "religion of the Father." The pre-Āryan aborigines already knew agriculture and urbanism (the Indus civilization) and, in general, adhered to the "religion of the Mother." Hinduism, as it has existed from the end of the Middle Ages, represents the synthesis of these two traditions, but with a marked predominance of the aboriginal factors; the contribution of the Indo-Europeans underwent a radical Asianization. Hinduism represents the religious victory of the soil.

Although the magical conception of the world is more accentuated among the Indo-Europeans, we may hesitate to make them the source of the magical tendency present in the Yoga complex and to give the entire credit for the mystical tendency to the aborigines. In our view, it seems more in agreement with the facts to find the Indo-European contribution in the considerable importance of ritualism and the speculations to which it gave rise, and to leave to the aborigines the tendency toward the concrete in religious experience, the need for a mystical devotion to personal or local divinities (Īśtadevatā, Gramādevatā). In so far as Yoga represents a reaction against ritualism and scholastic speculation, it adheres to the aboriginal tradition and stands against the Indo-European religious heritage. We have, in fact, frequently had occasion to stress the resistance to the various forms of Yoga on the part of orthodox circles—that is, of the tributaries of the Indo-European tradition. As we have pointed out, the absence of the Yoga complex from other Indo-European groups confirms the supposition that this technique is a creation of the Asian continent, of the Indian soil. If we are right in connecting the origins of yogic asceticism with the protohistorical religion of the Indus, we may justifiably conclude that in it we have an archaic form of mystical experience that disappeared everywhere else. For—to repeat—Yoga cannot be classed among the countless varieties of primitive mysticism to which the term shamanism is commonly applied. Yoga is not a technique of ecstasy; on the contrary, it attempts to realize absolute concentration in order to attain enstasis. In the universal history of mysticism, classic Yoga occupies a place of its own, and one that is difficult to define. It represents a living fossil, a modality of archaic spirituality that has survived nowhere else. (The concept "living fossils" has, of course, been profitably employed in various branches of biology—among others, in speleology. Certain forms of life that today flourish in caves belong to a fauna long since antiquated. "They are veritable living fossils," writes Father Racovitza, "and often represent very ancient periods of life—Tertiary and even Mesozoic." Thus, caves preserve an archaic fauna, of the greatest importance to an understanding of the primitive zoomorphic groups *that are unfossilizable*. It is in this sense that we can speak of certain archaic modalities of spirituality, which have remained in existence down to our day, as living fossils; they are of all the more interest for the history of the human mind because they leave no "documentary" traces, because they are, as we should express it, "unfossilizable.")

The archaism of Yoga is confirmed once again by its initiatory structure. We have called attention to the yogic symbolism of death and rebirth—death to the profane human condition, rebirth to a transcendent modality.[2] The yogin undertakes to "reverse" normal behavior completely. He subjects himself to a petrified immobility of body (*āsana*), rhythmical breathing and arrest of breath (*prāṇāyāma*), fixation of the psychomental flux (*ekāgratā*), immobility of thought, the "arrest" and even the "return" of semen. On every level of human experience, he does the *opposite* of what life demands that he do. Now, the symbolism of the "opposite" indicates both the post-mortem condition and the condition of divinity (we know that "left" on earth corresponds to "right" in the beyond, a vessel broken here below is equivalent to an unbroken vessel in the world of the afterlife and the gods, etc.). The "reversal" of normal behavior sets the yogin outside of life. But he does not stop halfway—death is followed by an initiatory rebirth. The yogin makes for himself a "new body," just as the neophyte in archaic societies is thought to obtain a new body through initiation.

At first sight the *rejection of life* demanded by Yoga might appear terrifying, for it implies more than a funerary symbolism—it entails experiences that are so many anticipations of death. Does not the arduous and complicated process by which the yogin detaches himself from and finally eliminates all the contents that belong to the psychophysiological levels of human experience recall the process of death? For, in the Indian view, death represents a brutal separation of the Spirit from all psychophysiological experiences. And, looking more closely, we see that the mystery of liberation, the return of the elements (*tattva*) to *prakṛti*, also signifies an anticipation of death. As we said,[3] certain yogico-tantric exercises are only an "anticipatory visualization" of the decomposition and return of elements in the circuit of nature, a process normally set in motion by death. Many of the experiences of the world beyond death that are described in the *Bardo Thödol*, the Tibetan Book of the Dead, are in strange correspondence with yogico-tantric exercises in meditation.

2 See above, pp. 5 ff.

3 Above, p. 272.

IX. *Conclusions*

We know now that this anticipatory death is an initiatory death—that is, that it is necessarily followed by a rebirth. It is for the sake of this rebirth to another mode of being that the yogin sacrifices everything that, on the level of profane existence, seems important. It is a sacrifice not only of his "life," but also of his "personality." In the perspective of profane existence, the sacrifice is unintelligible. But we know the answer of Indian philosophy: the perspective of profane existence is distorted. And it is so for two reasons: on the one hand, desacralized life is suffering and illusion; on the other, no final problem can be solved in its perspective. Let us recall the answer given by Sāṃkhya-Yoga to the problems concerning the cause and beginning of the pseudo slavery of Spirit in the circuit of matter and life. Sāṃkhya-Yoga answers: they are problems that are insoluble in our present human condition; in other words, they are "mysteries" for any intelligence that has not been liberated (we should say, for any "fallen" intelligence). He who would attain to comprehension of these "mysteries" must raise himself to another mode of being, and, to reach it, he must "die" to this life and sacrifice the "personality" that has issued from temporality, that has been created by history (personality being above all memory of our own history). The ideal of Yoga, the state of *jīvan-mukti*, is to live in an "eternal present," outside of time. "Liberated in life," the *jīvan-mukta* no longer possesses a personal consciousness—that is, a consciousness nourished on his own history—but a witnessing consciousness, which is pure lucidity and spontaneity. We shall not attempt to describe this paradoxical condition; indeed, since it is obtained by "death" to the human condition and rebirth to a transcendent mode of being, it cannot be reduced to our categories. Nevertheless, we will emphasize one fact, whose interest is chiefly historical. Yoga takes over and continues the immemorial symbolism of initiation; in other words, it finds its place in a universal tradition of the religious history of mankind: the tradition that consists in anticipating death in order to ensure rebirth in a sanctified life—that is, a life made *real* by the incorporation of the sacred. But India went particularly far on this traditional plane. For Yoga, the initiatory rebirth becomes the acquisition of immortality or absolute freedom. It is in the very structure of this paradoxical state, which lies outside of profane existence, that we must seek the explanation for the coexistence of "magic" and "mysticism" in Yoga. Everything depends upon what is meant by freedom.

ADDITIONAL NOTES

ADDITIONAL NOTES

[For full references, see the List of Works Cited.]

I, 1: *Sāṃkhya Texts and Bibliographies*

The word *sāṃkhya* has been variously interpreted. Richard Garbe (*Die Sāṃkhya-Philosophie*, pp. 131–34) derives it from *saṃkhyā* ("number") and takes it to mean "enumeration," "investigation," "analysis" (*Untersuchung, Prüfung, Unterscheidung, Erwägung*). Hermann Oldenberg (*Die Lehre der Upanishaden*, p. 351, n. 129) inclines to the meaning "examination," "calculation," "description by enumeration of constituents." Hermann Jacobi (reviewing the second edition of Garbe's book in the *Göttingische gelehrte Anzeigen*, CLXXXI [1919], 28) holds that *sāṃkhya* means defining a concept by enumerating its content; earlier (reviewing the first edition of Garbe's book, *Göttingische gelehrte Anzeigen*, CLVII [1895], 209; "Der Ursprung des Buddhismus aus dem Sānkhya-Yoga," especially pp. 47–53) he had held that the word refers to investigation of the categories of existence. It is not impossible that all these meanings were known and accepted in ancient India. However, the meaning "discrimination," "discernment," seems more probable, for the principal aim of the philosophy is to dissociate the soul from *prakṛti* (cf. also A. B. Keith, *The Religion and Philosophy of the Veda and Upanishads*, II, 535–51).

The earliest treatise is Īśvarakṛṣṇa's *Sāṃkhya-kārikā*. (The best edition is the one by S. S. Suryanarayana Śāstri, Madras, 1930. There are also a number of translations: H. T. Colebrooke, Oxford, 1837; J. Davies, London, 1881; R. Garbe, Leipzig, 1891; N. Sinha, Allahabad, 1915; cf. E. A. Welden, "I Metri delle *Sāṁkhya-Kārikās*.") The date of the work has not yet been established. In any case, it cannot be later than the fifth century, for the Buddhist monk Paramārtha translated it into Chinese in the sixth century. (Cf. J. Takakusu, "*Sāṃkhyakārikā* étudiée à la lumière de la version chinoise.") S. Radhakrishnan (*Indian Philosophy*, II, 254–55) holds that the *Sāṃkhya-kārikā* was composed c. A.D. 200, whereas S. K.

Belvalkar (*"Māṭhara-vṛtti,"* p. 168) is inclined to think that the date of its composition should be put in the first or second century of our era.

Whatever the precise date of the *Sāṃkhya-kārikā* may be, it is certain that Īśvarakṛṣṇa was not the first Sāṃkhya "author"; *kārikā* 70 says that the sage Kapila, mythical founder of the system, imparted the doctrine to Āsuri, who in turn transmitted it to Pañcaśikha, from whom Īśvarakṛṣṇa received it. On Kapila, see Garbe, *Die Sāṃkhya-Philosophie,* pp. 25–29; Jacobi's 1919 review of Garbe, p. 26; Radhakrishnan, pp. 254 ff.; V. V. Sovani, "A Critical Study of the Sāṅkhya System," pp. 391–92; G. Kaviraj, introd. to *Jayamaṅgalā,* ed. H. Sarma, p. 2 (Kapila regarded as a *siddha* in alchemical literature).

Some fragments of Pañcaśikha's work have come down to us: *Sāṃkhya-sūtras,* I, 127; VI, 68, etc. On Pañcaśikha himself, see: Garbe, "Pañcaśikha Fragmente"; Keith, *The Sāṃkhya System,* p. 48; Jacobi, "Sind nach dem Sāṅkhya-Lehrer Pañcaśikha die *Puruṣas* von Atomgrösse?"; E. W. Hopkins, *The Great Epic of India,* pp. 142–52. Chinese tradition (Takakusu, pp. 25 f.) makes Pañcaśikha the author of the *Ṣaṣṭitantra,* which Īśvarakṛṣṇa admits having summarized. On this treatise, see F. O. Schrader, "Das *Ṣaṣṭitantra*"; M. Hariyanna, "*Ṣaṣṭi-tantra* and Vārsaganya"; Keith, pp. 69–74.

Probably there were several "schools" of Sāṃkhya, differing in their theistic emphasis and their conception of the soul. Even the late commentators preserve the tradition of numerous Sāṃkhya "schools." Guṇaratna (fourteenth century), the commentator on the *Ṣaḍdarśanasamuccaya,* mentions two schools of Sāṃkhya: *maulikya* (original) and *uttara* (late). The former holds that there is a *prakṛti* (*pradhāna*) for each soul (*ātman*), whereas the latter, with the classic Sāṃkhya, believes that there is but one *pradhāna* for all individual souls (S. Dasgupta, *A History of Indian Philosophy,* I, 217; cf. Kalipada Bhattacharya, "Some Problems of Sāṅkhya Philosophy and Sāṅkhya Literature," p. 515; C. A. F. Rhys Davids, "Sāṅkhya and Original Buddhism"). Dasgupta (pp. 213–16) finds a preclassic Sāṃkhya doctrine in Caraka (but see Jean Filliozat, *La Doctrine classique de la médecine indienne,* p. 166); Otto Strauss in Vātsyāyāna ("Eine alte Formel der Sāṃkhya-Yoga-Philosophie bei Vātsyāyāna"). On preclassic Sāṃkhya, see E. H. Johnston, *Early Sāṁkhya.*

The earliest commentary on the *Sāṃkhya-kārikā* is the *Jayamaṅgalā,* attributed to Śaṅkara (ed. H. Sarma); its date is uncertain, but in any case it is earlier than Vācaspatimiśra (cf. Sarma, "*Jayamaṇgalā* and the Other Commentaries on *Sāṅkhya-Saptati*"). The work is not of much philosophical interest.

The *Sāṃkhya-tattva-kaumudī*, by Vācaspatimiśra (ninth century), attained wide circulation and has been one of the most consulted and discussed of Sāṃkhya treatises. (Sanskrit text and English translation by Gangānātha Jhā; German translation by Garbe, "Der Mondschein der Sāṃkhya-Wahrheit, Vācaspatimiśra's *Sāṃkhya-tattva-kaumudī*"; cf. A. Barth, *Œuvres*, II, 136–37.) There is a gloss on the *Sāṃkhya-tattva-kaumudī* by Nārāyaṇa (*Sāṃkhyacandrikā*).

The recently discovered *Māṭharavṛtti* (available in a not very satisfactory edition by Pandit Vishnu Prasad Sarma) has given rise to a series of controversies over its priority to another commentary on Īśvarakṛṣṇa, the *Gauḍapādabhāṣya*. According to Belvalkar ("*Māṭharavṛtti* and the Date of Īśvarakṛṣṇa," p. 172), who discovered the MS, the *Māṭharavṛtti* is the Sanskrit commentary translated into Chinese by Paramārtha between 557 and 569, which had previously been regarded as lost. Comparison of the *Māṭharavṛtti* with the French version of Paramārtha's commentary by Takakusu ("*Sāṃkhyakārikā*," pp. 978–1064) leads Belvalkar to believe that they are identical. The same scholar also considers the *Gauḍapādabhāṣya* (eighth century) to be a résumé of the *Māṭharavṛtti* (which he dates before the sixth century). A. B. Dhruva ("Trividham Anumānam," p. 275) puts the *Māṭharavṛtti* even earlier; arguing from a passage of the *Anuyogadvāra* that cites the *Māṭharavṛtti*, he maintains that the date of the latter must be put in the second to third century, if not in the first century. But his opinion has not been accepted.

The chronology proposed by Belvalkar for the various commentaries on Īśvarakṛṣṇa, as well as the priority of the *Māṭharavṛtti* over the *Gauḍapādabhāṣya*, has been disputed; see Belvalkar, "*Māṭhara-vṛtti*"; S. S. Suryanarayana Śāstri, "The Chinese *Suvarṇa-saptati* and the *Māṭhara-vṛtti*"; id., "Māṭhara and Paramārtha" (which brings out the differences between the two authors); Umesha Mitra, "*Gauḍapādabhāṣya* and *Māṭharavṛtti*" (rejects Belvalkar's thesis that the *Gauḍapādabhāṣya* is only a résumé of the *Māṭharavṛtti*, but places the latter between the tenth and thirteenth centuries, which seems improbable); Keith, "The *Māṭhara-Vṛtti*" (comes to the conclusion that Māṭhara, Paramārtha, and Gauḍapāda all used an earlier commentary, which is no longer extant).

Gauḍapāda, the commentator on Īśvarakṛṣṇa, cannot be the same person as the author of the *Māṇḍūkya-kārikā;* their philosophies are clearly too different. Cf. Amar Nath Ray, "The *Māṇḍūkya Upaniṣad* and the *Kārikās* of Gauḍapāda"; B. N. Krishnamurti Sarma, "New Light on the *Gauḍapāda-Kārikās.*" The *Gauḍapādabhāṣya* was translated into English, with a study, by H. H. Wilson (Oxford, 1837; frequently reprinted).

The *Sāṃkhya-pravacana-sūtra,* traditionally attributed to Kapila, is the second important classic treatise of the school. It probably dates from the fourteenth century, for neither Guṇaratna nor Mādhava, in his *Sarvadarśanasaṃgraha,* refers to it. Several commentaries: Aniruddha (fifteenth century) wrote the *Sāṃkhya-sūtra-vṛtti* (ed. Garbe; good English translation by the same: *Aniruddha's Commentary*). Mahādeva (after 1600) composed a gloss (*vṛttisāra*), which offers little of interest (the principal passages have been translated and edited by Garbe). The *Sāṃkhya-pravacana-bhāṣya,* by Vijñānabhikṣu (sixteenth century), is the most important commentary on the *Sūtras* (ed. Garbe, Cambridge [Mass.], 1895; German translation by the same, Leipzig, 1889; partial English translation by J. R. Ballantyne, *The Sānkhya Aphorisms of Kapila;* complete translation by N. Sinha, *The Sāṃkhya Philosophy*). Cf. Udaya Vīra Shāstri, "Antiquity of the *Sāṅkhya Sūtras.*"

The *Tattvasamāṣa,* a brief treatise containing only twenty-two *ślokas,* has been attributed to Kapila, although the text is quite late (fourteenth-fifteenth century). F. Max Müller (*The Six Systems of Indian Philosophy,* pp. 242 f.) wrongly supposed it the earliest text of the Sāṃkhya literature.

On Sāṃkhya, see also: Garbe, *Sāṃkhya und Yoga;* Paul Deussen, *Die nachvedische Philosophie der Inder,* pp. 408–506; Strauss, "Zur Geschichte des Sāṃkhya"; Oldenberg, "Zur Geschichte der Sāṃkhya-Philosophie"; Keith, *Religion and Philosophy,* pp. 535–51; Hopkins, *Great Epic,* pp. 97–157; Radhakrishnan, II, 249–353; Haraprasād Shāstri, "Chronology of Sāṃkhya Literature"; Abhay Kumar Majumdar, *The Sāṅkhya Conception of Personality;* Helmuth von Glasenapp, *La Philosophie indienne,* pp. 157 ff.; J. A. B. van Buitenen, "Studies in Sāṃkhya," I–III. On the relations between Sāṃkhya and Buddhism, cf. below, pp. 379–81.

I, 2: Patañjali and the Texts of Classic Yoga *

The identity of the two Patañjalis—the author of the *Yoga-sūtras* and Patañjali the grammarian—has been accepted by B. Liebich, Garbe, and

Dasgupta and denied by J. H. Woods (*The Yoga-System of Patañjali,* pp. xiii–xvii), Jacobi ("The Dates of the Philosophical Sūtras of the Brāhmans," especially pp. 26–27; "Über das ursprüngliche Yoga-system," especially pp. 583–84; "Über das Alter der Yogaśāstra"), and Keith (*Sāṃkhya System,* pp. 65–66; "Some Problems of Indian Philosophy," especially p. 433). Dasgupta refutes Woods' statement (p. xv) that the concept of substance (*dravya*) differed in the two Patañjalis. On the contrary, he finds numerous resemblances between the *Yoga-sūtras* and the *Mahābhāṣya;* for example, the *sphoṭa* doctrine, although it is a doctrine far from prevalent, appears in both books; both begin alike (*Yoga-sūtras: atha yogānuśāsanam;* and *Mahābhāṣya: atha śabdānuśāsanam*). Dasgupta believes that the first three books of the *Yoga-sūtras* were written by Patañjali the grammarian, and dates them in the second century B.C. The last book (IV), he considers a late addition. For one thing, it differs in terminology from the three preceding books; for another, it repeats what has already been said. Keith does not accept Dasgupta's interpretation. In his view, the *Yoga-sūtras* are the work of a single author, who, in any case, is not the same as the author of the *Mahābhāṣya.* Jacobi ("Über das Alter der Yogaśāstra"), comparing the vocabularies of the two works, concluded that they were not the same. Accepting these results, Jacobi and Keith find clear traces of anti-Buddhist polemics in Book IV of the *Yoga-sūtras,* whence it would follow that Patañjali's date can hardly be earlier than the fifth century. Jacobi had long before shown that if an Indian philosophical text refers to Vijñānavāda, it is later than the fifth century ("Dates," pp. 2, 25). Now, *Yoga-sūtras,* IV, 16, seems to refer to Vijñānavāda. Keith ("Some Problems," p. 433) and J. W. Hauer ("Das IV. Buch des *Yogasūtra,*" pp. 132–33) say that the reference is not to an indeterminate Vijñānavāda, but to the doctrines of Asaṅga and Vasubandhu.

Against these critiques, Jvala Prasad ("The Date of the *Yoga-sūtras*") attempts to prove that *sūtra* IV, 16, is not part of Patañjali's text, since it only repeats a line of Vyāsa's commentary (seventh-eighth century) in which he attacks the Vijñānavādins. Rāja Bhoja had long before remarked that this *sūtra* was an interpolation by Vyāsa, and hence did not comment on it. In addition, Dasgupta and Prasad point out that, even if the authors to whom *Yoga-sūtras,* IV, 16, refers are Vijñānavādins, we have no reason to believe that the reference is to Vasubandhu or Asaṅga. The text could equally well apply to some earlier idealistic school, such as those mentioned in the earliest Upaniṣads. "For example, the philosophy of such an early work as *Aitareya Āraṇyaka* is as good a Vijñānavāda as any other could be. All things of the world are described as knowledge (*prajñānam*) and having their existence only in and through knowledge" (Prasad, p. 371). However, Louis de la Vallée Poussin has repeatedly shown the dependence of the *Yoga-sūtras* on scholastic Buddhism (cf. "Notes bouddhiques" and "Le Bouddhisme et le Yoga de Patañjali"). See below, V, 1.

The best-known Sanskrit edition of the *Yoga-sūtras* is that published in the Ānandāśrama Sanskrit Series (No. CXLVII). With the commentary (*Yoga-bhāṣya*) by Veda-Vyāsa and the gloss (*Tattvavaiśāradī*) by Vācaspatimiśra, the *Yoga-sūtras* have been translated into English by Woods (*The Yoga-System of Patañjali*) and by Rāma Prasāda (*Patañjali's Yoga Sūtras*). Cf. also Hauer, "Eine Übersetzung der Yoga-Merksprüche des Patañjali"; Jhā, *The Yoga-Darśana.* King Bhoja (beginning of the eleventh century) wrote a commentary, the *Rājamārtaṇḍa*, on the *Yoga-sūtras* (edited and translated into English by Rājendralāla Mitra, *The Yoga Aphorisms of Patañjali*). Vijñānabhikṣu wrote a commentary on Vyāsa's *Yoga-bhāṣya*, the *Yogavārttika* (ed. Rāmakṛshṇa Śāstri and Keśava Śāstri), as well as a short treatise on Patañjali's doctrine, the *Yogasāra-saṃgraha* (ed. Jhā). The *Yoga-sūtras* were the subject of yet another commentary, the *Maṇiprabhā*, by Rāmānanda Sarasvatī (sixteenth century; tr. Woods, "The *Yoga Sūtras* of Patañjali as Illustrated by the Comment Entitled 'The Jewel's Lustre' "). On the other commentaries, cf. Theodor Aufrecht, *Catalogus Catalogorum*, I, 480. Of all these treatises, the most valuable are those by Vyāsa and Vijñānabhikṣu. Bhoja often contributes interesting interpretations. See also P. C. Divanji, "The *Yogayājñavalkya.*"

On the doctrines and practices of Yoga, see S. Dasgupta, *A Study of Patañjali;* id., *Yoga as Philosophy and Religion;* id., *Yoga Philosophy in Relation to Other Systems of Indian Thought;* id., *A History of Indian Philosophy* (I, 226 ff.); Radhakrishnan, *Indian Philosophy* (II, 336 ff.); Paul Oltramare, *L'Histoire des idées théosophiques dans l'Inde* (I, 290 ff., 300 ff.); Hauer, *Die Anfänge der Yogapraxis;* id., *Der Yoga als Heilweg;* Richard Roesel, *Die psychologischen Grundlagen der Yogapraxis;* Sigurd Lindquist, *Die Methoden des Yoga;* Alain Daniélou, *Yoga: the Method of Re-integration;* Jacques Masui, ed., *Yoga, science de l'homme intégral.* See also the bibliographies, given below, on Buddhism, tantrism, and Haṭha Yoga.

I, 3: On the Materialists

The best documentation on the subject of the Lokāyatas, and a philosophical refutation of their views, are found in Ch. I of the *Sarvadarśanasaṃgraha* and in Śāntarakṣīta's *Tattvasaṃgraha, ślokas* 1857–64 (with Kamalaśīla's commentary, tr. Jhā). See also: Giuseppe Tucci, "Linee di una storia del materialismo indiano"; Luigi Suali, "Matériaux pour servir à l'histoire du matérialisme indien"; Müller, *Six Systems*, pp. 94–104; Dakshinaranjan Shāstri, *Chārvākashashti*; id., *A Short History of Indian Materialism;* R. A. Schermerhorn, "When Did Indian Materialism Get Its Distinctive Titles?"; P. J. Abs, "Some Early Buddhistic Texts in Relation to the Philosophy of Materialism in India"; Walter Ruben, "Materialismus im Leben des alten Indien."

I, 4: The Self and Psychomental Experience

By its own nature (*svabhāva*), Spirit is eternal (*nitya*), pure (*śuddha*), illuminated (*buddha*), and free (*mukta*), says *Sāṃkhya-sūtras*, I, 19. And Vijñānabhikṣu, commenting on the passage, attempts to prove that the "relation" between Spirit and mental experience is illusory. Another passage (*Sāṃkhya-sūtras*, I, 58) adds that all the qualities attributed to Spirit (e.g., the faculty of comprehension, of will, etc.) are merely "verbal expressions," for they do not correspond to the reality (*tattva*). It is in this sense that we must understand *Sāṃkhya-sūtras*, III, 56, where Spirit is declared to be "omnipotent" (*sarvavit, sarvakartā*). Aniruddha, commenting on *Sāṃkhya-sūtras*, I, 97, explains that intelligence (*buddhi*), individuality (*ahaṃkāra*), and the senses (*indriyaṇi*) form an "empirical soul" (*jīva*), a "vital soul," capable of acting, but that the *jīva* must not be confused with the *puruṣa*. The same distinction is made by Śaṇkara, who postulates the existence of a "supreme soul" and of an empirical soul (*jīvātman*). Another passage (*Sāṃkhya-sūtras*, I, 160) declares that Spirit is of such a nature that we cannot say of it either that it is bound or that it is liberated (*vyāvṛtta-ubhayarūpah*); at least, this is what Vijñānabhikṣu takes the words to mean. See also Narendra, commenting on *Tattvasamāṣa*, 4; *Sāṃkhya-sūtras*, I, 96; I, 106; I, 162; III, 41, etc., and especially Vyāsa and Vācaspatimiśra ad *Yoga-sūtras*, I, 4, 5; III, 34; IV, 22. On *puruṣa* in preclassic Sāṃkhya, see Johnston, *Early Sāṁkhya*, pp. 52 ff.

I, 5: The Three Guṇas

There are many passages on the *guṇas* in all the Sāṃkhya and Yoga treatises and commentaries. We shall select a few: Īśvarakṛṣṇa, *Kārikā*, II, 16, with the commentaries by Māṭhara, Gauḍapāda, and Vācaspatimiśra; *Yoga-sūtras*, II, 15; II, 19 (Vyāsa's and Vācaspatimiśra's elucidations are important); IV, 13; IV, 32; Vācaspatimiśra, *Tattvavaiśāradī*, I, 16, etc. Émile Senart ("*Rajas* et la théorie indienne des trois *guṇas*") has attempted to explain the appearance of the *guṇas* in Indian thought by much earlier, post-Vedic intuitions. Victor Henry ("Physique védique") reduces the earliest speculations on the *guṇas* to the following schema: (mild) heat → (intense) heat → suffering → asceticism. In a more recent study ("La Théorie des *guṇas* et la *Chāndogya Upaniṣad*"), Senart resumes and completes his researches into the prehistory of the *guṇas*. Analyzing a passage from the *Chāndogya Upaniṣad* (VI, 2–4), he thus summarizes the Upaniṣadic conception of the constitution of the world: "Three cosmic elements combining in variable proportions to constitute the substance of the sensible world: *tejas, āpas, anna*" (p. 286). . . . "Three stages among which Vedic phraseology divides the perceptible universe. *Tejas*, to which a reddish luminosity (*rohita*) is attributed, the *āpases*, white in color (*śukla*), *anna*, which is black (*kṛṣṇa*), undoubtedly correspond to the upper region of the sun, the region of clouds, with its more tempered brightness, and the terrestrial region, with no luminosity of its own, which produces vegetation" (p. 287). Jean Przyluski ("La Théorie des *Guṇa*") finds analogies with the Iranian triad and believes that he can trace Semitic influences in the concept of the three *guṇas*. An excellent exposition and a penetrating philosophical interpretation in Dasgupta, *History of Indian Philosophy*, I, 243 ff.; id., *Yoga Philosophy*, pp. 70–111. Cf. also Garbe, *Sāṃkhya-Philosophie*, pp. 209–20; Radhakrishnan, *Indian Philosophy*, II, 263–65; Hopkins, *Great Epic*, pp. 119 ff., etc. On the history of the theory of the *guṇas* in preclassic India, Johnston, *Early Sāṁkhya*, pp. 25–41, should now be consulted.

I, 6: Logic and Theory of Knowledge in Sāṃkhya-Yoga

Sāṃkhya's logic and theory of knowledge are as summary as its contribution to cosmology is important and original. Although recognizing the need for a canon founding the validity of knowledge, Sāṃkhya and Yoga gave a secondary place to speculations on the syllogism (elaborated by Nyāya) or to the "evidence in itself" of perception (a theory cherished by the Mīmāṃsā school), and generally neglected the penetrating epistemological analyses inaugurated by the Buddhist philosophers. On Indian logic, see Satis Chandra Vidyābhūṣaṇa, *History of Indian Logic;* Keith, *Indian Logic and Atomism;* S. Sugiura, *Hindu Logic;* Hakuju Ui, *The Vaiśeṣika Philosophy;* Barend Faddegon, *The Vaiśeṣika-System;* Fyodor Ippolitovich Stcherbatsky, *Erkenntnistheorie und Logik nach der Lehre der späteren Buddhisten;* id., *Buddhist Logic;* Tucci, *Pre-Diṅnāga.* See also the bibliographical notes by La Vallée Poussin on recent publications in *MCB,* I (1931–32), 415–16.

Vyāsa (seventh century) and Vijñānabhikṣu (sixteenth century) grant a certain importance to logical problems, but it cannot be compared with the interest they show in metaphysics and psychology. Vyāsa (*bhāṣya* ad *Yoga-sūtras,* III, 52) outlines an analysis of time: for him, as for the Buddhist logicians, the real is only the *instant,* the "moment"; neither the succession of moments nor the arbitrary division of time into hours, days, fortnights, etc., possesses *objective reality;* they are mental constructions. This interpretation of Vyāsa's was probably inspired by the Buddhist philosophers, especially by Vasubandhu (cf. Stcherbatsky, *The Central Conception of Buddhism,* p. 43).

As in all other Indian systems, at the base of Sāṃkhya-Yoga logic stands the definition of *pramāṇa,* "proof," "mode of cognition"—in other words, the instruments that ensure the validity of a cognition. Īśvarakṛṣṇa repeats: "Perception [*dṛṣṭam, pratyakṣa*], inference [*anumāna*], and accurate testimony [*aptā vacanam*] are the three proofs" (*Sāṃkhya-kārikā,* 4). Perception is "knowledge through the senses" (ibid., 5). Vācaspatimiśra, interpreting this passage, adds that perception is the result of a mental process (*buddhi*) in which *sattva* predominates, which is obtained by attaching the perceptive sense to the object. In other words, perception is a sense activity, oriented toward objects, molded by them, and presenting their forms to the intellect (*buddhi*).

There is an identical definition in the *Sāṃkhya-sūtras* (I, 89): "*Pratyakṣa* is the knowledge that results from attachment (to objects) and represents their form." Vijñānabhikṣu (ad ibid.) adds: it is a "knowledge, a sort of modification of the intellect, which directs itself toward the object with which it is in relation." But the *puruṣa* is not influenced by this "modification" of the *buddhi.* Cf. also Woods, "La Théorie de la connaissance dans le système du Yoga."

To sum up, it is clear that by "perception" Sāṃkhya and Yoga understand a psychomental activity oriented toward objects, the latter existing as such and being regarded as neither sensations nor moments nor illusions. It is easy to understand why, with such premises, Sāṃkhya paid little attention to problems of perception, since it affirmed the validity of a datum obtained by direct intuition of external reality.

Inference or reasoning (*anumāna*) corresponds to the theory of the Nyāya school, and Sāṃkhya contributed nothing to its development. Buddhist influence does not appear here. It is a theory of inference in which perception is also implied (*Tattva-kaumudī,* 34). Īśvarakṛṣṇa gives the following definition (*Sāṃkhya-kārikā,* 6): "Inference is founded on the major term and on the minor term and is of three kinds"—a definition that is unintelligible without commentaries. But if the formula is so summary, that is because it refers to a universally known and universally accepted truth. Only the Cārvāka materialists denied *anumāna* as proof (*pramāṇa*), for the reason that the middle term (*vyāpti,* "permanent concomitance") is itself a truth requiring justification by inference, and thus a vicious circle is set up.

Inference is of three kinds: (1) a priori (*pūrvavat*), when the effect is inferred from the cause (rain is inferred from the presence of clouds); (2) a posteriori (*śeṣavat*), when the cause is inferred from the effect (rain is inferred from the flooded condition of the river); (3) *sāmānyatodṛṣṭa,* when the inference is from the general to the general (Vācaspatimiśra, *Tattva-kaumudī,* 35). Vijñānabhikṣu (ad *Sāṃkhya-sūtras,* I, 135) gives an example of this last variety of inference: the existence of the *guṇas* is inferred from the existence of the *mahat.* For Sāṃkhya, inference serves to prove the existence of principles (*tattva*) and is implied in the whole cosmic fabric that we have briefly described above (pp. 21 ff.). One of the special characteristics of the system, *the plurality of souls,* is likewise justified by inference. Sāṃkhya sets out from a truth universally accepted in India—that there have been men who have achieved liberation through knowledge, particularly the sages (Kapila, Āsuri, etc.) and the *ṛṣis.* If there had been but one universal soul, the first human being who liberated himself from the illusion of phenomena would inevitably have brought about the liberation of all souls, and there would be neither existence nor suffering in the universe today.

I, 7: *Sāṃkhya and the Critique of the Existence of God*

The arguments raised by the Sāṃkhya writers against the existence of God are rather feeble (as are Patañjali's and Vyāsa's contrary "proofs" to demonstrate the existence of Īśvara). There is no proof of the existence of God, says *Sāṃkhya-sūtras,* I, 92. God cannot exist, because he would necessarily be either free or bound (ibid., I, 93). A bound spirit could not be God, for he would be under the domination of *karma;* on the other hand, a free spirit could not be the Creator, for, being absolutely detached from matter, he could not have perceptions, nor desire for any kind of activity, and, finally, he would have no way of influencing matter (Aniruddha, ad ibid.). This argument is directed against the Nyāya school, for Aniruddha (ad ibid., III, 57) writes: "If God is conceived as a spirit accepted *by us,* we have nothing to object against his existence; but there is no proof of a God such as the Nyāya philosophy conceives him to be." Again in the *Sāṃkhya-sūtras,* we read (V, 10–11): "There is no proof of the existence of an eternal Īśvara; for to deduce his existence is impossible, a middle term [*vyāpti*] being lacking." This "middle term" should connect the creation and the Creator. But the creation is explained by *prakṛti;* hence the intervention of an exterior agent is unnecessary. Furthermore, the Sāṃkhya writers add, tradition itself, having its foundation in the Vedic revelation, speaks of *prakṛti* as the sole principle of the creation.

The same arguments are found in Vācaspatimiśra (commentary on *Sāṃkhya-kārikā,* 57). However, the *Sāṃkhya-kārikā* nowhere explicitly criticizes the existence of God. Īśvarakṛṣṇa's atheism is less pronounced than that of the *Sāṃkhya-sūtras;* as Śāstri puts it (p. xxix of the introduction to his edition of the *Sāṃkhya-kārikā*), "Īśvarakṛṣṇa was less concerned to deny the existence of God than to try to do without him." In any case, a "theistic" Sāṃkhya developed from the *Śvetāśvatara Upaniṣad* and was popularized by the *Bhagavad Gītā* (see below, pp. 394–95).

Cf. also Garbe, *Sāṃkhya-Philosophie,* pp. 191–95; id., *Sāṃkhya und Yoga,* p. 17; Dasgupta, *Yoga Philosophy,* pp. 231–58; Tucci, "Linee di una storia," pp. 42 ff.

I, 8: *Sāṃkhya and Buddhism*

There is an extensive bibliography on the relations between Sāṃkhya, Yoga, and Buddhism. We shall not repeat it here. (For the earlier publications, see Garbe's introduction to his translation of Aniruddha's *Sāṃkhya-sūtra-vṛtti*, pp. i–ii; the introduction is based on an earlier study, "Der Mondschein der Sāṃkhya-Wahrheit.") In any case, the problem has two distinct aspects: the influence of Sāṃkhya on Buddhism and the influence of Yoga on Buddhism. If certain Indianists deny that Sāṃkhya played a part in the philosophical formation of the Buddha or of primitive Buddhism, the majority of scholars nevertheless regard the influence of Yoga techniques as incontestable (see below, pp. 397–98).

Max Müller and Oldenberg were the first to reject the tradition—until then generally accepted—that Buddhism derives from Sāṃkhya. Garbe (in the study mentioned above and in *Sāṃkhya-Philosophie*, pp. 3–5) attempts to justify the tradition by indicating the eight points common to Sāṃkhya and Buddhism, among which he stresses the following: both Buddhism and Sāṃkhya are "enumerative philosophies"—that is, they make exaggerated use of classifications, enumeration, and schemata; both are pessimistic, antisacrificial, and antiascetic; both hold that Spirit must not be confused with psychomental experience; both regard liberation as the supreme goal of man. Garbe thinks that Sāṃkhya cannot have borrowed all its ideas and all its schemata from Buddhism, for it is difficult to imagine the creator of a philosophical system borrowing his elements from a religion that leaves all the important questions unsolved (for primitive Buddhism refused to discuss final problems, as unnecessary to the salvation of the soul).

Jacobi ("Der Ursprung des Buddhismus aus dem Sānkhya-Yoga") accepts Garbe's conclusions and gives them added support by bringing out the intimate relations between the *nidānas* and the "categories" of Sāṃkhya and calling fresh attention to the fact that Aśvaghoṣa, in the *Buddhacarita*, calls Buddha's first teacher, Arāḍa (Pāli, Aḷāra), "a partisan of Sāṃkhya" (p. 55). Jacobi is of the opinion that Aśvaghoṣa's testimony represents a genuine historical tradition (p. 57). He returns to the subject in his study, "Über das Verhältnis der buddhistischen Philosophie zu Sānkhya-Yoga und die Bedeutung des Nidānas," in which he makes his opinion explicit: "Buddhism appears not as a copy but as a personal reinterpretation of Sāṃkhya; the latter was not the model after which Buddhism was constructed, but rather the soil on which it grew" (p. 1). On Sāṃkhya as presented by Aśvaghoṣa (who lived—let us not forget—several centuries before Īśvarakṛṣṇa!), see Johnston, *The Buddhacarita*, I, lvi ff., 166 ff.; id., *Early Sāṁkhya*, pp. 35 ff., 54 ff.

Oldenberg, who in his *Buddha* had denied Sāṃkhya influence on Buddhism, criticizes Jacobi's statements ("Buddhistischen Studien," p. 693) and questions whether the Buddha, though steeped in Yoga ascetic practices, had also adopted the ideas of Sāṃkhya. He returns to the subject at greater length in his *Die Lehre der Upanishaden*, pp. 178–223, and in "Zur Geschichte der Sāṃkhya-Philosophie." As La Vallée Poussin has said, Oldenberg gradually convinced himself of the influence of Sāṃkhya on Buddhism. This view is shared by Richard Pischel (*Leben und Lehre des Buddha*, pp. 65 ff.). Cf. also: F. Lipsius, *Die Sāṃkhya Philosophie als Vorläuferin des Buddhismus*, pp. 106–14; Tucci, *Il Buddhismo*, pp. 58 ff.

Keith (*Sāṃkhya System*, pp. 23–33; cf. *Buddhist Philosophy*, pp. 38–43) chooses the middle road: "The only conclusion that can be drawn from the evidence is that some of the conceptions of Buddhism are very closely allied to those of the Sāṃkhya" (*Sāṃkhya System*, p. 29). Among the ideas common to Sāṃkhya and Buddhism, Keith includes the conception of the *saṃskāras*, the conception of causality, the correspondence between the four truths of the Buddha and the four stages of the doctrine of deliverance in Sāṃkhya-Yoga, the similarity between the experience of "liberation" in Buddhism and Sāṃkhya, etc. But he also finds numerous differences between the two systems. "It is, therefore, legitimate to conclude that the classical Sāṃkhya was not the source of Buddhism, and that any influence exercised on Buddhism by Sāṃkhya must have come from a system more akin to that of the Epic, unless we prefer the view that the influence should be regarded as coming from an earlier form of doctrine, which may be regarded as the common source of Buddhism and the Sāṃkhya of the Epic" (ibid., p. 31). "The proof of Sāṃkhya influence is obviously indirect, and not in itself complete" (*Buddhist Philosophy*, p. 42).

See also Eugen Hultzsch, "Sāṃkhya und Yoga in Siśupālayadha"; Walter Liebenthal, *Satkārya in der Darstellung seiner buddhistischen Gegner*; Hauer, *Das Laṇkāvatāra-Sūtra und das Sāṃkhya*; S. C. Vidyābhūṣaṇa, "Sāṃkhya Philosophy in the Land of the Lamas."

I, 9: Sāṃkhya's Critique of Buddhism

Sāṃkhya realism necessarily rejected the idealism and relativism of the medieval Buddhist schools. In late Sāṃkhya texts there are polemics with the Buddhist idealists. We shall examine the most important of them.

In discussing the reality of the external world, Vācaspatimiśra writes (*Tattvavaiśāradī*, I, 3): "Certainly, mother-of-pearl as such [*svarūpa*] *remains the same* whether the perception that refers to it is valid or false" —that is, whether one perceives it (rightly) as mother-of-pearl or (wrongly) as silver. For his part, the author of the *Sāṃkhya-sūtras* categorically states (I, 42): "(The world) is not a mere idea (since we have) direct apprehension of reality" (*na vijñānamātram bāhyapratīteh*). Commenting on this passage, Aniruddha explains the objectivity of the world (*jagat*) as follows: if it were a mere idea (*vijñāna*)— as the Buddhists maintain—we should not have the experience (*pratyaya*) that "*this* is a pot" but that "*I* am a pot" (*aham ghaṭaḥ iti pratyaya syāt, na tu ayam ghaṭaḥ iti*). If the opponent objects: the experience "*this* is a pot," although possessing the appearance of objective reality, is due to a "specific impression" (*vāsanāviśeṣa*), Aniruddha replies that these specific impressions must have had previous impressions that determined them; in which case, a substratum behind impressions is always accepted (for otherwise there would be a *regressus ad infinitum*), and this substratum can only be external reality. On the other hand, if the same Buddhist opponent objects that "the external object cannot exist, since a *whole* [*avayavin*] distinct from its *parts* [*avayava*] does not exist; the *parts* and the *whole* being one [*avayavāvayavinorekatvāt*], for they are perceived as one [*ekatvapratīteḥ*]"—the answer is that "the whole" often moves at the same time as the "parts" (a tree during a storm), but it sometimes happens that only the "parts" move, without the "whole" (the tree in a slight breeze).

However, certain idealists (the Śūnyavāda Buddhists, who postulate emptiness as the final substratum of reality) raise a new objection: "Since a knowledge without objects is impossible [*nirviṣayasya jñānasya adarśanāt*], knowledge cannot exist, if objects do not exist." To this Vijñānabhikṣu replies (ad *Sāṃkhya-sūtras*, I, 43): "From the nonexistence of the external world there would result only emptiness, not thought [*tarhi bāhyābhāve śūnyameva prasajyeta, na tu vijñānamapi*]. Why? Because the nonexistence of the external world equally implies the nonexistence of thought; and one can establish by induction [*anumānasambhavāt*] that, like the intuition of external reality, the intuition of thought is devoid of an object [*avastuviṣaya*]."

Vijñānabhikṣu, in his commentary on *Sāṃkhya-sūtras*, I, 45, finds another refutation for the Śūnyavādas, who postulate emptiness as the

Grund of existence. Those who say that "existence as such is perishable" declare a merely ignorant opinion. For "simple substances" cannot be destroyed, since no destroying causes exist. Only "compound substances" can be destroyed. Furthermore, it must be observed that time does not enter in as the destructive agent of external objects. To say, for example, "The jug no longer exists," is to record the new conditions in which that object now is. But Vijñānabhikṣu does not end his paragraph before raising a final objection: "If you admit that a proof of the existence of emptiness exists, then, by that very proof, emptiness is excluded; if you do not admit it, then, in the absence of proofs, emptiness is not proved; if you say that emptiness affirms itself, this would imply that it possesses intelligence, and so on." Another refutation of emptiness by Vijñānabhikṣu is eschatological: emptiness cannot be the goal of the soul, because the liberation (*mokṣa*) for which the soul languishes is a real thing.

To summarize, the Sāṃkhya arguments against the Buddhists protest (1) against the doctrine of "moments" (*kṣaṇa*), in the name of recognition of objects previously perceived; (2) against idealism, because of the perception of objects; (3) against emptiness (*Śūnyavāda*), by *reductio ad absurdum.*

Sāṃkhya realism was criticized both by Śaṇkara (*Brahma-sūtras,* II, 11, 1–10) and by the various idealistic schools (cf., for example, Vasubandhu's *Vijñaptimātratāsiddhi,* tr. La Vallée Poussin, I, 23–36).

II, 1: *The Obstacles to Concentration*

The nine obstacles to concentration are listed in *Yoga-sūtras,* I, 30. Vyāsa explains them as follows: (1) *vyādhi* (sickness) is disturbance of the physical equilibrium; (2) *styāna* (languor) is lack of mental disposition for work; (3) *saṃśaya* (indecision) is thought debating between the two sides of a problem: "it may be thus or thus"; (4) *pramāda* (heedlessness, insensibility) is the lack of initiative that prevents *samādhi;* (5) *ālasya* (softness) is inertia of mind and body owing to "heaviness" (*gurutva*); (6) *avirati* (sensuality) is the desire aroused when sensory objects possess the mind; (7) *bhrānti darśana* (false, invalid notion) is false knowledge; (8) *alabhdabhūmikatva* (inability to see reality because of psychomental mobility); (9) *anavasthitattva* (instability), which cannot maintain a continuity of thought, because the mind has not attained to *ekāgratā*. Additional obstacles are pain (*duḥkha*), despair (*dāurmanasya*), etc. (*Yoga-sūtras*, I, 31). "To prevent them, become accustomed to truth" (ibid., I, 32). Similarly, by cultivating universal friendliness (*maitrī*), compassion (*karuṇā*), content (*muditā*), and showing indifference to happiness, to unhappiness, to virtue or vices, one purifies the mind (ibid., I, 33). All this belongs to the common property of Indian ethics, and illustrations of it can be found in the literature of orthodoxy as well as in sectarian and popular literature.

II, 2: *On the* Āsanas

The technical term *āsana* is not among the oldest. It does not occur in the earliest Upaniṣads (it is first mentioned in *Śvetāśvatara Upaniṣad*, II, 10). It occurs in the *Bhagavad Gītā*, where it has the same meaning as in the *Kṣurikā Upaniṣad*, and in the *Buddhacarita* of Aśvaghoṣa (first century A.D.); cf. Deussen, *The Philosophy of the Upanishads*, pp. 387–88; Hopkins, "Yoga-Technique in the Great Epic," p. 348. There are numerous references to the *āsanas* in the *Śānti Parva* of the *Mahābhārata*, chs. 237, 241, 317. But there is no doubt about the antiquity of the practice; the Vedic texts sometimes refer to the yogic posture (cf. Hauer, *Die Anfänge der Yogapraxis*, pp. 21–31), and a number of the seals found at Mohenjo-daro represent divinities in the *āsana* position (see above, pp. 229 ff.). Among the yogic Upaniṣads that discuss *āsanas* at length, we shall mention the *Triśikhibrāhmaṇa Upaniṣad*, 34–52. The Haṭha-yogic *Gheraṇḍa Saṃhitā* describes thirty-two *āsanas;* the *Haṭhayogapradīpikā* defines fifteen, and the *Śiva Saṃhitā* eighty-four. For Haṭha Yoga, the postures have a very marked magical value; for example, *padmāsana* cures any kind of sickness (*Gheraṇḍa Saṃhitā*, II, 8), *muktāsana* and *vajrāsana* confer "miraculous powers" (ibid., II, 11–12), *mṛtāsana* calms mental agitation (ibid., II, 19), *bhujaṅgāsana* awakens the *kuṇḍalinī* (ibid., II, 42–43), etc. There are *āsanas* that "conquer death," a cliché common in Haṭha-yogic texts. Cf. Theos Bernard, *Haṭha Yoga*.

On *āsana* in the Pāli canon, cf. *The Yogāvacara's Manual of Indian Mysticism*, ed. T. W. Rhys Davids (tr. F. L. Woodward under the title *Manual of a Mystic*), p. 1, n. 2.

Cf. also Arthur Avalon, *The Serpent Power*, passim; Roesel, *Die psychologischen Grundlagen*, pp. 16–23.

II, 3: On Yogic Concentration

The first explicit reference in the Upaniṣads: *Kāṭhaka Upaniṣad*, VI, 11. The relevant passages in the *Mahābhārata* have been pointed out and discussed by Hopkins, "Yoga-Technique," pp. 351 ff. On the five *dhāraṇās* in Jainism, cf. Garbe, *Sāṃkhya und Yoga*, pp. 39 ff. The principal passages in the *Yoga-sūtras*, with the commentaries on them, are reproduced and analyzed by Lindquist, *Die Methoden des Yoga*, pp. 104 ff. —but it must be borne in mind that Lindquist reduces yogic meditation and concentration to various forms of self-hynotism.

For a personal experience of yogic concentration, see Bernard, *Haṭha Yoga*. Cf. also Filliozat's pertinent observations, "Sur la 'concentration oculaire' dans le Yoga," and Olivier Lacombe, "Sur le Yoga indien."

II, 4: Samādhi

On the meaning of *samādhi* in the didactic portions of the *Mahābhārata*, cf. Hopkins, "Yoga-Technique," pp. 337 ff.

The important passages from the *Yoga-sūtras* (especially I, 41–46), with the commentaries by Vyāsa, Vācaspatimiśra, and Bhoja, are conveniently reproduced and analyzed in Lindquist, *Die Methoden des Yoga*, pp. 118 ff., 144 ff.

On the identity of the terms *samādhi* = *samāpatti*, see especially Vyāsa, ad *Yoga-sūtras*, I, 43–44, and Vācaspatimiśra, ad I, 42–43.

On the parallelism between the four Buddhist *dhyānas* and the four varieties of *samprajñāta samādhi*, cf. Senart, "Bouddhisme et Yoga," pp. 349 ff.; La Vallée Poussin, "Le Bouddhisme et le Yoga de Patañjali," pp. 229–30. "Shall we raise the question: on which side, Yoga or Buddhism, were these common concepts and common doctrines first elaborated? Probability verging on certainty speaks for Yoga" (Oldenberg quoted by La Vallée Poussin, p. 230). See also below, pp. 397 ff.

II, 5: The Siddhis, *"Miraculous Powers"*

The classic Yoga texts are assembled in Lindquist, *Die Methoden des Yoga*, pp. 169–82; id., *Siddhi und Abhiññā*, in which he analyzes the Buddhist documents, especially Buddhaghoṣa's *Visuddhimagga*. Good bibliography of the sources for the *abhijñās* in Étienne Lamotte, *Le Traité de la Grande Vertu de sagesse de Nāgārjuna* (*Mahāprajñāpāramitāśāstra*), I, 329, n. 1.

On the *siddhis* in Haṭha-yogic literature, see, for example, *Śiva Saṃhitā*, III, 41 ff. On the *siddhis* in tantrism and in yogic folklore, see above, pp. 312 ff. Cf. also the legends of Siddhas, pp. 303 ff.

III, 1: *The* Vrātyas *and the Ecstatics of Vedic Times*

The problem of the *vrātyas* has been exhaustively treated by Moriz Winternitz, "Die Vrātyas," and especially by Hauer, *Der Vrātya.* On the *keśin* of *Ṛg-Veda,* X, 136, cf. Hauer, *Die Anfänge der Yogapraxis,* pp. 169 ff.; id., *Vrātya,* pp. 324 ff.

On asceticism and the literature of the *śramaṇas,* see La Vallée Poussin's bibliographical indications in his *Indo-Européens et Indo-Iraniens,* pp. 290 ff., 378 ff. There is an abundance of material on popular religion during the Vedic period in Ernst Arbman, *Rudra,* especially pp. 64 ff. On initiatory and ecstatic "male societies," see Stig Wikander's studies, *Der arische Männerbund* and *Vāyu.* On the shamanistic elements, cf. Ruben, "Schamanismus im alten Indien," and M. Eliade, *Shamanism,* pp. 403–441.

III, 2: *The Five Breaths*

The five "breaths" are the *prāṇa,* the *apāna,* the *samāna,* the *udāna,* and the *vyāna.* Arthur H. Ewing ("The Hindu Conception of the Functions of Breath") has made an exhaustive collection of references to them in Vedic literature. The gist of his conclusions is as follows: the *prāṇa* is the breath that moves upward from the umbilicus or the heart, and includes both inhalation and exhalation; *apāna* is a term with several meanings: the breath of the anus and the scrotum, of the large intestine, of the umbilicus; the *vyāna* is the breath that penetrates all the limbs; the *udāna* includes both eructation and the breath that carries the soul toward the head in the state of *samādhi* or of death; the *samāna* is the breath localized in the abdomen and is credited with ensuring digestion.

According to G. W. Brown ("Prāṇa and Apāna"), *prāṇa* is the thoracic breath, *apāna* the abdominal. Filliozat (*La Doctrine classique,* pp. 142 ff.) rejects Ewing's conclusions in part: even in the *Ṛg-Veda,* the *prāṇa* is already the breath of the upper part of the body, the *apāna* that of the lower, "and the connection between them is the *vyāna*, which circulates in the middle of the body" (p. 148). In any case, nothing justifies our translating *prāṇa* and *apāna* by "exhalation" and "inhalation," for the texts refer to the *prāṇa* and *apāna* "within the womb," to the role of the *prāṇa* in the development of the embryo (e.g., *Atharva Veda*, XI, 4, 14). "Now, of all conceivable organic breaths, the only ones that cannot possibly be involved in the case of the embryo are inhalation and exhalation" (Filliozat, p. 147). We must always bear in mind the homology breath=cosmic wind, documented from Vedic times (cf. *Ṛg-Veda*, X, 90, 13: wind was born from the breath of the cosmic man; *Atharva Veda*, XI, 4, 15: "the wind is called breath," etc.; cf. Filliozat, pp. 52 ff.). "Since the cosmic man's *prāṇa* or breath in general is wind, it is an inner breath, for it is inside the universe, the body of the cosmic giant, that the wind circulates" (ibid., p. 147). The inner breath is also known to Chinese traditions; see above, pp. 60 ff. For the Indo-Iranian mythology of the cosmic wind-breath, cf. Wikander, *Vāyu*, pp. 84 ff. and passim.

III, 3: Tapas *and the* Dīkṣā

See Oldenberg, *Die Religion des Veda*, pp. 397 ff.; Alfred Hillebrandt, *Vedische Mythologie*, I, 482 ff.; Hermann Güntert, *Der arische Weltkönig und Heiland*, pp. 347 ff.; Hauer, *Die Anfänge der Yogapraxis*, pp. 55 ff.; Keith, *The Religion and Philosophy of the Veda*, I, 300 ff.; Sylvain Lévi, *La Doctrine du sacrifice dans les Brāhmaṇas*, pp. 103 ff. Cf. also Eliade, *Shamanism*, pp. 412 ff. According to Barth, "nothing proves that the ceremony [of the *dīkṣā*] really goes back to the time of the Hymns . . . we shall search them in vain for either *dīkṣā*, or *dikṣita*, or any equivalent term, or for specific allusions to anything of the kind"; see also La Vallée Poussin, *Indo-Européens*, pp. 368 ff. However, the conception is archaic: it is difficult to see why it should not have been known to the Vedic Indians, since the mythology and the technique of sweating—which, moreover, are found everywhere—are documented among the Germans, the Scythians, and the Iranians.

III, 4: *Hinduization of Autochthonous Religion*

The assimilation of aboriginal gods is a process that is still going on. We shall confine ourselves to citing a few observations recorded by Indian folklorists, especially Sarat Chandra Mitra, for the literature on the subject is immense. The "conversion" to Hinduism is, however, more superficial than otherwise; there is always a residue of elements betraying the "primitive" character of new gods or new cults. Thus, for example, when the original tribes were converted, they accepted the Hindu divinities (for the most part, female divinities) but did not employ Brāhmans to perform the rituals; see Mitra, "On the Conversion of Tribes into Castes in North Bihār," on an Orāon tribe adoring the goddess Bhagavatī under an old tree; id., "On the Cult of the Jujube Tree," on the vegetation demon Itokumāra, the ceremonies of whose worship are performed only by unmarried girls, without the participation of Brāhmans.

There are cases, too, in which Hindu temples, built on sites formerly consecrated to pre-Āryan cults, are served by *priests who are pariahs;* it was the sacredness of the site that counted (a well-known phenomenon in the history of religions; see our *Patterns*, pp. 199 ff., on the continuity of sacred sites). During the festival of the Mother-Goddess (Ammāl or Āttal), which continues for sixteen days, a pariah is kept and fed in the temple as the fiancé of the Goddess. A pariah ties the *tāli* around the neck of Egāttāla, tutelary goddess of Madras. In the province of Mysore, a Holiya is regarded as the priest of the local goddess, and the pariah chief of the village as the master of the village (Gustav Oppert, *On the Original Inhabitants of Bharatavarṣa or India*, p. 52). Elsewhere, too, pariahs rather than Brāhmans perform the ritual of the Goddess (cf. William Crooke, *An Introduction to the Popular Religion and Folk-lore of Northern India*, I, 47). The pariahs belong to pre-Āryan tribes; they know the secrets of the Goddess; they represent the "masters of primordial sacrality."

Even when the aboriginal tribes are dogmatically and juridically incorporated into Hinduism, having assimilated the Brāhmanic mythology, the caste system, etc., they usually do without the services of Brāhmans. Like the ancient autochthonous divinities, the ancient religious ceremonies survive, but under different names and sometimes with a changed meaning. The tribes still venerate the sacred places—a tree, a lake, a spring, a cave—haunted by their tutelary divinities. In order to assimilate them, Hinduism identified these tutelary divinities with the many manifestations of Śiva or Kālī (Durgā); as for the ancient cult sites, they were validated by episodes from Hindu mythology. An example is the goddess Kālijai, who is the tutelary divinity of Lake Chilka (Orissa), and whose aboriginal structure is further confirmed by the fact that fowls are sacrificed to her; cf. S. C. Mitra, "The Cult of the Lake-Goddess of Orissa." See also Nanimadhab Chaudhuri, "Rudra-Śiva—as an Agricultural Deity" (the cult of Śiva among semi-Hinduized tribes, pp. 185 ff.); Mitra, "Notes on Tree-Cults in the District of Patna in South Bihār"; id., "On the Worship of the Pipal Tree in North Bihār." The cult of the pipal is treated in an immense literature; for references in the epic and the Purāṇas, cf. J. J. Meyer, *Trilogie altindischer Mächte und Feste der Vegetation*, II, 132–34; for the earliest period, cf. Chaudhuri, "A Prehistoric Tree Cult."

The goddess Durgā-Kālī, who was to play a decisive role in tantrism (see pp. 202 ff.), was very probably an aboriginal divinity of vegetation and agriculture. The symbiosis tantrism-vegetation cult is still traceable in Bengal: cf. Chintaharan Chakravarti, "The Cult of Bāro Bhāiyā of Eastern Bengal," on the cult of the "twelve brothers," Bāro Bhāiyā, and of their mother Vanadurgā, in the districts of Kotalipada and Faridpur. Their worship is conducted near an *aśvatha* or *sheora* tree, on Tuesday or Friday, days favorable for the tantric liturgy; goats, sheep, and buffaloes are sacrificed. According to the *mantras* recited, Vanadurgā corresponds to the Durgā of tantric iconography.

The cosmico-vegetable structure of Durgā, documented in the Purāṇas and in tantric literature, made her especially popular among aboriginal tribes in process of Hinduization. The *Devī-Māhātmya*, XCII, 43–44 (= *Mārkaṇḍeya Purāṇa*, 81–93), celebrates the goddess' great victory over the demons of drought, Mahiṣa, Sumbha, and Nisumbha: "Then, O Gods, I will nourish [lit., I will support] the whole universe by these vegetables that maintain life and that grow from my body during the season of rains. Then shall I become glorious on earth like Sākamharī ["she who bears herbs" or "who nourishes herbs"] and, in that same season, I shall disembowel the great *asura* named Durgammā"; for the liturgical context of this myth, cf. Mitra, "On the Cult of the Tree-Goddess in Eastern Bengal"; for the myth, Heinrich Zimmer, *Myths and Symbols in Indian Art and Civilization*, pp. 190 ff. An important rite, the *navapatrikā* (the "nine leaves"), shows the vegetational character of Durgā: "O, O leaf [*patrikā*], O nine forms of Durgā! You are the darling of Mahādeva; accept all these offerings and protect me, O queen of heaven. *O, adoration to Durgā dwelling in the nine plants*" (Mitra, pp. 232–33).

As a tree divinity, Durgā is found chiefly in the districts of Mymensingh and Tippera, where she is known by the name of Bana Durgā. She lives in the *sheora* tree (*Streblus asper*), sometimes in the roots of the *uduma* tree (*Ficus glomerata?*). Bana Durgā is worshiped before the ceremony of investiture with the sacred thread, before the marriage ceremony, and in general before any auspicious ritual. At Comilla, in the Tippera district, she is worshiped in the root of the *Kāmini* tree (*Murraya exotica*) with the formula: "(Submission to the goddess) Durgā who dwells in the *sākota* tree." Pigs are usually sacrificed to her; on the occasion of the *pūjā*, the sacrifice consists of twenty-one cocks. This detail is valuable evidence for her non-Āryan origin and character. Mitra ("On the Worship of Dakshina Rāya as a Rain-God") compares the sacrifice of duck eggs spotted with vermilion to the offering of drakes made in southern Bengal to a non-Āryan divinity, Dakshina Rāya, who has the form of a tiger. Non-Āryan customs in connection with the goddess Kālī are also found in the popular Kālī-Nautch festival, during which bands of masked dancers go through the streets, after having worshiped the goddess at midnight, three days earlier, under a banyan tree (see Dhirendra Nath Majumdar, "Notes on Kālī-Nautch"). We shall have occasion to return to the relations between Durgā and popular vegetation cults (see pp. 373 ff.). What must be emphasized now is the tireless power of absorption shown by Hinduism, which even in our day still transforms aboriginal tribes into castes and subcastes and their divinities into epiphanies of Śiva and Durgā.

III, 5: *The Upaniṣads*

On *brahman*, see Jarl Charpentier, *Brahman;* Georges Dumézil, *Flamen-Brahman;* Keith, "New Theories as to *Brahman*"; B. Heimann, *Studien zur Eigenart indischen Denkens*, pp. 40 ff.; H. G. Narahari, *Ātman in Pre-Upaniṣadic Vedic Literature*, pp. 22 ff.; Louis Renou, "Sur la notion du *brahman*"; Jan Gonda, *Notes on Brahman.*

Upaniṣads: For editions, translations, and critical studies published up to 1931, refer to Renou, *Bibliographie védique*, secs. 96–116. Of particular interest are: R. D. Ranade, *A Constructive Survey of Upanishadic Philosophy;* Oldenberg, *Die Lehre der Upanishaden;* Deussen,

Die Philosophie der Upanishads; Oltramare, *L'Histoire des idées,* I, 63 ff.; B. Barua, *A History of Pre-Buddhistic Philosophy;* S. Dasgupta, *Indian Idealism,* pp. 20 ff.; id., *History of Indian Philosophy,* vol. I; Keith, *Religion and Philosophy,* pp. 534 ff.; Maryla Falk, "Il Mito psicologico nell' India antica," especially pp. 346–97, 421–569; Ruben, *Die Philosophen der Upanishaden;* Renou, "Le Passage des Brāhmaṇa aux Upaniṣad."

On mystical speculations in regard to sleep (*Bṛhadāraṇyaka Upaniṣad,* IV, 3, 9 ff.), cf. Heimann, pp. 130 ff.

Kaṭha Upaniṣad, French tr. L. Renou; cf. Ananda K. Coomaraswamy, "Notes on the *Kaṭha Upaniṣad.*"

Śvetāśvatara Upaniṣad, French tr., with commentary, Aliette Silburn; see also R. G. Bhāndārkar, *Vaiṣṇavism, Śaivism and Minor Religious Systems,* pp. 106–11; Richard Hauschild, *Die Śvetāśvatara-Upaniṣad;* Hauer, "Die *Śvetāśvatara-Upaniṣad*"; id., *Glaubensgeschichte der Indogermanen,* I, 208 ff.; Johnston, "Some Sāṁkhya and Yoga Conceptions of the *Śvetāśvatara Upaniṣad.*" *Śvetāśvatara Upaniṣad,* VI, 13, definitely refers to the soteriological validity of Sāṃkhya philosophy in combination with Yoga practice.

Māṇḍūkya Upaniṣad, French tr. E. Lesimple; cf. Zimmer, *Philosophies of India,* pp. 372 ff., and the translation, with commentary, by Alex Wayman, "Notes on the Sanskrit Term *Jñāna,*" pp. 263–64.

Maitrī Upaniṣad, French tr., with commentary, Anne Marie Esnoul. Cf. Hopkins, *Great Epic,* pp. 33 ff.; Dasgupta, *Yoga Philosophy,* pp. 65–66; Hauer, *Der Yoga als Heilweg,* pp. 26 ff.; E. A. Welden, "The Sāṁkhya Teachings in the *Maitrī Upaniṣad.*"

Deussen has attempted a schematic presentation of Yoga practice, as found in the middle-period Upaniṣads—from *Maitrāyaṇī* to *Haṃsa*—by tracing each *aṅga.* His list of citations is reasonably complete, so that we need not repeat it; cf. *Philosophy of the Upanishads,* pp. 387–95. *Yama* and *niyama* do not appear in the classic lists; *āsana* is first mentioned in the *Śvetāśvatara* (II, 10); the three moments of *prāṇāyāma* (*recaka, pūraka, kumbhaka*) appear in the *Khurika* (5, etc.); *pratyāhāra,* as we have seen, is mentioned as early as the *Chāndogya* (VIII, 15), and *dhāraṇā* in the *Maitrāyaṇī* (VI, 34); *dhyāna* and *samādhi* do not have the same meaning in the classic Upaniṣads as they have in the *Yoga-sūtras.* The current edition of the yogic Upaniṣads is A. Mahādeva Śāstri, *Yoga Upaniṣads,* English tr. T. R. Śrīnivāsa Ayyaṅgār.

III, 6: "Mystical Sounds"

The *Bṛhadāraṇyaka Upaniṣad* (V, 9) speaks of the "noise . . . that one hears on covering the ears thus. When one is about to depart, one hears not this sound" (tr. R. E. Hume, *The Thirteen Principal Upanishads*, p. 153). The *Vaikhānasasmārtasūtra*, V, 1 (ed. W. Caland, pp. 68–69) says that the dying man hears "the sound of a bell," which gradually diminishes until the moment of death. The Pāli canon attributes the same signal to the voices of divinities; according to *Dīgha-nikāya*, I, 152, "the voices of the Devas and *yakṣas* are said to be like the sound of a golden bell." Bell sounds are heard in certain tantric bodily postures and meditations; for example, in the *anāhata cakra* (cf. *Mahānirvāṇa-tantra*, V, 146). The *Nādabindu Upaniṣad* (31 ff.) describes all the mystical sounds heard by the yogin when he meditates in the *siddhāsana* position, during the practice of the *vaiṣṇavīmudrā*. Similarly, the *Dhyānabindu*, whose principal meditation begins with mystical concentration on the syllable *OṂ*, mentions several strange sounds: "The *nāda* is localized in the *vīṇādaṇḍa* [spine]; the sound . . . is like that of sea shells, etc. When it has reached the cavity (corresponding to the element) *ākāśa*, it is like the cry of the peacock" (102). See also *Haṭhayogapradīpikā*, IV, 79 ff., and *Gheraṇḍa Saṃhitā*, V, 78 ff.

There is today in India a religious sect, the Rādhā Soāmis, which meditates on "mystical sound." The meditation is called *śabd-yoga*, "the yoga of sound." The center of the Rādhā Soāmis is at Beas, near Kapurthala, where the sect owns a quite beautiful temple. In the course of a visit I made to Beas in November, 1930, my informers described this meditation as having to be begun by concentration "on the space between the eyebrows"; when the sound of a bell is heard, it is the first sign that the *shabd* meditation is valid. One of the phases of the meditation is a sensation of ascent. Cf. Myron H. Phelps, ed., *Discourses on Radha-Swami Faith* (of no interest, for it contains hardly any information on technique).

Of course, mystical auditions were susceptible of various evaluations. Fo-T'u-Têng, a Buddhist monk of Kucha, who had visited Kashmir and other parts of India, arrived in China in 310 and exhibited various magical accomplishments; in particular, he prophesied from the notes of bells; cf. A. F. Wright, "Fo-T'u-Têng. A Biography," pp. 337 ff., 346, 362.

The author of the *Dabistān* also speaks of meditation on "absolute sound" (in Arabic, *sant mutluk;* in Hindī, *anahid*)—a meditation commonly called *azad awa,* or "free voice" (*Dabistān,* tr. D. Shea and A. Troyer, I, 81; the *Dabistān,* a copious treatise on Indian religions, was compiled by Muḥsin-i-Fāni in the seventeenth century). According to him, meditation on mystical sounds was also familiar to Muḥammad (revelation of the "bell tones," *sant mutluk*), and Ḥāfiẓ refers to them in the quatrain: "No person knows where my beloved dwells; this much only is known, that the sound of the bell approaches."

The *Dabistān* describes auditory meditation as follows: "The devotees direct the hearing and understanding to the brain, and whether in the gloom of night, in the house, or in the desert, hear this voice, which they esteem as their *dhikr. . . .*"

According to some of the Arabic mystical writers, *dhikr* actualizes sounds or voices audible "in the circumference of the head"; sounds "of trumpets and cymbals," "sounds of water, sound of the wind, voice of a very hot fire, voices of mills, tread of horses, voices of the leaves of trees when the wind blows on them" (Ibn 'Aṭa' Allāh, cited by Louis Gardet, "La Mention du nom divin (*dhikr*) dans la mystique musulmane," p. 667).

On similar mystical auditions, cf. W. Y. Evans-Wentz, *Tibet's Great Yogī Milarepa,* p. 37, etc. Discussion in Roesel, *Die psychologischen Grundlagen,* pp. 67–68.

III, 7: Lists of Ascetics

The following list, cited by Varāhamihira, is said by his commentator Utpala to have been composed by the Jaina master Kālakācārya (see the extracts from Utpala in D. R. Bhāndārkar, "Ājīvikas," p. 287): *śākya* ("wearer of a red robe"); *ājīvika; bhikṣu* (or *sannyāsi*); *caraka* ("wearer of a skull"); *nigganthа* ("naked ascetic," Jaina); *vanyāsana* ("hermit"). We have two other lists (Georg Bühler, "Barābar and Nāgārjuni Hill-Cave Inscriptions of Aśoka and Daśaratha," p. 362; cf. A. Govindacarya Svāmin, "The Pāñcarātras or *Bhāgavat-Śāstra,* p. 960). The first mentions: *tāvasia* (*tāpasika,* "hermit"); *kāvālia* (*kāpālika,* "wearer of a skull"); *rattavada* (*raktapata,* "wearer of a red robe"); *cadardi* (*ekadaṇḍi,* "the ascetic with a staff," *ājīvika*); *jai* (*yati*); *caraa* (*caraka*); *khavanai* (*kṣapaṇaka*). The second list includes: *jalana* (*jvalana, sāgnika*); *hara* (*īśvarabhakta*, "worshiper of the divinity"); *sugaya* (*sugata*, "Buddhist"); *keśava* (*keśavabhakta*, "worshiper of Keśava," *bhāgavata*); *sui* (*śrutimārgarata*, "adherent of the *śruti*"—i.e., *mīṃāṃsaka*); *brahma* (*brahmabhakta*, "worshiper of Brahmā," *vanāprastha*); *nagga* ("naked"). All these lists mention the tantric sects (Kāpālika, *ūrdhvaśravaka*). See also below, pp. 421 ff.

IV, 1: *The* Mahābhārata

See: Oldenberg, *Das Mahābhārata;* Jacobi, *Mahābhārata;* Hopkins, *Great Epic;* Joseph Dahlmann, *Das Mahābhārata als Epos und Rechtsbuch* (see the discussion in Barth, *Œuvres*, IV, 347–403). An ample bibliography in Winternitz, *Geschichte der indischen Literatur*, I, 263 ff.; III, 623. Ethnological interpretation of the traditions preserved by the *Mahābhārata*, in G. J. Held, *The Mahābhārata*, and Charles Autran, *L'Épopée hindoue*. Wikander has elucidated the Vedic mythology underlying the legend of the Pāṇḍavas: "La Légende des Pāṇḍava et la substructure mythique du *Mahābhārata*" (see also Dumézil, *Jupiter, Mars, Quirinus: IV*, pp. 55–85); cf. Wikander, "Sur le fonds commun indo-iranien des épopées de la Perse et de l'Inde."

IV, 2: *Sāṃkhya in the* Mokṣadharma

Verses 11,039–11,040 are a veritable *crux translatoris*. Regarded by Hopkins (*Great Epic*, pp. 104 ff.) as proof of an atheistic Sāṃkhya in the *Mokṣadharma*, they have been interpreted in the completely opposite sense by Franklin Edgerton ("The Meaning of Sānkhya and Yoga," especially pp. 27–29).

Hopkins translates *anīśvaraḥ katham mucyed* by "How can one be freed when one is without a personal God?" and regards the question as put by the adherents of Yoga. Edgerton translates *anīśvara* by "supreme, without a master," which, according to him, excludes any allusion to the atheism of Sāṃkhya. Edgerton's interpretation confirms Dahlmann's views in regard to the original meaning of preclassic Sāṃkhya (cf. *Die Sāṃkhya-Philosophie*, pp. 5 ff.), but his translation of *anīśvara* has been rejected by Hopkins and Keith (*Religion and Philosophy*, II, 543–44). See also Oldenberg, "Zur Geschichte der Sāṃkhya-Philosophie," p. 231.

As for the "plurality of souls"—a characteristic mark of the classic Sāṃkhya—it is mentioned in the *Mokṣadharma:* "According to the teachings of Sāṃkhya and Yoga, there are many souls in the world; they do not admit that but one soul exists" (*Mahābhārata,* XII, 11,714). But if the context is read attentively, it becomes clear that the reference is to a plurality of empirical souls, *anima,* nucleuses of psychic experiences, limited and individualized—in short, to the "unilluminated" soul spellbound by the illusion of being individuated and isolated. It is the old illusion against which the Upaniṣads fought—the illusion of being limited by one's psychomental experiences. In the *Mokṣadharma,* empirical souls are emanations of the Universal Soul, the Unique, the Brahman, and, by illumination, they return to it. But Īśvarakṛṣṇa, in denying God (Īśvara) as the unique and creating soul, had to accept an infinite plurality of *puruṣas,* of souls completely isolated from one another, without any possibility of communication between them. In the summary of Sāṃkhya doctrine given in the Tamil epic poem *Maṇimēkalai,* it is said that but one *puruṣa* exists. This conception of Sāṃkhya in the *Maṇimēkalai* closely resembles that in the *Mokṣadharma* (cf. S. S. Suryanarayana Śāstri, "The *Maṇimēkalai* Account of the Sāṃkhya"). On this problem, see Johnston, *Early Sāṁkhya,* pp. 9 ff., 27, etc.

IV, 3: The Art of Entering Another's Body

See Maurice Bloomfield, "On the Art of Entering Another's Body." In Hemacandra's *Yogaśāstra* (VI, 1) the art of entering another's body (*parapurakāyapraveśa*) is preceded by the "art of separating soul from body," called *vedhaviddhi.* See also Lindquist, *Methoden des Yoga,* pp. 13 ff. Religious and secular folklore abounds in examples of "entering into another's body," especially into corpses; cf. Theodor Benfey, ed., *Pantschatantra,* I, 123 (the body of King Candragupta was occupied, after his death, by a *yakṣa*); C. H. Tawney, tr., *Prabandhacintāmaṇi,* p. 170 (the king enters the body of his dead elephant); N. M. Penzer, ed., *Somadeva's Kathā-sarit-sāgara,* I, 37, etc.; Jacques Bacot, *La Vie de Marpa, le "traducteur,"* p. 70 (Marpa performed the "translation of life" into the dead body of a pigeon; the pigeon revived, while the Lama's body was "like a corpse"). Interesting details of the technique of *parapurakāyapraveśa* in Evans-Wentz, ed., *Tibetan Yoga and Secret*

Doctrines, pp. 26 ff. Tantrism has some knowledge of this technique; cf. *Kaulajñāna-nirṇaya*, IV, 2; VII, 31 ff.

IV, 4: *The* Bhagavad Gītā

The *Bhagavad Gītā* has given rise to an immense literature. Cf. Winternitz, *Geschichte der indischen Literatur*, I, 365 ff.; III, 625 (for bibliography of the polemics occasioned by Garbe's thesis); a short exposition in J. E. Carpenter, *Theism in Medieval India*, pp. 249–67; philosophical interpretations in Belvalkar, *Vedānta Philosophy*, pp. 84–134, and S. Dasgupta, *History of Indian Philosophy*, II, 437–552. The most frequently cited translation, made from the Indian point of view, remains K. T. Telang's. On W. D. P. Hill's translation, see Charpentier, "Some Remarks on the *Bhagavadgītā*." Cf. Edgerton's edition and translation. For a psychological interpretation of Yoga practice in the *Bhagavad Gītā*, see Hauer, *Der Yoga als Heilweg*, pp. 61 ff. To be added to Winternitz's bibliography: Lamotte, *Notes sur la Bhagavadgītā;* F. Otto Schrader, *The Kashmir Recension of the Bhagavadgītā;* R. Otto, *Die Urgestalt der Bhagavad-Gītā;* id., *Die Lehr-Traktate der Bhagavad-Gītā* (Otto distinguishes eight texts added to the original nucleus, to the *Ur-Gītā*); Belvalkar, "The So-called Kashmir Recension of the *Bhagavad Gītā*." The *Anugītā* (*Mahābhārata*, XIV, 16–51) forms a sort of appendix to the *Bhagavad Gītā;* the amalgamation of Sāṃkhya-Yoga and Vedānta is carried even further.

IV, 5: *The Pāñcarātras* *

The idea of Yoga that we find in the *Bhagavad Gītā*—a means of delivering the soul wholly to Kṛṣṇa—is especially prominent in the literature of the *Pāñcarātras*—that is, of the Viṣṇuist sect based on the cult of Kṛṣṇa. Thus, for example, in the *Ahirbudhnya Saṃhitā* (chs. 21–32, devoted to Yoga), Yoga is called "adoration in the heart" (*hridaya-ārādhana*) or "outward sacrifice" (*bāhyayajñā*). The soul, in its original purity—that is, separated from matter—is still in contact with all things; it is described in the same terms as in *Bṛhadāraṇyaka-Upaniṣad*, IV, 3, 23 ff., and in *Iśā Upaniṣad*, 5. Yoga is defined as a "union of the human soul with the supreme soul" (*jivātmaparamātmanoḥ saṃyoga*). Through Yoga meditation, it is possible to gain, even in this life, the experience of union with God, accessible only to the "liberated."

The history of the Pāñcarātra or Bhāgavata sect remains quite obscure, despite the work of Bhāndārkar, Grierson, and Schrader. However, it can safely be said that the sect arose from autochthonous theistic nucleuses (Āryan or non-Āryan), and not under the influence of Christianity, as A. Weber thought. Its "philosophy," deriving from Sāṃkhya, is highly eclectic, and its mystical practices are based upon the cult of Viṣṇu-Vāsudeva. The *Bhagavad Gītā* has remained the sacred book of these sects, while their doctrines and message have been circulated by the Saṃhitās, treatises that have for the most part been preserved in southern India, the study of which began only with the publication, by Schrader, of a critical edition of the *Ahirbudhnya Saṃhitā* (1916). A Saṃhitā comprises four subjects: *jñāna*, or philosophy; *yoga*, or mystical practice; *kriyā*, or building of temples and dedication of images, and *caryā*, or social and ritual activity. Each Saṃhitā deals principally with one or another of these subjects, neglecting or even passing over the others. The critical bibliography on Bhāgavata literature and history is immense. See the archeological documents collected and discussed by Rāmaprasād Chanda, *Archaeology and Vaishnava Tradition*. On Bhāgavata chronology and philosophy, Schrader, *Introduction to the Pāñcharātra and the Ahirbudhnya Saṃhitā*. Discussions and opinions in G. A. Grierson, "The Nārāyanīya and the Bhāgavatas," pp. 253–54; A. Govindacarya Svāmin, "The Pāñcarātras or *Bhāgavat-Śāstra*"; R. G. Bhāndārkar, *Vaiṣṇavism*, pp. 38–41, 100; Hemchandṛa Ray Chaudhuri, *Materials for the Study of the Early History of the Vaishnava Sect* (abundant documentation and bibliography); S. K. De, "Bhāgavatism and Sun-worship." On the celebrated passage of Patañjali the grammarian in which he treats of the iconographic representation of Kṛṣṇa, see Sten Konow, *Das indische Drama*, p. 44; Lévi, *Le Théâtre indien*, I, 314; in general, the bibliography on this subject is very large (cf. La Vallée Poussin, *L'Indȩ aux temps des Mauryas*, pp. 187–88). Further on the subject of the Bhāgavatas: Carpenter, *Theism in Medieval India*, pp. 220–21; Hopkins, *Great Epic*, pp. 144–45; Belvalkar, *The Brahmā-Sūtras of Bādarāyaṇa*, pp. 129–32; D. L. De, "Pāñcarātra and the Upaniṣads"; L. Silburn, in Renou and Filliozat, *L'Inde classique*, I, 747 ff.

V, 1: *Yoga and Buddhism*

The essentials of the biography of the Buddha and of Buddhist doctrines and techniques will be found in: E. J. Thomas, *The Life of Buddha as*

Legend and History; Lamotte, "La Légende du Buddha"; Bacot, *Le Bouddha;* A. Foucher, *La Vie du Bouddha;* André Bareau, "La Date du Nirvāṇa"; Tucci, *Il Buddhismo;* Edward Conze, *Buddhism, Its Essence and Development;* La Vallée Poussin, *Nirvāṇa;* id., *La Morale bouddhique;* id., *Le Dogme et la philosophie du bouddhisme;* Keith, *Buddhist Philosophy in India and Ceylon;* Coomaraswamy, *Hinduism and Buddhism.* See, since 1930: *Bibliographie bouddhique,* published under the direction of Marcelle Lalou. See also *Hôbôgirin,* Paul Demiéville editor in chief.

On the Buddha as "king of physicians" and Buddhism as the "new medicine": *Hôbôgirin,* III, 230 ff. On the relations between Yoga and Buddhism: Senart, "Bouddhisme et Yoga"; Lindquist, *Die Methoden des Yoga,* pp. 73 ff.; C. A. F. Rhys Davids, "Religiöse Übungen in Indien und der religiöse Mensch"; La Vallée Poussin, "Le Bouddhisme et le Yoga de Patañjali."

On *nirvāṇa* and its yogic essence there is a copious literature; see especially: La Vallée Poussin, *Nirvāṇa;* Stcherbatsky, *The Conception of Buddhist Nirvāṇa;* Keith, "The Doctrine of the Buddha"; Stcherbatsky, "The Doctrine of the Buddha"; Przyluski and Lamotte, "Bouddhisme et Upaniṣad": "*Nirvāṇa* is derived from the root *va* 'to blow.' Strictly, it designates a state in which the breath ceases to move: this notion must have been borrowed from the theory of deep sleep, as it appears in the Upaniṣads" (p. 154). Cf. also Coomaraswamy, "Some Pāli Words," pp. 156–63.

On the mystical structure of the *asaṃskṛta,* see André Bareau, "L'Absolu en philosophie bouddhique."

V, 2: Buddhist Samādhi *and the* Jhānas

For the Buddhists, *samādhi* was only a state preliminary to certain higher stages that are passed through before the attainment of *nirvāṇa.* Through *samādhi* one can obtain the five kinds of supreme wisdom and even arhatship. "Being in perfect *samādhi*" is the fifth of the "eight thoughts of the great man," says the Chinese *Ekottarā* (Przyluski, "Le Parinirvāṇa et les funérailles du Buddha," p. 438). Buddhaghoṣa (*Aṭṭhasālinī,* 118) says that *samādhi* is identical with *cittass' ekaggatā,* "concentration of mind," "fixation of the mental flux on a single point." "This concentration of mind called *samādhi* has as its characteristic mark the absence of wandering, of distraction; as its essence the binding together of the states of mind that arise with it . . . as its condition precedent calmness; as its sustenance wisdom (for it is said: 'He who is at peace he knows and sees'). . . . It must be understood as steadiness of mind" (quoted in T. W. Rhys Davids, ed., *The Yogāvacara's Manual*, p. xxvi). According to Rhys Davids, the term *samādhi* does not occur either in Sanskrit or Pāli before the Piṭakas. The *Mahāvyutpatti* gives a list of 118 *samādhis* (Oltramare, *La Théosophie bouddhique*, p. 357, n. 2). *Aṅguttara-nikāya*, I, 229 (*sutta* 163), *Saṃyutta-nikāya*, IV, 363, and *Vinaya*, III, 93, list three kinds of *samādhi: suññata* (characterized by emptiness), *appanihita* (without aim), and *animitta* (without signs). Buddhaghoṣa explains them as follows: devoid of appetites, of evil desires, of stupidity; without aim, because the aim of rebirth in heaven is renounced; without signs, because devoid of the three signs, *lakṣaṇa* (Rhys Davids, p. xxvii). But such explanations are external, scholastic. The negative meaning of these three higher *samādhis* (*samyak samādhi*) is to be understood as their refusal to submit to any classification and delimitation. See also *Abhidharmakośa*, VIII, 183; La Vallée Poussin, "Musīla et Nārada," pp. 203 ff. (Harivarman on the seven *samādhis*); Lamotte, *Traité*, I, 321 (Nāgārjuna on the three *samādhis*); ibid., II, 1028 ff. (on the *dhyānas*), 1035 ff. (the *dhyānas* and the *samāpattis*); *Hôbôgirin*, III, 283 (the *jhānas*); Coomaraswamy, "Some Pāli Words," pp. 138 ff. (*jhāna, samādhi*).

V, 3: Non-Buddhist Dhyāna *and Buddhist Pseudo* Dhyāna

"Poṭṭhapāda said: '. . . But long ago, Sir, on several occasions, when various teachers, Samaṇas and Brāhmans, had met together, and were seated in the debating hall, the talk fell on trance [*abhisaññānirodho*, "the cessation of consciousness"], and the question was: "How then, Sirs, is the cessation of consciousness brought about?" . . . Another said: " . . . There are certain Samaṇas and Brāhmans of great power and influence. It is they who infuse consciousness into a man, and draw it away out of him. When they infuse it into him he becomes conscious, when they draw it away he becomes unconscious." Thus do others explain the cessation of consciousness' " (*Poṭṭhapāda Sutta, Dīgha-nikāya*, I, 179 f.; tr. T. W. Rhys Davids, *Dialogues of the Buddha*, I, 246). "Buddhaghoṣa explains that the ground for this view is the way in which sorcerers work charms (*athabbanikā athabbannaṃ payojenti—*

perhaps "Atharva priests work out an Atharva charm") which make a man appear as dead as if his head had been cut off; and then bring him back to his natural condition" (Rhys Davids' note, I, 246–47). On the trances and ecstasies of the Buddha's teachers, cf. *Majjhima-nikāya*, I, 164; see also Keith, *Buddhist Philosophy*, pp. 124, 139, 144, and La Vallée Poussin, *Nirvāṇa*, p. 77, n. 2.

In contrast, there was also pseudo *dhyāna*, and those monks who claimed to have attained arhatship and to possess *alama-riya-ñaṣia-dassanaṃ* (superknowledge) ceased to be members of the community (it is to this pseudo *dhyāna* that the fourth Pārājika rule refers). See the case of the four pseudo *dhyānas*—i.e., "lay" *dhyānas*, probably mere hypnotic states—in Przyluski, *La Légende de l'empereur Açoka*, pp. 390–91. The venerable Upagupta proves to a young man of Mathurā, who believes that he has realized the four stages of arhatship, that he is mistaken and has realized only illusory trances.

V, 4: *Paths and Stages of Meditation*

The canonical texts dealing with the *jhānas* and *samāpattis* are listed in Lamotte, *Traité*, II, 1023, n. 3. On the *samāpattis* in the *Abhidharmakośa*, cf. La Vallée Poussin, "Musīla et Nārada," pp. 215 ff. (especially *Abhidharmakośa*, II, 212 ff.); id., *La Morale bouddhique*, pp. 74 ff. For Nāgārjuna's interpretation, cf. Lamotte, II, 1023–95. There is a significant correspondence between the four stages of the career of a Buddhist saint (*śrotāpanna, sakṛdāgāmin, anagāmin, arhat*) and the four *dhyānas*. As Przyluski observes, this tetrad belongs to Indian thought in general. The triadism of the earlier Upaniṣads (three states of consciousness, three worlds, three *guṇas*, three Vedas, etc.) was replaced by the tetrad. The fourth psychic "state" is *turīya* or *caturtha*, which expresses the notion of absolute, infinite, unlimited, and which was also borrowed by the Buddhists (Przyluski and Lamotte, "Bouddhisme et Upaniṣad," especially pp. 160 ff.).

V, 5: Siddhis *and* Abhijñās

The sources for the *abhijñās* are given in Lamotte, *Traité*, I, 329, n. 1. Among recent studies, we shall mention: La Vallée Poussin, "Le Bouddha et les Abhijñās"; Lindquist, *Die Methoden des Yoga*, pp. 169–

87; id., *Siddhi und Abhiññā;* P. Demiéville, "Sur la mémoire des existences antérieures."

Some texts refer to six or even seven superknowledges; cf. *Mahāvyutpatti*, sec. 14.

On the shamanistic character of some *siddhis*, see our *Shamanism*, pp. 407 ff., and above, pp. 321 ff.

On the popular elements, see Joseph Masson, *La Religion populaire dans le canon bouddhique pāli.*

V, 6: *Paribbājakas, Ājīvikas*

On ascetics and monks contemporary with the Buddha, cf. T. W. Rhys Davids, *Buddhist India*, pp. 141–48; Bimala Charan Law, "A Short Account of the Wandering Teachers at the Time of the Buddha"; id., "Influence of the Five Heretical Teachers on Jainism and Buddhism"; id., "Gautama Buddha and the Paribrājakas." Law believes that the *paribbājakas* can be regarded as the precursors of a political science, and he notes a number of coincidences with the *Arthaśāstra* (cf. "Wandering Teachers," pp. 402–06). In reality, all that is involved is certain antisacerdotal opinions that are manifestations of the general trend of the period. The few elements that it is possible to deduce in regard to the doctrines of the heterodox teachers have been systematized by Barua, *Pre-Buddhistic Philosophy*, and Law, "Influence." Cf. also Jacobi, "On Mahāvīra and His Predecessors"; A. L. Basham, *History and Doctrines of Ājīvikas*, pp. 11 ff., 80 ff., 94 ff.; I. B. Horner, "Gotama and the Other Sects."

On the Ājīvikas and on Makkhali Gosāla, see A. F. R. Hoernle, "Ājīvikas" (cf. K. B. Pathak, "The Ājīvikas," and D. R. Bhāndārkar, "Ājīvikas"); Charpentier, "Ājīvika"; Barua, "The Ājīvikas"; id., *Pre-Buddhistic Philosophy*, pp. 297–318; Basham, *History*, an excellent monograph, which also employs the Tamil sources. Makkhali Gosāla's biography has been preserved, with the inevitable distortions, in the *Bhagavatī Sūtra* of the Jains (XV, 1 ff.; tr. Hoernle in the appendix to *Uvāsagadasāo;* tr. E. Leumann in W. W. Rockhill, *Life of the Buddha*, pp. 251–54).

VI, 1: *On the Literature of Tantrism* *

Not long ago it was still thought that the beginnings of tantric literature must be put in the seventh century (cf., for example, Winternitz,

Geschichte der indischen Literatur, I, 482, etc.). A manuscript of the *Kubjikāmata-tantra* in Gupta characters cannot be earlier than the seventh century (H. Shāstri, *Catalogue of Palm-Leaf and Selected Paper Mss.,* I, 87). A manuscript of the *Parameśvaramata-tantra* is dated 858, although the original is earlier (Shāstri, I, 52, 87; II, 21). Other tantric texts, in the existing manuscripts, are of the eighth to ninth century. But they were composed much earlier. In addition, without bearing the name of tantra, certain works are strictly tantric in content—e.g., the *Mahāmeghasūtra* (sixth century) deals with *dhāraṇīs* and *mantras;* cf. C. Bendall, "The *Megha-sūtra,* Text and Translation." And Tucci has proved ("Animadversiones Indicae") that some tantric schools existed several centuries earlier; for example, the *Suvarṇaprabhāṣasūtra* was translated into Chinese in the first half of the fifth century. The same is true of the *Mahāmāyurīvidyārajnī,* translated by Kumārajīva as early as c. A.D. 405. The *Tattvasiddhiśāstra* of Harivarman (fourth century A.D.) and the *Madhyāntānugamaśāstra* of Asaṇga—the original of which is lost and which exists only in a Chinese translation—mention the name of a tantric school, *na ya sin mo* (Nyāyasauma, Nayasamya, Nayasauma). Tucci, studying the history of this school, proves that its antiquity is beyond question. (See also Chakravarti, "The Soma or Sauma Sect of the Śaivas"; the Saumas have connections with tantrism.) The *Āryamañjusśrīmūla-tantra,* which is certainly earlier than the fifth century A.D., contains chapters devoted to the goddesses, to the *mudras,* to the *mantras,* and to *maṇḍalas* (Tucci, p. 129; Przyluski, "Les Vidyārāja," pp. 306 ff.). In the *Mahāyāna-samparigraha-śāstra* (Nanjio, No. 1183; R. Kimura, "A Historical Study of the Terms Mahāyāna and Hinayāna," p. 40) there are passages on repetition of the name of Buddha as a means of salvation that strongly resemble later tantric texts.

A passage in the *Mahāyānasūtrālaṃkāra* (IX, 46), treating of *maithunasya parāvṛttau,* has chiefly instigated the controversy over the antiquity of sexual practices in Buddhism: Lévi translated *parāvṛtti* as "revolution," and, in his view, the reference was to the mystical pairs of Buddhas and Bodhisattvas. But Winternitz ("Notes on the *Guhyasmāja-Tantra* and the Age of the Tantras") proposed taking *parāvṛtti* as "turning aside," "discarding." Bagchi rightly observes ("A Note on the Word *parāvṛtti*") that Winternitz's interpretation is inadequate: *parāvṛtti* literally means "turning (the functions of the mind) round to an opposite point." Cf. also Coomaraswamy, "Parāvṛtti: Transformation,

Regeneration, Anagogy," and La Vallée Poussin, "Notes de bibliographie bouddhique," pp. 400–01.

Certain Orientalists tend to exaggerate the antiquity of the tantras. Thus Braja Lal Mukherjī ("Tantra Shastra and Veda") and Chakravarti ("Antiquity of Tāntricism") attempt to prove perfect agreement between tantrism and the Vedas. B. Bhattacharyya believes that the practices and doctrines of tantrism were introduced by the Buddha himself; cf. *An Introduction to Buddhist Esoterism*, p. 48, and the introduction to his edition of the *Sādhanamālā*, I, xvi-xvii. All these opinions go too far; tantrism contains certain very old elements, some of which belong to the religious protohistory of India, but their introduction into Buddhism and Hinduism began comparatively late—in any case, not before the first centuries of our era.

Bhattacharyya, in his edition of the *Guhyasamāja Tantra* (p. xxxvii), proposes to date the text (which he attributes to Asaṇga) in the third century. According to Winternitz ("Notes") there are no clear grounds for this attribution to the great philosopher Asaṇga. However, many Buddhistic tantras make the attribution; cf. S. B. Dasgupta, *An Introduction to Tāntric Buddhism*, p. 46, n. 4. The importance of the *Guhyasamāja* is shown by the large number of commentaries on it: cf. Marcelle Lalou, *Répertoire du Tanjur*, p. 13, and George N. Roerich, tr., *The Blue Annals*, I, 356–74; for Tson-kha-pa's commentaries, cf. E. E. Obermiller, "Tson-kha-pa le Pandit," pp. 335–37. See also Tucci, "Some Glosses upon the *Guhyasamāja*," and Wayman, "Notes," pp. 258 ff.

On the origin and spread of tantrism, see Sarat Chandra Roy, "Caste, Race, and Religion in India," pp. 92 ff.; Wilhelm Koppers, "Probleme der indischen Religionsgeschichte," pp. 773 ff. and passim; Rajendra Chandra Hazra, "Influence of Tantra on the Tattvas of Raghunandana"; Lévi, "On a Tantrik Fragment from Kucha"; Bagchi, "On Some Tāntrik Texts Studied in Ancient Kambuja"; id., "Further Notes on Tāntrik Texts Studied in Ancient Kambuja"; id., "On Foreign Element in the Tāntras"; Bhattacharyya, "The Cult of Bhūtaḍāmara."

The following may also be consulted on tantrism: Eugène Burnouf, *Introduction à l'histoire du bouddhisme indien*, pp. 465 ff.; Barth, *Œuvres*, I, 178 ff.; H. H. Wilson, *Sketch of the Religious Sects of the Hindus*, pp. 159 ff.; R. Mitra, *The Sanskrit Buddhist Literature of Nepāl*, pp. 17 ff.; W. Wassilieff, *Le Bouddhisme*, pp. 162 ff.; La Vallée Poussin, *Boud-*

dhisme: Études et matériaux, pp. 118 ff.; id., *Bouddhisme: Opinions sur l'histoire de la dogmatique*, pp. 378 ff.; J. H. C. Kern, *Der Buddhismus*, II, 521 ff.; Winternitz, *Geschichte*, I, 482; R. G. Bhāndārkar, *Report on the Search for Sanskrit Manuscripts*, pp. 87 ff.; H. Shāstri, *Notices of Sanskrit Manuscripts*, pp. xxiv ff.; Kern, *Manual of Indian Buddhism*, pp. 133 ff.; L. A. Waddell, *The Buddhism of Tibet*, pp. 147 ff.

On the Vajrayāna, see also: H. Shāstri, "The Discovery of a Work by Āryadeva in Sanskrit"; cf. id., "Buddhism in Bengal since the Muhammadan Conquest"; B. Bhattacharyya, "Origin and Development of Vajrayāna"; cf. id., "Buddhists in Bengal"; id., "Glimpses of Vajrayāna"; id., "The Home of Tantric Buddhism"; S. K. De, "The Buddhist Tantric Literature (Sanskrit) of Bengal"; Rāhula Sānkṛtyāyana, "Recherches bouddhiques"; Tucci, "Animadversiones Indicae"; id., *Tibetan Painted Scrolls*, pp. 209–49 (pp. 211 ff., comparison with Gnosticism); id., "Buddhist Notes"; Glasenapp, "Tantrismus und Śaktismus"; id., "Die Entstehung des Vajrayāna"; id., *Buddhistische Mysterien;* id., "Ein buddhistischer Initiationsritus des javanischen Mittelalters" (on the *Sang hyang kamahāyānam mantrānaya*, a tantric text translated into Javanese in the thirteenth century, edited by J. Kats in 1910 and re-edited by K. Wulff in 1935); La Vallée Poussin, "Notes de bibliographie bouddhique," pp. 277 ff.

On tantrism in China and Tibet: Lin Li-kouang, "Puṇyodaya (Na-T'i), un propagateur du tantrisme en Chine et au Cambodge"; Chou Yi-liang, "Tantrism in China"; Joseph Needham, *Science and Civilisation in China*, II, 425–30; Li An-che, "Rñin-ma-pa: the Early Form of Lamaism," and especially Tucci, *Tibetan Painted Scrolls*, passim (see also *Indo-Tibetica*, I, 93–135; III, 75, on the *Tattvasaṃgraha*).

On Nāgārjuna: good bibliography in Nalinaksha Dutt, "Notes on the Nāgārjunikoṇḍa Inscriptions"; add the bibliographies indicated by La Vallée Poussin, "Notes et bibliographie bouddhiques," pp. 383, n. 2, 393 ff.; "Notes de bibliographie bouddhique," pp. 365, 374 ff., 270. See especially Lamotte, *Traité*, and Demiéville's review, *JA*, CCXXXVIII (1950), 375–95. For the medical and alchemical traditions relating to Nāgārjuna, see Filliozat, *Doctrine classique*, pp. 9 ff., 12 ff. Cf. also Lévi, "Un Nouveau Document sur le bouddhisme de basse époque dans l'Inde," pp. 420–21, and our Note VIII, 2.

Recent editions of Buddhist tantric texts include: B. Bhattacharyya, ed., *Sādhanamālā;* id., *Two Vajrayāna Works* (contains the *Prajño-*

pāyaviniścayasiddhi and the *Jñānasiddhi*); Louis Finot, "Manuscrits sanskrits de Sādhana's retrouvés en Chine" (edition and translation of short tantric texts); Bagchi, ed., *Kaulajñāna-nirṇaya and Some Minor Texts of the School of Matsyendranātha* (three short treatises, *Akulavīra-tantra, Kulānanda-tantra, Jñānakārikā*); Mario Carelli, ed., *Sekoddeśatīkā of Naḍapāda*. For the origin and history of the *Kālacakra-tantra*, see Roerich, *Blue Annals*, II, 753–838.

The Hindu tantras can be consulted in the Tantrik Texts series, published under the direction of Arthur Avalon (Sir John Woodroffe), 1913 *et sqq.* (twenty vols. in 1952). The most important are: *Kulārṇava-tantra* (ed. Tārānātha Vidyāratna), the chief text for the Kaulā school; *Kālīvilāsa-tantra* (ed. P. C. Tarkatīrtha); *Mahānirvāṇa-tantra* (tr. Woodroffe, *Tantra of the Great Liberation*); *Tantratattva* (tr. Woodroffe, *The Principles of Tantra*); *Ṣaṭcakranirūpaṇa* and *Pādukāpañcaka* (tr. Woodroffe, *The Serpent Power*). See also B. Bhattacharyya, ed., *Śakti-saṇgama-tantra;* Arthur H. Ewing, "The *Śāradā-tilaka Tantra.*"

General works on tantrism: Woodroffe, *Shakti and Shākta;* id., *The Garland of Letters;* P. H. Pott, *Yoga en Yantra;* G. C. Evola, *Lo Yoga della potenza;* S. B. Dasgupta, *Introduction to Tāntric Buddhism;* id., *Obscure Religious Cults as Background of Bengali Literature.*

The following may be profitably consulted: Woodroffe, "Kuṇḍalinī Śakti"; Zimmer, "On the Significance of the Indian Tantric Yoga"; Coomaraswamy, "The Tantric Doctrine of Divine Biunity."

VI, 2: On Tantrism and Iconography

As we know, the Vedic ritual demanded neither temples nor statues of the gods. The cult of images is not documented in the texts until quite late (fourth century B.C.); according to Indian tradition, it developed among the Śūdras. J. N. Farquhar ("Temple and Image Worship in Hinduism") sees in the Śūdras Āryanized aboriginals who, admitted into the Vedic society, brought their own rituals with them. This is a probable hypothesis, in view of the structure of the aboriginal religions (see below, pp. 428 ff).

On the influence of tantric ideas upon Buddhist art, see Ludwig Bachofer, "Zur Geschichte der chinesischen Plastik vom VIII.–XIV. Jahrhundert," pp. 74 ff. Tantrism elaborated an original conception of the nature of the gods. Advayavajra's *Mahāsukhaprakāṣa* (cf. H. Shāstri, ed., *Advayavajrasaṃgraha*, pp. 50–51) declares that the gods are manifestations of the universal void (*śūnya*) and that hence they have no ontological existence. The *Sādhanamālā* explains the evolution of the gods from the "void" by a process comprising four stages: (1) right perception of the *śūnyatā;* (2) its connection with the *bīja-mantra;* (3) conception of an iconic image; (4) external representation of the god (Bhattacharyya, ed., *Sādhanamālā*, introd., II, 122 ff.). On tantric iconography, see Foucher, *Étude sur l'iconographie bouddhique de l'Inde* (second "Étude," pp. 59 ff., 101 ff.); T. A. Gopīnātha Rao, *Elements of Hindu Iconography;* Alice Getty, *The Gods of Northern Buddhism;* B. Bhattacharyya, *The Indian Buddhist Iconography;* A. K. Gordon, *The Iconography of Tibetan Lamaism;* id., *Tibetan Religious Art.*

For an understanding of Indian architectonic and iconographic symbolism, the reader can usefully consult Paul Mus's great work, *Barabuḍur;* Coomaraswamy's studies: *Elements of Buddhist Iconography,* "The Philosophy of Mediaeval and Oriental Art," and *Figures of Speech or Figures of Thought;* Tucci's *Indo-Tibetica* series (especially vol. III, pts. 1 and 2, *I Templi del Tibet occidentale*). See also: Lalou, *Iconographie des étoffes peintes (paṭa) dans le Mañjuśrīmūlakalpa;* Jeannine Auboyer, *Le Trône et son symbolisme dans l'Inde ancienne;* Marie Thérèse de Mallmann, *Introduction à l'étude d'Avalokiteçvara;* Stella Kramrisch, *The Hindu Temple.*

On the cult of Tārā, cf. Waddell, "The Indian Buddhist Cult of Avalokita and his Consort Tārā."

VI, 3: On the Ascetic Practices and the Yoga of the Jainists *

Śubhadra's *Jñānārṇava:* Yoga (ch. XXII, pp. 232–38), *dhyāna* (ch. XXV, pp. 253 ff.), *prāṇāyāma* (ch. XXIX, pp. 284 ff.), *maṇḍala* (pp. 287 ff.). Contains a curious classification of the phases of respiration: exhalation through the right nostril and inhalation through the left nostril are bad; exhalation through the left nostril and inhalation through the right nostril are good (pp. 292 ff.).

Hemacandra's *Yogaśāstra* and Haribhadra's treatises (*Yogabindu, Yogadṛṣtisamuccaya, Yogaviṃśikā,* and *Soḍaśaka*) contain a great many technical details and even elements of yogic folklore. See an exposition of their doctrines in Nathmal Tatia, *Studies in Jaina Philosophy,* pp. 289 ff.; cf. also Garbe, *Sāṃkhya und Yoga,* pp. 39 ff.

The essentials of the philosophy and religion of the Jainas will be found in Glasenapp, *Der Jainismus;* A. A. Guérinot, *La Religion djaïna;* Walther Schubring, *Die Lehre der Jainas;* C. J. Shah, *Jainism in North India, 800* B.C.–A.D. *526.*

On *siddhis,* Yoginis, etc., in Jaina tradition, see Kalipada Mitra, "Magic and Miracle in Jaina Literature." Adris Banerji ("Origins of Jain Practices") compares the presentation of the *tīrthaṇkara* in Jaina art "with arm falling above the knees" (*ājānu-lambita-bāhu-dvayaṃ*) with the figures found at Harappā, of which the arms also fall above the knees (cf. M. S. Vats, *Excavations at Harappā,* pl. XCIII, pp. 331–32, figs. 300 and 318). Banerji believes that he can establish a relation between the nudity of the Jaina ascetics and the nudity of the protohistorical figures from Harappā (cf. Vats, figs. 307–08, 317–18; and figs. 13–14, 18–19, and 22 from Mohenjo-daro). On this problem, see also below, Note VIII, 11. On the archaic elements, see Bagchi, "Primitive Elements of Jainism." On the iconographic symbolism, cf. Coomaraswamy, "The 'Conqueror's Life' in Jaina Painting."

VI, 4: *On the* Mudrās *

The sources for the meaning of the term *mudrā* have been assembled by Otto Stein, "The Numeral 18," p. 21 n., and pertinently analyzed by Przyluski, "Mudrā." As early as 1892, R. Otto Francke ("Mudrā = Schrift") proposed translating *mudrā* by "writing or art of reading"; cf. Coomaraswamy's criticism in "Mudrā, muddā." Fritz Hommel ("Pāli muddā = babylonisch musarū und die Herkunft der indischen Schrift") believes that *mudrā* (Pāli *muddā,* "writing," "seal") is derived from the Babylonian (*musarū,* "writing," "seal") through Old Persian, which changed *z* into *d* (*musarū* > *muzrā* > *mudrā*).

In India, *mudrā* is related to: (1) the dance (cf. A. M. Meerwarth, "Les *Kathākalis* du Malabar"; R. Vasudeva Poduval, *Kathākali and Diagram of Hand Poses*); (2) symbolic language (Penzer, ed., *Somadeva's Kathā-sarit-sāgara,* I, 46, 80–82, with a good bibliography; from which we select: Alice Dracott, *Simla Village Tales,* pp. 47–50; James H. Knowles, *Folk-tales of Kashmir,* pp. 215, 220; Crooke, "Secret Messages and Symbols Used in India"; to these should be added Auboyer, "*Moudrā* et *hasta* ou le langage par signes"); (3) iconography (see especially Coomaraswamy, *The Mirror of Gesture*); (4) ritual, properly speaking

(Tyra de Kleen, *Mudrās;* Aisaburo Akiyama, *Buddhist Hand-Symbol,* valuable especially for the illustrations).

According to the *Śabdastomamahāniddhi,* p. 488 (cited by Oppert, *Original Inhabitants,* p. 414, n. 170), *mudrā* seems to have yet another meaning: to eat "fried grain."

Mudrās play an important part in the rituals of the Japanese Buddhist sects of tantric origin (cf. *Si-do-in-dzou: Gestes de l'officiant dans les cérémonies mystiques des sectes Tendai et Singon,* pp. 3–5, 15, 23, 31–32, 38, etc.). We shall not enter into the symbolism of gestures in other religions (see, for example, S. H. Langdon, "Gesture in Sumerian and Babylonian Prayer," and the Iranian parallels pointed out by J. J. Modi, *Asiatic Papers,* III, 170–94). But it is interesting to note that symbolical valorization of ritual gestures remains current even in the most highly evolved mysticisms. According to a Persian tradition earlier than the fourteenth century, al-Ḥallādj was the author of a short text on the symbolism of the fifteen attitudes required in the course of canonical prayer: "to rinse the mouth is to gain sincerity; to snuff up water is to deny pride; to stand is to participate in the divine permanence; or, inside the curtains of one's tent, to prostrate oneself is to enter into union with the divine," etc. (Louis Massignon, *La Passion d'al-Hallâj, martyr mystique de l'Islam,* II, 782). See also Gardet, "Mention du nom divin," p. 665.

On *mudrā* in tantric rituals, cf. *Mahānirvāṇa-tantra* (*Tantra of the Great Liberation,* ed. Avalon), III, 4 ff. (*karanyāsa* and *aṇganyāsa*); V, 48, 74 (*yonimudrā*); V, 86, 112 (*jñānamudrā*), etc.; *Śāradātilaka-tantra,* VI, 75–111; *Kāmaratna-tantra* (ed. Hemchandra Goswami Tattabhusan), pp. 5 ff. See also R. H. van Gulik, *Hayagrīva,* pp. 51 ff.; S. B. Dasgupta, *Introduction to Tāntric Buddhism,* pp. 113, 177–78, 187 ff.

In "left-hand" tantrism, *mudrā* is the term applied to the partner in the sexual rite (see pp. 261 ff.). It is not easy to see how this designation was arrived at; Przyluski points out that *mudrā,* literally "seal," also means "womb." But, as we shall see later, the real meaning of sexual union in tantric ritual is "immobilization" of the *bodhicitta* (which, in contexts of this nature, designates the *semen virile*). The *bandhas* and *mudrās* employed by Haṭha Yoga are bodily positions through which the adept is able to control the nerves and muscles of the genital region; now, according to the texts, this control is related to control of the breaths. The adept becomes able to control his semen as he controls his breaths; he can "arrest" it, "immobilize" it, just as he arrests breathing during *kumbhaka*. We must bear in mind that "immobilization" of the semen through *prāṇāyāma* is always connected with a similar immobilization of the states of consciousness (see p. 253).

VI, 5: Mantras *and* Dhāraṇīs *

On *mantras* in Vedism and Brāhmanism, cf. Winternitz, *Geschichte*, I, 148 ff., 236 ff.; in Buddhism, ibid., II, 275; in the tantras, ibid., I, 481 ff. *Dhāraṇīs* in the pre-Buddhist period, ibid., I, 94 ff., 103 ff.; the term first appears in Buddhism with the *Lalitavistara* and the *Saddharmapuṇḍarīka* (ibid., II, 380); Waddell ("The Dhāraṇī Cult in Buddhism") believes that the technique existed from the beginnings of Buddhism (see also id., " 'Dhāraṇī,' or Indian Buddhist Protective Spells"). Comprehensive studies: Wassilieff, *Bouddhisme*, pp. 144 ff.; La Vallée Poussin, *Bouddhisme: Études*, pp. 119 ff.; Hauer, *Die Dhāraṇī im nördlichen Buddhismus;* Woodroffe, *Garland of Letters* (treats chiefly of the speculations of late tantrism); Evola, *Yoga della potenza*, pp. 234 ff. Mahāyānic lists of *dhāraṇīs*, texts, and interpretations: *Vijñaptimātratāsiddhi*, tr. La Vallée Poussin, II, 613–14; *Traité*, tr. Lamotte, I, 318 ff.; R. Tajima, *Étude sur le Mahāvairocana-sūtra*, p. 103, etc. *Mantras* and *dhāraṇīs* in the Hayagrīva cult: Gulik, *Hayagrīva*, pp. 48 ff.; in Japan: M. W. de Visser, *Ancient Buddhism in Japan*, II, 520 ff.; cf. also Lucian Scherman, "Siddha."

Almost every tantra includes the presentation of a number of *mantras:* see especially the *Śāradātilaka-tantra*, chs. VI–XXIII. *Tantrābhidāna, with Vījanighaṇṭu and Mudrānighaṇṭu* (ed. Tārānātha Vidyāratna) constitutes a sort of dictionary giving the tantric meanings of the vowels and consonants. Important and extremely useful: *Dakṣiṇāmūrti, Uddhārakoṣa. A Dictionary of the Secret Tantric Syllabic Code*, ed. Raghu Vira and Shodo Taki.

For the theory of sound, the doctrines of the Mīmāṃsā are especially to be consulted. See Umesha Mitra, "Physical Theory of Sound and Its Origin in Indian Thought."

For Zen practices, cf. D. T. Suzuki, *Essays in Zen Buddhism*, III, 195 ff.

An important text of Kashmirian Śivaism, Abhinavagupta's *Tantra-*

sāra (ed. M. R. Shāstri, pp. 12–17), translated, with commentary, by Tucci, *Teoria e pratica del maṇḍala*, pp. 66–68.

On the mythical personification of *mantras*, cf. Przyluski, "Les Vidyārāja," especially pp. 308 ff.

VI, 6: Dhikr *

T. P. Hughes (*A Dictionary of Islam*, pp. 703 ff.) summarizes the technique of *dhikr* after Maulawī Shāh Waliyu'llāh, of Delhi. Cf. Massignon, *Passion d'al-Hallâj*, II, 696 ff.; id., "Le Souffle dans l'Islam." Gardet ("Mention du nom divin") should now be consulted. The author compares the "*dhikr* of the tongue" with *dhāraṇā* and the "*dhikr* of the heart" with *dhyāna* (pp. 670, 205). "If our analysis of the experience of *dhikr* is correct, it follows that this experience, by its successive ascendancy over all the zones of the individual, proves to be a 'milder' but to some degree a more indirect and risky, less reliable method of attaining the explicit goal of yoga" (ibid., p. 207).

On the relations between Islamic mysticism and India, see Massignon, *Essai sur les origines du lexique technique de la mystique musulmane*, pp. 75 ff., 86 ff.; M. M. Moreno, "Mistica musulmana e mistica indiana" (*samādhi*, pp. 125 ff.; artificial ecstasies, pp. 136 ff., *fanā'* and *nirvāṇa*, pp. 156 ff.). See also Émile Dermenghem, "Techniques d'extase en Islam."

VI, 7: Maṇḍala *

Each tantra has a *maṇḍala* proper to it. See Tucci ("Some Glosses," pp. 342 ff.) on the *maṇḍala* of the *Guhyasamāja-tantra;* cf. Carelli, ed., *Sekoddeśaṭīkā*, pp. 25 ff.; B. Bhattacharyya, *Niṣpannayogāvalī* (text by Abhayākaragupta, of the Vikramaśīla monastery), for a description of twenty-six *maṇḍalas*. See Foucher, *Étude*, II, 8 ff.; Coomaraswamy, *Elements of Buddhist Iconography;* Visser, *Ancient Buddhism in Japan*, I, 159–75; Finot, "Manuscrits sanskrits," pp. 13 ff.; Zimmer, *Kunstform und Yoga im indischen Kultbild*, pp. 54 ff., 94 ff.; Mus, *Barabuḍur*, I, 320 ff.; Pott, *Yoga en Yantra; Hôbôgirin*, III, 279 (*chakuji*, "choosing the ground"); B. L. Suzuki, "The School of Shingon Buddhism. Pt. II: The Mandara"; Chou Yi-liang, "Tantrism in China"; W. E. Clark, ed., *Two Lamaistic Pantheons*, I, xv–xviii; Lin Li-kouang, "Puṇyodaya."

On the symbolism of the *maṇḍala* and its relations with architectonic symbolism, cf. Mus, passim; Tucci, *I Templi del Tibet*; id., *"Mc'od rten" e "Ts'a-ts'a" nel Tibet indiano ed occidentale.* On the symbolism of the circumambulation of temples, see Gisbert Combaz, "L'Évolution du stūpa en Asie," pp. 124 ff. On the relations between the symbolism of painted stuffs (*paṭa*) and of *maṇḍalas*, see Lalou, *Iconographie des étoffes peintes.*

On the problem in general, see Tucci, *Teoria e pratica.*

On the symbolism of the center, cf. Eliade, *Patterns*, pp. 374 ff.; id., *The Myth of the Eternal Return*, pp. 12 ff.; id., *Images and Symbols*, pp. 37 ff. On the psychological symbolism of the *maṇḍala*, see C. G. Jung, *Psychology and Alchemy*, pars. 122 ff.; id., "Concerning Mandala Symbolism," in *Archetypes and the Collective Unconscious*, pars. 627 ff.

VI, 8: *On the Literature of Haṭha Yoga* *

See Farquhar, *An Outline of the Religious Literature of India*, p. 384; G. W. Briggs, *Gorakhnāth and the Kānphaṭā Yogīs*, pp. 251–58; Mohan Singh, *Gorakhnāth and Mediaeval Hindu Mysticism*, pp. 8 ff. See also below, Note VIII, 3.

There are several editions of the *Gorakṣa Śataka* with its commentaries (*Gorakṣa Paddhati*, etc.); edition and translation of the *Śataka* by Briggs, pp. 284–303. On the *Gorakṣa Saṃhitā*, see also Tucci, "Animadversiones Indicae," pp. 134–36.

Haṭhayogapradīpikā: Sanskrit edition with the commentary of Brahmānanda and the glosses of Śrīdhara (1889); German translation with notes, by Hermann Walter, "Svātmarāna's *Haṭhayogapradīpikā*"; editions with English translations by Brahmānanda Bhaba (1889), Śrīnivāsa Ayyaṇgār (1893), and Pañcam Sinh (1915); the numeration of stanzas sometimes differs in these editions.

Gheraṇḍa Saṃhitā: ed. Bhuvanana Chandra Vasaka; English translation by Rai Bahadur Śrīśa Chandra Vasu; German translation by Richard Schmidt, *Fakire und Fakirtum im alten und mondernen Indien.*

Śiva Saṃhitā: edition and English translation by Rai Bahadur Śrīśa Chandra Vidyarṇava.

A considerable number of extracts from these three treatises will be found in Bernard, *Haṭha Yoga*, and Daniélou, *Yoga*. See also Zimmer, "Lehren des Haṭhayoga, Lehrtexte."

Tantric anatomy and physiology have been interpreted in medical terms in a number of studies, among which we cite: Baman Das Basu, "Hindu System of Medicine." Cf. also Roesel, *Die psychologischen Grundlagen*, pp. 39 ff.; V. G. Rele, *The Mysterious Kuṇḍalinī.*

Scientific observations on Haṭha yogins: Charles Laubry and Thérèse Brosse, "Documents recueillis aux Indes sur les 'yogins.'" See also Hubert Risch, "Le Haṭha Yoga"; Filliozat, "Les Limites des pouvoirs humains dans l'Inde" (with additional bibliographical references).

VI, 9: Cakras, Ādhāras, *etc.*

For the doctrine of the *cakras: Ṣaṭcakranirūpaṇa* and *Pādukāpañcaka* (ed. and tr. Woodroffe, *The Serpent Power*); *Kūlārṇava-tantra* (ed. Tārānātha Vidyāratna), ch. VIII; *Gorakṣa Śataka* (repr. in Briggs, *Gorakhnāth*, pp. 284–304).

On the *ādhāras*, see Briggs, pp. 317 ff. Description and interpretation of the *cakras* in Evola, *Yoga*, pp. 311 ff. It should be remembered in this connection that, according to some authors, the Hesychastic tradition (see above, p. 63) distinguishes four "centers" of concentration and prayer: (1) the cerebrofrontal cranial center (located in the space between the eyebrows); (2) the buccolaryngeal center (corresponding to "the commonest thought: that of the intelligence, expressed in conversation, correspondence, and in the first stages of prayer"—A. Bloom, "L'Hésychasme, Yoga chrétien?" pp. 185 ff.); (3) the pectoral center ("situated in the upper and median region of the chest." "Stability of thought, already manifestly colored by a thymic element, is much greater than in the preceding cases, but it is still thought that defines the emotional coloring and that is modified by it"—ibid.); (4) the cardiac center (situated "near the upper part of the heart, a little below the left breast," according to the Greek Fathers; "a little above," according to Theophanes the Recluse and others. "It is the physical site of perfect attention"—ibid.).

VI, 10: *On the "Intentional Language"* *

H. Shāstri, in his *Bauddha Gān O Dohā*, explained *sandhyā-bhāṣā* as follows: "All the works of the Sahajayāna are written in the *Sandhyā-bhāṣā*; [this] is a *bhāṣā* (language) of light and darkness (*ālo-ā-dhāri*), partly light, partly darkness; some parts can be understood while others cannot. In other words, in these discourses on *dharma*, which are of a high order, there are references also to different things." According to Vidhushekar Shāstri ("Sandhābhāṣā"), "the word *sandhāya* of the Buddhists is nothing but *abhisandhāya* found in Brāhmanic and Buddhist works." Chinese sources warrant the conclusion that *sandhā-bhāṣya* means *ābhiprāyika vacana*—that is, "intentional speech." The same interpretation of the term is upheld by Bagchi ("The Sandhābhāṣā and Sandhā-vacana"), who cites other supporting passages from the Chinese sources, especially from ch. XIII of the *Hevajra-tantra*, devoted to *sandhā-bhāṣā*. A number of poetic and mystical texts composed in "intentional speech" have been collected by S. B. Dasgupta in an appendix to his *Obscure Religious Cults* (pp. 477 ff.: "Enigmatic Language of the Old and Mediaeval Poets").

On the *Dohās*, see M. Shahidullah, ed., *Les Chants mystiques de Kānha et de Saraha;* B. Bhattacharyya, "The Date of the Bauddha Gān O Dohā"; Dasgupta, pp. 61 ff., 93 ff., 423 ff., and passim; Bagchi, *Materials for a Critical Edition of the Old Bengali Caryāpadas;* cf. also Anath Nath Basu, "Tattvasvabhāvadṛṣṭigītikā dohā"; C. Bendall, "*Subhāṣitasaṃgraha,*" pp. 71 ff.

VI, 11: "By the same acts . . ." *

The *Prajñopāyaviniścayasiddhi* (I, 15) of Anaṇgavajra, the master of Indrabhuti, repeats the same saying. In this treatise, as in Indrabhuti's *Jñānasiddhi*, *maithuna* is insistently recommended (B. Bhattacharyya, ed., *Two Vajrayāna Works*, pp. 20–29, 33–35, etc.). The *mudrā* (ritual marriage partner) must be presented to the *guru*, and the rite cannot take place until after an initiation performed by the *guru*. In addition to *maithuna* with the *mudrā* consecrated for the purpose, the yogin may enjoy as many women as he wishes, drink alcoholic beverages, steal, even kill, without committing a "sin." At the end of his treatise Indra-bhuti explains that the doctrine must be kept secret and be communicated only to initiates, otherwise great evils would result.

The *Subhāṣitasaṃgraha* (ed. Bendall, p. 38) cites some verses from Āryadeva's *Cittaviśuddhiprakaraṇa* to the same purport as the saying in the *Jñānasiddhi: yena yena hi badhyante jantavo raudrakarmaṇā, sopāyena tu tenaiva mucyante bhavabandanāt*, etc. Moreover, the *Su-*

trālaṃkāra (XIII, 11–13) had already affirmed that "it is by *kleśa* ["passion," "impurity"] that one can emerge from *kleśa*" (*kleśata eva kleśaniḥsaranaṃ;* cited by La Vallée Poussin, "À propos du *Cittaviśuddhiprakaraṇa* d'Āryadeva," p. 413). On Āryadeva's treatise, cf. Prabbhubhai Patel, "*Bodhicittavivaraṇa*"; id., "*Cittaviśuddhiprakaraṇam*"; the same scholar has edited the Sanskrit text and the Tibetan translation (cf. his *Cittaviśuddhiprakaraṇa of Āryadeva*); see also Glasenapp, *Mystères bouddhistes*, pp. 32 ff.

VI, 12: *Retention of Breath and Arrest of Semen in China* *

Henri Maspéro, in his "Les Procédés de 'Nourrir le principe vital' dans la religion taoïste ancienne," has studied the Chinese theories and techniques of respiration (see above, pp. 59 ff.). We must here note certain resemblances with the tantric methods for simultaneously arresting breath and the emission of semen. We quote a passage from the "Biography of the Real Man of Pure Transcendence, Master P'ei," a "short hagiographic tale," which Maspéro dates as of the fifth century: the text puts the method for the "return of semen" among the five recipes of the Immortal Master Chiang: "By perfect meditation (every external) thought must be banished; then men and women can practice the method of Eternal Life. This procedure is absolutely secret: transmit it only to sages! . . . Each time that one practices (this procedure), he must enter into meditation: he must first lose consciousness of his body and lose consciousness of the outer world. After that he must grind his teeth for seven series and say this prayer: May the Original White Essence of Metal spread life among my Five Flowers (the five viscera). May the Lord Yellow Old Man of the Center harmonize my souls and put my Essence in order. May the Great Essence of the August Supreme, coagulating the humors, make the Transcendent hard as a bone. May the six breaths of the Great Real Without Superior coil within! May the Mysterious Old Man of Superior Essence bring back the Essence to repair my brain! Let me unite (the *yin* and the *yang*), let the Embryo be melted and the Jewel kept!

"When the prayer is finished, the men will keep (their minds fixed on) their loins, firmly preserving the Essence and distilling the Breath, which follows the spinal column and rises to the Ni-huan against the current; this is what is called 'causing to return to the Origin,' *huan-yüan;* the women will keep (their minds fixed on) their hearts, nourishing the spirits, distilling an unchanging fire, making the Breath descend from the two breasts to the loins, whence it again mounts through the spinal column and also goes to the Ni-huan: this is what is called 'transforming the real,' *hua-chen*. After a hundred days, one reaches Transcendence. If one practices (this procedure) for a very long time, one spontaneously becomes a Real Man, and, living eternally, one traverses the centuries. This is the method of not dying" (tr. after Maspéro, pp. 386–87).

We must note the alchemical symbolism of respiration and the sexual act. Gulik (*Erotic Colour Prints of the Ming Period, with an Essay on Chinese Sex Life*) has brought out the homologies between alchemical and sexual terminology in the Taoist treatises (pp. 115 ff.: the woman is assimilated to the crucible, etc.). See also Max Kaltenmark, *Le Lie-sien tchouan* (*Biographies légendaires des Immortels taoïstes de l'antiquité*), pp. 57–58.

We cite another text: "A Book of the Immortals says: the principle of making the Essence return to repair the brain consists in copulating in order to agitate the Essence violently; (then) when it is about to be emitted, one quickly seizes (the penis) with the two middle fingers of the left hand behind the scrotum and in front of the anus, one presses hard, and slowly expels the Breath through the mouth, at the same time grinding the teeth several tens of times without holding the Breath. Then, when one emits the Essence, the Essence cannot emerge, but it returns from the Jade Stem (the penis) and rises to enter the brain. This procedure is transmitted from Immortal to Immortal; drinking blood, they swear not to transmit it at random" (*Yü-fang chih-yao*, I b, tr. after Maspéro, p. 385). See also Gulik, p. 78.

These sexual techniques probably represent a tantric influence; the conception of sexual union as a spiritual union between the male and female principles represented by the sun and the moon is curiously reminiscent of Haṭha Yoga and Sahajīyā. For the same practices in Japan, see Gulik, pp. 85 ff.

VI, 13: *Sahajīyā and Viṣṇuism*

On Sahajīyā, see Manindra Mohan Bose, "An Introduction to the Study of the Post-Chaitanya Sahajiā Cult"; id., *The Post-Caitanya Sahajiā Cult of Bengal;* S. B. Dasgupta, *Obscure Religious Cults*, pp. 131 ff.

On Viṣṇuist mystical literature, cf. Dinesh Chandra Sen, *History of*

Bengali Language and Literature; id., *The Vaiṣṇava Literature of Mediaeval Bengal*; id., *Chaitanya and His Age*; id., *Chaitanya and His Companions*; Melville T. Kennedy, *The Chaitanya Movement.*

On the "emotion" (*rasa*) to be cultivated in one's relations with the divinity, see Abhayakumar Guha, "Rasa-Cult in the *Chaitanya Charitāmṛta.*" S. K. De has devoted an erudite study to the problem of the rhetorical classifications of mystical feelings, "The Bhakti-Rasa-Śāstra of Bengal Vaiṣṇavism." We quote a list of *anubhāvas* ("results") that pursue and fortify a mystical emotion aroused by love of Kṛṣṇa (ibid., p. 662): "*nṛtya* (dancing), *viluṭhita* (rolling on the ground), *gītā* (singing), *krośana* (loud crying), *tanu-moṭana* (twisting of the body), *huṃkāra* (shouting), *jṛmbhā* (yawning), *śvasa-bhūman* (profusion of sighs), *lokānapekṣita* (disregard for popular opinion), *lālāsrava* (foaming at the mouth), *aṭṭa-hāsa* (loud laughter), *ghūrṇā* (giddiness), *hikkā* (hiccough)." All these rhetorical classifications correspond to concrete experiences.

VII, 1: *Alchemists, Yogins, and "Magical Flight"*

The *Rasārṇava*, cited by Mādhava in his *Sarvadarśanasaṃgraha* (Ānandāśrama Series edn., p. 80; tr. E. B. Cowell and A. E. Gough, p. 140), mentions the yogic process of *dehavedha* by which one can "fly about in the sky" (see also P. C. Rāy, *A History of Hindu Chemistry*, introd., I, 75). This is the well-known *siddhi,* characteristic of both Yoga and shamanism. India possesses a considerable stock of legends about flying kings and magicians (cf., for example, Penzer, ed., *Somadeva's Kathā-sarit-sāgara*, II, 62 ff.; III, 27, 35; V, 33, 35, 169 ff.; VIII, 26 ff., 50 ff., etc.). Anavatapta, the miraculous lake, could be reached only by those who possessed the supernatural power of flight; Buddha and the arhats reached it in a wink, just as, in Hindu legend, the *ṛṣis* soared through the air to the divine and mysterious country of the north named Śvetadvīpa: cf. W. E. Clark, "Śākadvīpa and Śvetadvīpa"; Kasten Rönnow, "Some Remarks on Śvetadvīpa"; on Anavatapta, cf. Thomas Watters, *On Yuan Chwang's Travels in India*, I, 35; Visser, *The Arhats in China and Japan*, pp. 24 ff.; on Śvetadvīpa, cf. Eliade, *Shamanism*, pp. 409 ff.; Otto Maenchen-Helfen, "Śvetadvīpa in Pre-Christian China"; on the flight of arhats, cf. Visser, pp. 172 ff.; Lévi and Édouard Chavannes, "Les seize Arhats protecteurs de la loi," pp. 23, 263 ff.

On "magical flight" in China, cf. Eliade, *Shamanism*, pp. 448 ff.; Berthold Laufer, *The Prehistory of Aviation*, pp. 14 ff.; in Tibet, cf. Bacot, *Vie de Marpa*, pp. 13 ff.

On the legend of the three supernatural mountains that stand in the middle of the sea, which no one can approach, see Chavannes, *Les Mémoires historiques de Se-ma-Ts'ien*, II, 152–53. See also E. W. Hopkins, "The Fountain of Youth."

VII, 2: Nāgārjuna as Alchemist

For Nāgārjuna's biography, see Albert Grünwedel, *Tāranātha's Edelsteinminne*, pp. 14 ff.; Max Walleser, "The Life of Nāgārjuna from Tibetan and Chinese Sources," and above, Note VI, 1, p. 404. On his relations with alchemy, P. C. Rāy, *Hindu Chemistry*, introd., I, 92 ff., Grünwedel, "Die Geschichten der vierundachtzig Zauberer," pp. 221–22; Filliozat, "Nāgārjuna et Agastya, médecins, chimistes et sorciers"; id., *La Doctrine classique*, p. 10. It is quite possible that, besides tantric alchemy, properly speaking, certain mineralogical observations were incorporated into the alchemical tradition and transmitted under the name of Nāgārjuna: the symbiosis between "mystical" (or metaphysical) "truth" and "observational truth" (rudiments of scientific thought and chemical experiment) is a phenomenon documented throughout the history of alchemy. Thus, for example, in the *Rasopaniṣat* (ed. K. S. Śāstri; see L. D. Barnett's review, *Journal of the Royal Asiatic Society* [1930], pp. 445–46), we have the following: "The sage Nāgārjuna had the vision of this magical procedure: in the southern kingdom of Kerala where there are so many forests, not far from the sea, in a village named Affection [*prīti*], thence they extract rocks in the shape of *pippalis* that have deposits of gold. They are taken and reduced to soft powder. This powder is treated with horse blood; it is liquefied seven times by means of human blood; it is ground again in the water of the basilisk with the five products of the cow; then it is dried in accordance with the rules so that it forms a sort of paste, which is passed through a sieve; into the liquid obtained, a hundredth part [?] of copper is put; each part of this copper thus treated is doubled; the whole is melted together and combined with a portion of gold; it is mixed with honey, milk, etc.; thus one obtains a magnificent gold, as brilliant as river gold" (tr. after Lévi,

"Kaniṣka et Śātavāhana," pp. 104 ff.; Lévi had previously used this text in his article "Un Nouveau Document," p. 421).

VII, 3: On Indian Alchemy

Cf. Arthur Waley, "References to Alchemy in Buddhist Scriptures." Further references to alchemy are found in the *Mahāyāna-saṃgraha-bhāṣyā* (Nanjio, No. 1171; tr. into Chinese by Hsüan Tsang, c. 650) and in the *Abhidharma-mahāvibhāṣā-śāstra* (Nanjio, No. 1263; tr. into Chinese by Hsüan Tsang, 656–59). Some information concerning Nāgārjuna as alchemist in Lamotte, *Traité*, I, 383, n. 1. See also Stein, "References to Alchemy in Buddhist Scriptures," and Note VII, 2.

For Indian alchemy and prechemistry, see Rāy, *Hindu Chemistry;* cf. also Rasacharya Kaviraj Bhudeb Mookerjee, *Rasa-jala-nidhi; or, Ocean of Indian Chemistry and Alchemy* (a worthless compilation, but containing many citations from traditional alchemical works). On the role of mercury in Indian alchemy, Rāy, introd., I, 105; Edmund von Lippmann, *Entstehung und Ausbreitung der Alchemie*, I, 435; II, 179; Julius Jolly, "Der Stein der Weisen," p. 98. On the Tamil *sittars*, cf. Barth, *Œuvres*, I, 185; Filliozat, review of Mookerjee's *Rasa-jala-nidhi*, pp. 111–12: the *sittars* divided *sarakkus* ("substances," "ingredients") into *ān* and *peṇsarakku*, male and female ingredients, a grouping that suggests the binomial *yin-yang* of Chinese speculation. Léon Wieger (*Histoire des croyances religieuses et des opinions philosophiques en Chine*, p. 395) believes that the Taoist alchemist Ko Hung (Pao P'u Tzŭ) of the third century imitated the *Rasaratnācara*, attributed to Nāgārjuna. In this case, the *Rasaratnācara*, which had been held to belong to the seventh or eighth century (cf. Lamotte, *Traité*, I, 383, n. 1), "might really go back to the period of the Buddhist Nāgārjuna of the second century" (Filliozat, *Doctrine classique*, p. 10). But it is also possible that Tamil alchemy underwent Chinese influence (cf. Filliozat, "Taoïsme et Yoga," especially p. 120).

On the alchemical MSS of the Cordier collection, see Filliozat, "Liste des manuscrits de la collection Palmyr Cordier."

Summary of research on Greco-Egyptian alchemy, in R. P. Festugière, *La Révélation d'Hermès Trismégiste*, p. 217.

On the psychology of alchemical symbolism, cf. Jung, *Psychology and Alchemy;* id., "Psychology of the Transference." On the metaphysics of alchemy, cf. Evola, *La Tradizione ermetica.*

VII, 4: Chinese Alchemy

For translations of alchemical texts and progress achieved, see the following: Lippmann, *Entstehung*, I, 449–61; II, 65–66; O. S. Johnson, *A Study of Chinese Alchemy;* Waley, "Notes on Chinese Alchemy"; W. A. P. Martin, *The Lore of Cathay*, pp. 41–71; Alfred Forke, *The World-Conception of the Chinese*, pp. 227–300; Eliade, *Alchimia asiatica*, pp. 9–44; Tenney L. Davis and Lu-ch'iang Wu, "Chinese Alchemy"; id., "T'ao Hung-ching"; id., "An Ancient Chinese Treatise on Alchemy, Entitled *Ts'an T'ung Ch'i*"; Laufer, review of Johnson, *Isis*, XII (1929), 330–32; J. R. Partington, "Chinese Alchemy"; id., "The Relationship Between Chinese and Arabic Alchemy"; B. F. Read, "Chinese Alchemy"; Masumi Chikashige, *Alchemy and Other Chemical Achievements of the Ancient Orient;* William H. Barnes, "Possible References to Chinese Alchemy in the Fourth or Third Century B.C."; Davis, "The Dualistic Cosmogony of Huai-nan-tzŭ and Its Relations to the Background of Chinese and of European Alchemy"; Barnes and H. B. Yuen, "T'ao, the Recluse (A.D. 452–536), Chinese Alchemist"; Homer H. Dubs, "The Beginnings of Alchemy."

On Ko Hung (Pao P'u Tzŭ) see: Wieger, *Histoire*, pp. 385–406; Forke, "Ko Hung, der Philosoph und Alchimist"; Johnson, pp. 133–34; Davis, "Ko Hung (Pao-P'u Tzŭ), Chinese Alchemist of the Fourth Century"; Davis and Wu, "Ko Hung on the Gold Medicine and on the Yellow and the White" (this article contains a translation of chs. IV and XVI of Ko Hung's treatise; chs. I–III are translated by Eugen Feifel, "*Pao-p'u Tzŭ*"; ibid., a new translation of ch. IV; chs. VII and XI are translated by Davis and Ch'ên Kuo-fu, "The Inner Chapters of *Pao-p'u-tzŭ*"). Now see further, Needham, *Science*, II, 437–41.

Dubs (pp. 80 ff.) believes that the origin of alchemy is to be sought in the China of the fourth century B.C. He argues that alchemy could not arise except in a civilization in which gold was unfamiliar and methods of assaying gold unknown; but in Mesopotamia these methods were current from the fourteenth century B.C., which makes the Mediterranean origin of alchemy unlikely. But this view appears not to have been accepted by the historians of alchemy (see F. Sherwood Taylor, *The Alchemists*, p. 75). Dubs (p. 84) thinks that alchemy reached the West through Chinese travelers. However, the possibility remains that "scientific" alchemy in China represents a foreign influence (cf. Laufer, review in *Isis*, XII [1929], 330–31). We know that An Shih-kāo, the famous Parthian translator of Buddhist scriptures, who visited China in the second century, was well acquainted with Iranian magic and astrology (Maspéro, "Communautés et moines bouddhistes chinois aux IIe et IIIe siècles"; Bagchi, *Le Canon bouddhique en Chine*, I, 8, 23; Paul Pelliot, "Meou-tseu ou les doutes levés"). But we do not know if he was also acquainted with alchemy (Waley, "Notes," p. 23). Chinese astrology was influenced by Iranian astrology (Léopold de Saussure, *Les Origines de l'astronomie chinoise*, passim). Moreover, commercial and cultural relations between China and Iran were already of considerable antiquity (cf. Laufer, *Sino-Iranica*, pp. 189 ff.). The role of the Parthian kingdom in Sino-Roman commerce has been well elucidated, from Chinese sources, by Friedrich Hirth, *China and the Roman Orient*, pp. 42, 70, 173, 174. For the role of the Arabs, see Hirth and W. W. Rockhill, *Chau Ju-kua: His Work on the Chinese and the Arab Trade*, pp. 2–15. See also Eliade, *Alchimia asiatica*, pp. 42–44. On the importation of Mediterranean ideas into China, see Dubs, pp. 82–83, nn. 122–23.

VII, 5: *Metallurgy and Alchemy*

We have elsewhere studied the relations between shamans and smiths; see *Shamanism*, pp. 470 ff. Chinese mythological traditions link the founders of dynasties with the "secrets" of metallurgy; see Marcel Granet, *Danses et légendes de la Chine ancienne*, II, 609 ff., and passim. Furnaces for smelting metals were assimilated to the cosmic principles: Yu put five of his furnaces in correspondence with *yang* and four with *yin*, for the Chinese divided the metals into male and female (Granet, II, 496; Fernand de Mély, "L'Alchimie chez les chinois et l'alchimie grecque"—an article to be consulted with caution—pp. 330 ff.). Furnaces became a sort of judge simply by the fact that a highly sacred operation was performed in them; they could recognize virtue, and the greatest penalty inflicted on a criminal was to boil him in this kind of furnace. To construct a furnace was an act of virtue, to be performed by a pure man who knew the "rites of the art" (Granet, II, 491, 496).

The *Ṛg-Veda* (X, 72, 2) still preserves the tradition of certain vegetable drugs (*jaratībhiḥ oṣadhībhiḥ*) in the possession of smiths; on this problem, cf. Manindra Nath Banerjee, "Iron and Steel in the Ṛgvedic Age"; id., "On Metals and Metallurgy in Ancient India."

We shall not dwell on the infinitely complex relations between the Cyclopes, the Dactyls, the Curetes, the Telchines, and metalworking; cf. Robert Eisler, "Das Quainzeichen und die Queniter" (smiths, dancers, sorcerers); Bengt Hemberg, *Die Kabiren*, pp. 286 ff.; id., "Die Idaiischen Daktylen."

It is probable that the minerals extracted from a mine were assimilated to embryos; the Babylonian word *kubu* has been translated by some scholars as "embryo," by others as "abortion"; see the bibliography and summary of the controversy in Eliade, *Metallurgy, Magic and Alchemy*, pp. 30 ff., and *The Forge and the Crucible*, pp. 71 ff., 186 f. In any case, there is a secret correspondence between metallurgy and obstetrics: the sacrifice that was sometimes performed in proximity to the furnaces in which minerals were prepared resembles obstetric sacrifices; the furnace was assimilated to a womb; within it, the "embryo-minerals" were to complete their growth, and in a period very much shorter than would have been required had they remained hidden in the ground. In his turn, the alchemist takes up and completes the work of nature, at the same time working to "make" himself: he dreams of "completing" the growth of metals, of transmuting them into gold.

VIII, 1: *On the Aghorīs, the Kāpālikas, and the Cult of Skulls*

See Crooke, "Aghorī"; id., *The Tribes and Castes of the North-western Provinces and Oudh*, I, 26 ff.; Henry Balfour, "The Life History of an Aghorī Fakir"; H. W. Barrow, "On Aghorīs and Aghorapanthīs." Barrow's study, based on documents collected by E. T. Leith, is the most reliable and the richest as yet written. It contains a complete bibliography and much oral information. See also F. Buchanan, in R. M. Martin, *History of the Antiquities of Eastern India*, II, 492 ff. On the Aghorīs at the end of the nineteenth century, see J. C. Oman, *The Mystics, Ascetics, and Saints of India*, pp. 164–67. Passages from two unpublished commentaries on the *Prabhoda Chandrodaya* have been published by Tucci, "Animadversiones Indicae," p. 131. The same author (p. 129) prints a list of the twenty-four Kāpālikas after the *Śabaratantra;* an identical list, given in the *Gorakṣasiddhāntasaṃgraha*, adds that these twenty-four Kāpālikas were created by Nātha (Śiva) to fight against the twenty-four avatārs of Viṣṇu. On the coalescence between the

Kāpālikas and the Lokāyatikas, cf. Dakshinaranjan Shāstri, "The Lokāyatikas and the Kāpālikas."

On the role of skulls in Lamaism, cf. Rockhill, "On the Use of Skulls in Lamaist Ceremonies"; Laufer, *Use of Human Skulls and Bones in Tibet,* who suggests (p. 5) an influence from Śivaist tantrism. But the Indian influences are probably superimposed on an ancient corpus of local beliefs, for skulls play a religious and divinatory role in Siberian shamanism; cf. Eliade, *Shamanism*, pp. 245, 434 ff., etc. On the protohistorical relations between the cult of skulls and the idea of renewal of the life of the cosmos in China and Indonesia, cf. Carl Hentze, "Zur ursprüngliche Bedeutung des chinesischen Zeichens *t'ôu* = Kopf."

For the cult of skulls in western India and the adjacent regions, see Robert Heine-Geldern, "Kopfjagd und Menschenopfer in Assam und Birma"; id., "Mutterrecht und Kopfjagd im westlichen Hinterindien"; P. Wilhelm Schmidt, "Mutterrecht und Kopfjagd im westlichen Hinterindien."

For human sacrifices to Śiva and Kālī in Kāmarūpa (Assam), the tantric country par excellence, cf. E. A. Gait, "Human Sacrifices in Ancient Assam"; Koppers, "Probleme der indischen Religionsgeschichte," pp. 775 ff.

VIII, 2: On the "Orgies" of the Vallabhācāryas

On the *rāsamaṇḍalīs* (lit., "circles of play"), often degenerating into orgies, cf. Wilson, *Sketch*, p. 119; F. S. Growse, *Mathurā*, pp. 283, 295, etc.; Carpenter, *Theism in Medieval India*, pp. 434 ff.; Bhāndārkar, *Vaiṣṇavism*, p. 76; Farquhar, *Outline*, pp. 312 ff.; Glasenapp, "Die Lehre Vallabhācāryas."

The erotic excesses of Mahārājas practicing the *rāsamaṇḍalī* to the point of pathological turpitude were denounced in a violent pamphlet, *History of the Sect of Mahārājas, or Vallabhāchāryas, in Western India,* from whence all later writers on the subject have drawn their information. Similar orgies, which took place in Śaktic and tantric circles in the Himālayan region, especially at Garhwāl, were the *coli-mārgs* (*coli* = breast cloth), so named because each man received as partner in the rite the woman whose breast cloth he had drawn by lot (W. Ward, H. H. Wilson, and E. T. Atkinson, cited by Briggs, *Gorakhnāth*, pp. 173 ff.). It is interesting to note that John Fryer (*A New Account of East India and Persia*, I, 294; II, 255) describes orgies much like those of the Vāmacārīs and attributes them to the Parsees of India. On sacred orgies in Moslem Persia, see S. G. W. Benjamin, *Persia and the Persians*, pp. 353–55; C. J. Wills, *In the Land of the Lion and Sun, or Modern Persia*, pp. 154, 339, etc. Similar practices are found in the Chirāgh-Kush, "the extinction of lamps"; cf. Ney Elias, ed., *A History of the Moghuls of Central Asia*, p. 218 n. E. A. Westermarck (*The History of Human Marriage*, pp. 51 ff.) and, after him, Crooke (Fryer, II, 255, n. 1) are inclined to contest the authenticity of these accounts.

However, from what we know of the Russian sects (K. K. Grass, *Die russischen Sekten;* discussion in Robert Hertz, *Mélanges de sociologie religieuse et folklore*, pp. 229 ff.) and also of the sect of Innocentists of Bessarabia, such orgies are not at all improbable.

VIII, 3: Gorakhnāth, Matsyendranāth, and the Eighty-four Siddhas *

For Gorakhnāth and the Kānphaṭa Yogīs, see Dalpatrām Prānjivan Khakhar, "History of the Kānphaṭās of Kachh"; G. S. Leonard, "Notes on the Kānphaṭā Yogīs"; Crooke, *Tribes and Castes*, III, 153–59; L. P. Tessitori, "Yogīs (Kānphaṭā)"; Mohan Singh, *Gorakhnāth and Mediaeval Hindu Mysticism;* Briggs, *Gorakhnāth;* S. B. Dasgupta, *Obscure Religious Cults*, pp. 219–87, 442–60. On the cult of Gorakṣanāth in Bengal, see S. C. Mitra, "On the Cult of Gorakshanātha in Eastern Bengal." The god is the protector of cows; cf. also Mitra, "On the Cult of Gorakshanātha in the District of Rangpur in Northern Bengal"; Briggs, *The Chamārs*, pp. 149 ff.

For Matsyendranātha, cf. Tucci, "Animadversiones Indicae," pp. 133 ff.; Lévi, *Le Népal*, I, 347 ff.; Bagchi, ed., *Kaulajñāna-nirṇaya*, introd., pp. 8–32; Dasgupta, *Obscure Religious Cults*, pp. 442 ff.

For the eighty-four Siddhas, see Grünwedel, "Die Geschichten": Guru Udhili (pp. 205–06); Indrapāla and Lui-pā (pp. 215–16); Guru Luipa (pp. 143 ff.); Līlapāda (p. 144); Virupa (pp. 145–47); Ḍombī (pp. 147–48); Gorakhnāth (pp. 153–54); Capari (pp. 201–02); Vyāli (pp. 221–22); Karuni and Nāgārjuna (pp. 165–67), etc. Cf. Tucci, "Animadversiones Indicae," p. 138; Waddell, *The Buddhism of Tibet*, p. 42; Lévi, "Un Nouveau Document" (on Nāgārjuna, pp. 420–21); Rāhula Sānkṛtyāyana, "Recherches bouddhiques"; Bagchi, *Kaulajñāna-*

nirṇaya, pp. 20 ff.; Briggs, *Gorakhnāth*, pp. 136 ff.; Dasgupta, *Obscure Religious Cults*, pp. 232 ff.; V. V. Ramana Śāstri, "The Doctrinal Culture and Tradition of the Siddhas"; S. K. De, "Buddhist Tantric Literature," pp. 15 ff. (Kukkurīpāda, Lui-pā, Matsyendranāth, Gorakhnāth, Kāṇhu-pā, etc.). On connections with alchemy, see above, p. 280.

VIII, 4: *The Burial of Ascetics*

The custom of burying ascetics and yogins, instead of burning their corpses, is quite old in India; cf. Keith, *Religion and Philosophy*, p. 417, n. 3. The *Vaikhānasasmārtasūtra* (V, 8) mentions the funeral ceremonies of yogins and *yatis* (whose bodies are buried near a stream) and *sannyāsis* (X, 8). It was natural not to commit to the fire the bodies of those who had gained liberation, whose souls were already identified with God. Ascetics were buried in the posture of meditation, and *liṅgas* were set up on their tombs. Many of these tombs later became temples. William Simpson ("Some Suggestions of Origin in Indian Architecture") finds the origin of Indian religious architecture in this custom. "Towards the South-West corner of the outer wall of the monastery there is a cemetery, also attached to the monastery. The dead bodies of the monks, unlike those of other Hindus, are buried, and the cemetery contains the graves of about two hundred persons. The body is buried in a sitting posture, and in the case of mere neophytes a small circular mound, of solid brickwork, from three to four feet high, is all that is deemed necessary for a covering for the grave. For men of greater consequence, a temple is held essential, and in it, immediately over the corpse, a *liṅgam* is invariably consecrated. . . . It would seem that even for a neophyte a *liṅgam* was held essential" (R. Mitra, *Buddha Gayā*, p. 4, quoted by Simpson, p. 56).

Ascetics are buried seated or in the yogic position that secured them their liberation. Their identification with Śiva is attested by the *liṅgam* set up on their tombs. Cf. also Archaeological Survey of India, Southern Circle, *Annual Report*, 1911–12, p. 5: "*Sannyāsins* are not cremated, but buried, *liṅga* shrines or *brindāvāna* being raised to mark the spot"; ibid., 1915–16, p. 34. "In the case of *sannyāsins* . . . a raised masonry platform is sometimes set up over the place of burial, on which a *tulsi* plant is grown, or a stone *liṅgam* is set up as though to proclaim to the world that the body buried below has attained to the sacred form of Śiva-*liṅga*" (Coomaraswamy, "Indian Architectural Terms," p. 264).

In some places the yogin's skull is broken, to allow "the soul and the breath" to escape. Oman (*Mystics*, p. 157) describes the ceremony, which he had witnessed in the Madras Presidency: "The dead *saddhu* was placed in a sitting position on his grave, a quantity of salt was piled up about him, and earth thrown in till the body was nearly covered up. Then upon the top of the shaven head, still exposed to view, a large number of cocoanuts were broken in order to crack the skull and afford the imprisoned soul a means of exit from the now useless body. The fragments of the cocoanuts which had been used for the liberation of the dead man's soul were, I remember, eagerly sought for by the bystanders" (cf. also J. A. Dubois, *Mœurs, institutions et cérémonies des peuples de l'Inde*, pt. II, ch. 36). Breaking the skull is a funeral custom that is also found elsewhere. In Malaysia, the soul is supposed to leave the body through the top of the head. The *hala*, the Semang medicine man, is buried with his head protruding from the grave; cf. Paul Schebesta, *Les Pygmées*, p. 154.

VIII, 5: *Yogins and Fakirs*

It would be interesting to trace the earliest accounts of yogins and of fakirs' "miracles" to reach Europe. Garbe refers to a few of them (*Sāṃkhya und Yoga*, pp. 47–48). Cf. also id., "Über den willkürlichen Scheintod indischer Fakirs." An account of the yogin Haridas, who buried himself for four months, is reprinted from J. M. Honigberger, *Thirty-five Years in the East*, as an appendix to Rai Bahadur Śrīśa Chandra Vidyarṇava, *An Introduction to the Yoga Philosophy*, pp. 64–70. Wilson (*Sketch*, p. 133 n.), following the *Asiatic Monthly Journal* of March, 1829, tells of a yogin who could remain suspended in air for a considerable time (twelve to forty minutes). The yogin willingly repeated the performance anywhere, "not for money but for courtesy." He could also remain under water for several hours. "He declines to explain how he does it, merely saying he has been accustomed to do so." Sir Monier Monier-Williams ("A Case of *Samādh* in India") describes several cases of yogic miracles of which he had heard or which he had seen himself. The "rope trick" has been treated in an abundant bibliography: cf. R. Schmidt, *Fakire und Fakirtum*, pp. 167 ff.; Massignon, *La Passion d'al-Hallâj*, I, 80 ff. (the "rope trick" in Moslem hagiographic legends); Sir Henry Yule, ed., *The Book of Ser Marco Polo*, I, 318 ff.; Hayes

O'Grady, ed., *Silva Gadelica*, p. 321 (the "rope trick" attributed to the sea god Manannan Mac Lir). Oman (*Mystics*, pp. 183–84) quotes from the *Civil and Military Gazette* (Lahore, May, 1895) the case of a yogin who buried himself and revived after ten days, giving a perfect description of heaven. Cf. also Alfred Lehmann, "Einige Bemerkungen zu indischen Gauklerkunststücken." Levitation, incombustibility, and other fakirs' miracles are also known from other geographical regions (cf. Olivier Leroy, *La Lévitation*; id., *Les Hommes salamandres*).

Descriptions of tantric yogins and ascetics are found in the narratives of Arabian, Persian, and Chinese travelers. "A people known by the name of *baykardjy* are conspicuous in India. These men go naked, and their long hair covers their bodies and privy parts; they let their nails grow until they become like spikes; they remove only the parts that break. They live after the manner of wandering monks; each of them wears around his neck a cord to which is attached a human skull" (Abu-Zeyd al-Ḥassan of Syraf, tr. after J. T. Reinaud, *Relations de voyages faits par les arabes et les persans dans l'Inde et à la Chine*, I, 133–34; other descriptions in Reinaud, *Mémoire . . . sur l'Inde antérieurement au milieu du XI*e *siècle*). Ma Huan, in his description of Cochin, speaks of the "*chokis* (yogis) who lead a life as austere as the Taoists of China, but who are married" (George Phillips, "Mahuan's Account of Cochin, Calicut, and Aden," p. 343). On the yogins of Cochin, see further Rockhill, "Notes on the Relations and Trade of China with the Eastern Archipelago and the Coast of the Indian Ocean During the Fourteenth Century" (pp. 450–51), where texts by ibn Baṭūṭah, Niccolò de' Conti, and Duarte Barbosa on the yogins of Malabar are mentioned. Other descriptions in Fryer, *New Account*, I, 138; II, 35 (ascetic wearing a gold ring on his penis); II, 77 (on the Lingayats); II, 104.

We must bear in mind that the yogins and *saddhus* contributed to the spiritual unification of India, both by their journeys throughout the country and by their monasteries and sacred places. Although they were divided into countless sects, their ascetic techniques and mystical itineraries differed very little. The Indian religious orders were "militarized" during the Middle Ages. India, too, knew orders of knights-ascetics, probably organized to defend the monks against the Moslems. In course of time, these "militarized" orders, in some districts, became real "gangs," which terrorized the villages. British rule suppressed and disarmed them; yet even today, we still find the arms of these "military orders" in some temples, and at the Kumbh Melā festival the *sannyāsis* march in procession, carrying wooden lances, emblems of the arms of former times. Cf. Farquhar, "The Fighting Ascetics of India"; id., "The Organization of the Sannyāsīs of the Vedānta." A number of previously unpublished documents on the activities of the knights-ascetics in the eighteenth century have been published by Jamini Mohan Ghosh, *Sannyāsī and Fakir Raiders in Bengal.*

VIII, 6: *On Late Buddhism and Crypto-Buddhism*

Haraprasād Shāstri was one of the first to call attention to late Buddhism; cf. a sketch of his work and the bibliography of his publications in an article on him by Narendra Nath Law, "Mm. Dr. Haraprasād Śāstri," especially pp. 356–69. Notable among his studies are "Buddhism in Bengal since the Muhammadan Conquest" (especially pp. 57 ff.) and *The Discovery of Living Buddhism in Bengal.* Copious material (including important extracts from the *Śūnya Purāṇa*) in Nagendra Nath Vasu, *Modern Buddhism and Its Followers in Orissa:* survivals of *śūnya* and *dharma*, pp. 45 ff.; cult of *dharma*, pp. 14, 21, 111, etc. See also Maheswar Neog, "The Worship of Dharma in Assam." The survival of popular Buddhism can be followed in the building of *stūpas* and *caityas*, which have continued to be erected down to recent times (Vasu, pp. 139 ff.; cf. also R. Chanda, *Bhanja Dynasty of Mayurbhanj and Their Ancient Capital Khiching*, a report of the archeological excavations of 1922–25). On decadent Buddhism, cf. Benoy Kumar Sarkar, *The Folk-Element in Hindu Culture*, pp. 169, 181 ff., etc.; Bagchi, "Decline of Buddhism in India and Its Causes." The *Śūnya Purāṇa* was edited by N. N. Vasu; a new edition has been published by Charuchandra Banerjee, with important studies by Shahidullah, Basant Kumar Chatterjee, and Charuchandra Banerjee. On the cult of Dharma, cf. S. B. Dasgupta, *Obscure Religious Cults*, pp. 297–358, 461–78.

On the implantation of crypto-Buddhism among the people, cf. S. C. Mitra, "The Cult of the Tortoise-shaped Deities of Midnapur and Bankura in Western Bengal."

On late Buddhism (fourteenth century), observed in the travels of an Indian priest, Dhyāna Ghadra, in provinces other than Bengal and Orissa (Madras, Punjab, Coromandel, etc.), cf. Waley, "New Light on Buddhism in Medieval India."

VIII, 7: *Yoginīs, Ḍākinīs, Yakṣas, Durgā*

On the influence of aboriginal and exotic cults upon tantrism, see: Tucci, "Tracce di culto lunare in India," p. 423, n. 1; id., "Animadversiones Indicae," pp. 156 ff.; Bagchi, "On Foreign Element in the Tāntras"; on possible Iranian influences on Buddhist iconography, cf. Grünwedel, *Alt-Kutscha*, pt. I, pp. 54 ff.

On vegetation cults in India, see the copious data given by Meyer, *Trilogie*, and Odette Viennot, *Le Culte de l'arbre dans l'Inde ancienne.* On Durgā, cf. also Pratāpachandra Ghosha, *Durgā Pūjā;* E. A. Payne, *The Śāktas;* Sten Konow, "A European Parallel to the Durgāpūjā"; Koppers, "Probleme," passim. On the relations between tantrism and witchcraft, cf. S. N. Roy, "The Witches of Orissa," and Koppers, pp. 783 ff.

On Yakṣas, Yakṣinīs, Ḍākinīs: Noël Péri, "Hārītī, la mère-de-démons," especially pp. 38 ff., 81 ff. (the tantric cult, degenerate forms of magic, etc.); see also Filliozat, *Étude de démonologie indienne;* Eliade, "Notes de démonologie"; Coomaraswamy, *Yakṣas;* Raymonde Linossier, "Les Peintures tibétaines de la collection Loo," especially pp. 53 ff.; Jitendra Nath Banerjea, "Some Folk Goddesses of Ancient and Mediaeval India"; Przyluski and Lalou, "Notes de mythologie bouddhique: 1. Yakṣa et Gandharva"; Joseph Masson, *La Religion populaire dans le canon bouddhique pāli,* pp. 126–31; Autran, *L'Épopée hindoue,* pp. 170–90. On the motif "woman and tree": J. P. Vogel, "The Woman and Tree or *śālabhañjikā* in Indian Literature and Art"; on Yakṣas as guardians of *stūpas,* cf. Chanda, "Medieval Sculpture in Eastern India," p. 236.

On the *caitya:* V. R. Ramchandra Dikshitar, "Origin and Early History of Caityas"; in southern India, K. R. Subramanian, *Buddhist Remains in Āndhra,* pp. 24 ff.; N. Venkata Ramanayya, *An Essay on the Origin of the South Indian Temple,* pp. 53 ff.; in Tibet, Tucci, *"Mc'od rten" e "Ts'a-ts'a,"* pp. 24 ff.

On Yakṣas and Yakṣinīs in Jain iconography, see James Burgess, "Digambara Jaina Iconography," p. 464.

On *pīṭhas,* see Dines Chandra Sirkar, "The Śākta Pīṭhas."

VIII, 8: *The Dravidian Contribution*

Not long ago, the transformations of Indo-Āryan were explained by the influence of Dravidian; see, for example, Robert Caldwell, *A Comparative*

Grammar of the Dravidian or South-Indian Family of Languages; Konow, in *Linguistic Survey of India,* IV, 278 ff.; cf. S. K. Chatterji, *The Origin and Development of the Bengali Language,* I, 174 ff. Caldwell in particular maintained that the inflections of Sanskrit and the appearance of the cerebrals was explained by Dravidian, but the tendency toward cerebralization was already present in Indo-Āryan; cf. Jules Bloch, "Sanskrit et dravidien"; id., "Some Problems of Indo-Āryan Philology," pp. 730–44; id., *L'Indo-aryen du Véda aux temps modernes,* pp. 321–31. The phenomenon of cerebralization also occurs in the Muṇḍa languages; cf. Bloch, "Some Problems," pp. 731–32; Przyluski, "Un Ancien Peuple du Penjab: les Udumbara." As to aboriginal influences on Sanskrit, Jules Bloch stresses Muṇḍa influences, especially on vocabulary (see Note VIII, 10).

It has been suggested that there are connections between Dravidian and Etruscan, Dravidian and Uralian; cf. Schrader, "Dravidisch und Uralisch"; Thomas Burrow, "Dravidian Studies, IV: The Body in Dravidian and Uralian."

On the anthropology and ethnology of the Dravidians, cf. G. Montadon, *La Race, les races,* pp. 174–77; id., *Traité d'ethnologie culturelle,* pp. 180 ff.; A. L. Kroeber, *Anthropology,* pp. 478 ff.

For the religious life of the Dravidian populations and the *grāmadevatās,* material and bibliographies will be found in: Oppert, *Original Inhabitants;* W. T. Elmore, *Dravidian Gods in Modern Hinduism;* Henry Whitehead, *The Village Gods of South India.* Cf. also S. C. Roy, *Orāon Religion and Customs;* J. S. Chandler, "Names of God in the Tamil Language Which Denote His Oneness"; O. R. von Ehrenfels, "Traces of a Matriarchal Civilization among the Kolli Mailayālis."

The contribution made to Hinduism by Dravidian religious sentiment has been considerable; we should, however, hesitate to follow G. W. Brown ("The Sources of Indian Philosophical Ideas") when he claims a Dravidian origin for all the great intuitions and fundamental concepts of Indian thought.

On *pūjā,* see: Jarl Charpentier, "The Meaning and Etymology of Pūjā"; Przyluski, "Totémisme et végétalisme dans l'Inde."

The *grāmadevatās* can assume any form: among their countless "forms," the *Grāmadevatāpratiṣṭhā* mentions the skull of Brahmā, the head of Viṣṇu, the skull of Renukā, the face of Draupadī, the body of Sītā, the Pramāthas (the train who follow Śiva), the Pāriṣadas (companions of Viṣṇu), demons of all kinds, the *yoginīs*, various kinds of idols of the Śakti in wood, stone, or clay, etc. (Oppert, p. 455).

VIII, 9: *Snakes*, *Dragons*, Nāgas

On the cult and symbolism of the snake, see: Vogel, "Serpent Worship in Ancient and Modern India," especially pp. 305 ff. on *nāgas* in Kashmir and the Punjab (cf. B. R. Beotra, "Gods and Temples in the Suket State," especially pp. 170 ff.); Vogel, *Indian Serpent-Lore*, pp. 35 ff.; Winternitz, "Der Sarpabali, ein altindischer Schlangencult." We may dismiss C. F. Oldham's hypothesis (*The Sun and the Serpent*) that the *nāgas* were human beings who believed themselves descended from the sun. Kern was the first to see that the *nāgas* were connected with the waters. Dragons and snakes are identified with the "masters of the soil," the "autochthons"; cf. Autran, *L'Épopée hindoue*, pp. 66–169. On the metaphysical symbolism of the snake—which represents the pre-formal modality of the universe, the unfragmented "one" that precedes all creation—cf. Coomaraswamy, *The Darker Side of the Dawn;* id., "Sir Gawain and the Green Knight: Indra and Namuci."

The only instance of Indian ophiolatry with human sacrifice as yet known has been found among the Khāsīs of Assam: the snake divinity is named U Thlen. On myths of U Thlen, see P. R. T. Gurdon, *The Khāsīs*, pp. 175–78; K. U. Rafy, *Folktales of the Khāsīs*, pp. 58–64. A recent case of such a sacrifice, dating from 1924, is reported by S. C. Mitra, "On a Recent Instance of the Khāsī Custom of Offering Human Sacrifices to the Snake-Deity."

On the different iconographic representations of the *nāga*-gods, see Combaz, *L'Inde et l'Orient classique*, pp. 56 ff.; cf. id., "Masques et dragons en Asie" (pp. 102 ff., the dragon; pp. 136 ff., the *makara* in India; pp. 172 ff., the dragon in China).

Przyluski ("La Princesse à l'odeur de poisson et la nāgī dans les traditions de l'Asie orientale") studied a group of legends that reflect some aspects of the maritime civilization of the Southwest: "The underlying idea: one of the magico-religious forces that make heroes resides in water. . . . Sharply opposed to the continental Indo-Āryan and Chinese peoples, for whom the gods dwell on the summits of mountains and in the upper atmosphere. In China, divine power and authority come from above; the Emperor is the Son of Heaven" (p. 281). Another idea, complementary to the sacredness of water: sovereignty appertains to women and is transmitted through women. Cf. also Przyluski, "Dragon chinois et Nāga indien"; id., "Le Prologue-cadre des *Mille et une Nuits* et le thème du *svayaṃvara*" (traces of matriarchy in Indian tales, in Cambodia, in Chinese folklore, etc.).

On aquatic symbolism, see Eliade, *Patterns*, pp. 188 ff., and id., *Images and Symbols*, pp. 125 ff.

VIII, 10: *Muṇḍa, Proto-Muṇḍa*

A bibliography of the essential studies down to 1933 will be found in Constantin Régamey, "Bibliographie analytique des travaux relatifs aux éléments anaryens dans la civilisation et les langues de l'Inde." The point of departure for all research into the Muṇḍas is found in the studies of P. Wilhelm Schmidt, in which he established clear connections between the Mon-Khmer linguistic group and the languages of Malaysia; cf. "Die Mon-Khmer Völker." Description of the Muṇḍa languages, Grierson, *Linguistic Survey of India*, IV, 1–275; cf. also I, 32–38. S. K. Chatterji ("The Study of Kōl") prefers to call this linguistic group "Kōlarian" (from *kōl*, Āryan pronunciation of an old Muṇḍa word meaning "man").

On the influences exercised by the Austroasiatic languages and cultures upon Sanskrit and the Indo-European culture, see: Lévi, "Pré-aryen et pré-dravidien dans l'Inde"; Przyluski, "De quelques noms anaryens en indo-aryen"; id., "Emprunts anaryens en indo-aryen," *BSL*, XXIV (1924), 118–23 (Skr. *lāṅgala*, "plow"; *laguḍa*, "rod"; *liṅga;* common Austroasiatic root, *lak*); ibid., 255–58 (the names of the betel in Austroasiatic); ibid., XXV (1925), 66–71 (Skr. *bāṇa*, "arrow"; Austroasiatic words of the type *panah*); ibid., XXVI (1926), 98–103 (the name of the elephant, etc.); ibid., XXX (1930), 196–201; id., "La Numération vigésimale dans l'Inde"; id., "Bengali Numeration and non-Āryan Substratum"; F. B. J. Kuiper, "An Austro-Asiatic Myth in the *Rig-Veda*" (Indra and the boar that he kills with an arrow shot through a mountain); id., "Proto-Mūṇḍā Words in Sanskrit"; id., "Mūṇḍā and Indonesian."

As to Austroasiatic migrations into India, Paul Rivet holds ("Les Océaniens," p. 250) that "at an extremely early epoch, a series of human migrations set out from the south of Asia or from the Indian

Archipelago; they spread fanwise across the Pacific and the Indian Ocean, and, having peopled all the islands of these two oceans, reached the New World in the east, Japan in the north, Europe in the west, and Africa." He considers that the first wave was Australian, the second Melanesian. Petroglyphs identical with Australian petroglyphs have been found in the vicinity of Benares. The use of the boomerang has survived in Celebes, in southeastern India, and in Gujarāt (p. 236). "I am more and more convinced that, through the entire Mediterranean basin and a greater or lesser part of Africa, there was an Oceanian substratum that acted upon the peoples of various origins who invaded these regions in the course of the ages" (Rivet, *Sumérien et Océanien*, p. 8). The center of dispersion was doubtless southern Asia or the Indian Archipelago (ibid., p. 9). For Heine-Geldern, on the contrary, the arrival of the Dravidians in India preceded that of the Austroasiatics: cf. "Ein Beitrag zur Chronologie des Neolithikums in Südostasien" (on the Muṇḍa migrations, pp. 814–30); id., "Urheimat und früheste Wanderungen der Austronesier." Cf. also C. Tauber, *Entwicklung der Menschheit von den Ur-Australiern bis Europa.*

Excellent study of the cultural stratigraphy of the various Indian populations in Hermann Niggemeyer, "Totemismus in Vorderindien."

On Polynesian influences in southern India, see: James Hornell, "The Origins and Ethnological Significance of Indian Boat Designs"; id., "The Boats of the Ganges." Parallels between Sumatra and India: H. C. Das-Gupta, "A Few Types of Indian Sedentary Games"; id., "On a Type of Sedentary Game Prevalent in Shahpur" (the *sher-bakr*, "tiger-goat," a game attested in Orissa, Tibet, and Sumatra).

See also Ruben, "Über die Literatur der vorarischen Stämme Indiens."

VIII, 11: *Harappā and Mohenjo-daro* *

Sir John Marshall (and others), *Mohenjo-Daro and the Indus Culture;* Ernest Mackay, *The Indus Civilization;* Vats, *Excavations at Harappā;* Heinz Mode, *Indische Frühkulturen und ihre Beziehungen zum Westen* (pp. 165–71, bibliography); Henry Heras, "More about Mohenjo Daro"; F. Gelpke, "Induskultur und Hinduismus"; Viktor Golubev, "Essais sur l'art de l'Indus. I: L'Homme au châle de Mohenjo-Daro" (on the statue that has been supposed to represent a yogin in meditation; the author believes it to be the effigy of a priest; influence of the statuary art of earlier Asia). On all these problems, see the admirable synthesis by Stuart Piggott, *Prehistoric India* (Harappā and Mohenjo-daro, pp. 132–213).

We shall not list the innumerable attempts to decipher the Indus inscriptions: cf., for example, Wilhelm von Hevesy, "The Easter Island and the Indus Valley Scripts" (but see also Heine-Geldern, "Die Osterinselschrift"; Bedřich Hrozný, "Inschriften und Kultur der Proto-Inder von Mohenjo-Daro und Harappā." On the cult of vegetation in the Indus civilizations, see Viennot, *Le Culte de l'arbre*, pp. 7–19.

IX, 1: *Dissemination of Yogic Techniques and Cultural Contacts Between India and the World* *

On Tibetan Yoga, see: Waddell, "Lamaism in Sikhim," especially pp. 305 ff. (on the "positions of meditation" and respiratory techniques); Alexandra David-Neel, "L'Entraînement psychique chez les thibétains"; id., *Mystiques et magiciens du Thibet*, pp. 245 ff. See also: Bacot, *Le Poète tibétain Milarépa*, pp. 200 ff.; Evans-Wentz, *Tibet's Great Yogī Milarepa*, pp. 194 ff.; id., *Tibetan Yoga and Secret Doctrines*, passim; Grünwedel, *Die Legenden des Nā-ro-pa* (but see also Tucci, "À Propos the Legend of Nāropā"); Siegbert Hummel, "Die Lamaistischen Tempelfahnen und ihre Beziehung zu Yoga." On Yoga in Mongolia, A. M. Pozdnejev, "Dhyāna und Samādhi im mongolischen Lamaismus." On *dhyāna* (*ch'an*) in China, cf. Conze, *Buddhism*, pp. 201 ff.; John Blofeld, tr., *The Path of Sudden Attainment;* on Zen, cf. D. T. Suzuki, *Essays in Zen Buddhism;* id., *An Introduction to Zen Buddhism;* id., *Manual of Zen Buddhism* (translations of texts).

On the dissemination of Indian spiritual techniques in Indonesia, everything has been said in Paul Mus's monumental work, *Barabuḍur.* See also Przyluski, "Le Bouddhisme tantrique à Bali d'après une publication récente": Javanese tantrism approaches that of the Japanese Shingon sect, but represents an earlier stage (p. 160). On cultural contacts between India and China, cf. Elmer H. Cutts, "Chinese-Indian Contacts Prior to the Latter Half of the First Century"; Bagchi, *India and China: a Thousand Years of Cultural Relations* (pp. 221–22, bibliography).

On cultural contacts between India and the West, the essential materials and bibliographies will be found in Henri de Lubac, *La Rencontre du bouddhisme et de l'Occident;* Lamotte, "Les Premières Relations entre l'Inde et l'Occident"; on Indian influences, cf. *Mémorial Sylvain Lévi,* pp. 190, 206–07, 210–12, etc.; Marcel Mauss, "Rapports historiques entre la mystique hindoue et la mystique occidentale": "Lassen had already pointed out that, in Plotinus, the procedures preparatory to ecstasy were remarkably similar to those of Buddhism and various Brāhmanic systems. . . . And in a magical papyrus of the second century we find certain Hindu beliefs mentioned (cf. Norden, *Geburt des Kindes,* 1924, p. 112); Isis is compared to Māyā, name and personification of the Buddha's mother and also of the Great Illusion." But see also Lubac, "Textes alexandrins et bouddhiques"; Filliozat, "La Doctrine des brâhmanes d'après saint Hippolyte"; id., "Les Échanges de l'Inde et de l'Empire romain aux premiers siècles de l'ère chrétienne"; id., *La Doctrine classique,* pp. 205 ff.

The problem of Indian influences on Christian theology and mysticism has been approached as a whole by Ernst Benz, "Indische Einflüsse auf die frühchristliche Theologie" (see especially pp. 197 ff., Ammonius Saccas and the dissemination of Indian philosophy among the Neoplatonic and Christian circles of Alexandria). But we must not lose sight of the fact that the influence was also exerted in the opposite direction: in the *Īśvara Gītā,* a late, Śivaist imitation of the *Bhagavad Gītā,* Yoga, interpreted as union of the human soul with God (Īśvara = Śiva), is referred to as *sunaphā;* the term also occurs in the astrological work of Varāhamihira (sixth century A.D.). Now, it is of Greek origin (Winternitz, *Geschichte,* III, 567, 569, 571): Plotinus and Proclus use the word *synaphé* in the sense of mystical union between soul and spirit; see P. E. Dumont, "Sunaphā. Note sur un passage de l'*Īśvaragītā* du *Kūrmapurāṇa.*" Cf. also Lacombe, "Note sur Plotin et la pensée indienne."

LIST OF WORKS CITED

ABBREVIATIONS

A	*Anthropos* (Salzburg)
ABAW	*Abhandlungen der königlichen Bayerischen Akademie der Wissenschaften* (Munich)
ABORI	*Annals of the Bhāndārkar Oriental Research Institute* (Poona)
AJP	*American Journal of Philology* (Baltimore)
AO	*Acta orientalia* (Leiden)
AUS	*Allahabad University Studies*
BB	Bibliotheca Buddhica
BCLS	*Bulletin de la Classe des lettres et des sciences morales et politiques, Académie royale de Belgique* (Brussels)
BEFEO	*Bulletin de l'École française d'Extrême-Orient* (Hanoi)
BI	Bibliotheca Indica
BS	Bollingen Series
BSL	*Bulletin de la Société de Linguistique* (Paris)
BSOS	*Bulletin of the School of Oriental and African Studies* (University of London)
EJ	*Eranos-Jahrbuch* (Zurich)
FMNH	Field Museum of Natural History
GOS	Gaekwad's Oriental Series
HJAS	*Harvard Journal of Asiatic Studies* (Cambridge, Mass.)
HOS	Harvard Oriental Series
IA	*Indian Antiquary* (Bombay)
IHQ	*Indian Historical Quarterly* (Calcutta)
JA	*Journal asiatique* (Paris)
JAOS	*Journal of the American Oriental Society* (New Haven)
JASB	*Journal of the Anthropological Society of Bombay*
JBORS	*Journal of the Bihār and Orissa Research Society* (Bankipore)

JCE	*Journal of Chemical Education* (Easton, Pa.)
JDL	*Journal of the Department of Letters* (University of Calcutta)
JISOA	*Journal of the Indian Society of Oriental Art* (Calcutta)
JOR	*Journal of Oriental Research* (Madras)
JRAS	*Journal of the Royal Asiatic Society* (London)
JRASB	*Journal of the Royal Asiatic Society of Bengal* (Calcutta)
MAGW	*Mitteilungen der anthropologischen Gesellschaft zu Wien*
MCB	*Mélanges chinois et bouddhiques* (Brussels)
MI	*Man in India* (Ranchi)
MO	*Le Monde oriental* (Uppsala)
MRANL	*Memorie delle Reale Accademia nazionale dei Lincei*, Classe di scienze morali, storiche e filologiche (Rome)
MS	*Monumenta serica* (Peking)
NGWG	*Nachrichten von der königlichen Gesellschaft der Wissenschaften zu Göttingen*
NIA	*New Indian Antiquary* (Bombay)
OZ	*Ostasiatische Zeitschrift* (Berlin)
PAAAS	*Proceedings of the American Academy of Arts and Sciences* (Boston)
PTS	Pāli Text Society Translation Series
RHR	*Revue de l'histoire des religions* (Paris)
SBB	Sacred Books of the Buddhists
SBE	Sacred Books of the East
SBH	Sacred Books of the Hindus
TT	Tantrik Texts
ZB	*Zeitschrift für Buddhismus* (Munich)
ZDMG	*Zeitschrift der deutschen morgenländischen Gesellschaft* (Leipzig)
ZII	*Zeitschrift für Indologie und Iranistik* (Leipzig)

LIST OF WORKS CITED

For items preceded by an asterisk, see p. 480.

ABHAYĀKARAGUPTA. *See* BHATTACHARYYA, BENOYTOSH.

ABHINAVAGUPTA. *See* SHĀSTRI, MUKUNDA RĀMA.

ABS, P. J. "Some Early Buddhistic Texts in Relation to the Philosophy of Materialism in India." In *Actes du XVIIIe Congrès international des Orientalistes*, pp. 157–59. Leiden, 1932.

ABŪ'L FAḌL, 'ALLĀMI. *See* BLOCHMANN, H., and JARRETT, H. S.

ADVAYAVAJRA. *See* SHĀSTRI, HARAPRASĀD.

AIYAṆGĀR, ŚRĪNIVĀSA. *See* AYYAṆGĀR, T. R. ŚRĪNIVĀSA.

AKIYAMA, AISABURO. *Buddhist Hand-Symbol.* Yokohama, 1939.

ANIRUDDHA. *See* GARBE, RICHARD, and SINHA, NANDALAL.

ARBMAN, ERNST. *Rudra: Untersuchungen zum altindischen Glauben und Kultus.* Uppsala, 1922.

ARCHAEOLOGICAL SURVEY OF INDIA, SOUTHERN CIRCLE. *Annual Report.* Madras, 1911–12; 1915–16.

ASAṆGA. *See* WOGIHARA, UNRAI.

AUBOYER, JEANNINE. "*Moudrā* et *hasta* ou le langage par signes," *Oriental Art* (PARIS), III (1950–51), 153–61.

———. *Le Trône et son symbolisme dans l'Inde ancienne.* PARIS, 1949.

AUFRECHT, THEODOR. *Catalogus catalogorum: an Alphabetical Register of Sanskrit Works and Authors.* Leipzig, 1891–1903. 3 pts.

AUNG, S. Z. *See* DAVIDS, C. A. F. RHYS.

AUTRAN, CHARLES. *L'Épopée hindoue: étude de l'arrière-fonds ethnographique et religieux.* Paris, 1946.

AVALON, ARTHUR. *See* WOODROFFE, SIR JOHN.

AYYAṆGĀR, T. R. ŚRĪNIVĀSA, tr. *Haṭhayogapradīpikā of Svātmārāma Svāmin.* Bombay, 1893. Last repr., Adyar, 1933.

———, tr. *The Yoga Upaniṣads*, ed. G. ŚRĪNIVĀSA MURTI. Adyar, 1938. 2nd edn., Adyar, 1952.

BACHOFER, LUDWIG. "Zur Geschichte der chinesischen Plastik vom VIII.–XIV. Jahrhundert," *OZ*, XXIV, n.s. XIV (1938), 65–82.

BACOT, JACQUES. *Le Bouddha.* Paris, 1947.

———. *Le Poète tibétain Milarépa: ses crimes, ses épreuves, son nirvāṇa.* Paris, 1925.

BACOT, JACQUES. *La Vie de Marpa, le "traducteur."* Paris, 1937.

BĀDARĀYAṆA. *See* BELVALKAR, SHRIPAD KRISHNA.

BAGCHI, PRABODH CHANDRA. *Le Canon bouddhique en Chine: les traducteurs et les traductions.* Paris, 1927–38. 2 vols.

———. "Decline of Buddhism in India and Its Causes." In *Sir Asutosh Mookerjee Silver Jubilee Volumes*, vol. III, pt. 2, pp. 405–21. Calcutta, 1921–27. 3 vols. in 5.

———. "Further Notes on Tāntrik Texts Studied in Ancient Kambuja," *IHQ*, VI, 1 (1930), 97–107. (Reprinted in his *Studies in the Tāntras*, pp. 16–26.)

———. *India and China: a Thousand Years of Cultural Relations.* 2nd edn., Bombay, 1950.

———, ed. *Kaulajñāna-nirṇaya and Some Minor Texts of the School of Matsyendranātha.* Calcutta, 1934. (Calcutta Sanskrit Series III.)

———. *Materials for a Critical Edition of the Old Bengali Caryāpadas: a Comparative Study of the Text and the Tibetan Translation.* Pt. I. Calcutta, 1938.

———. "A Note on the Word *parāvṛtti*," in his *Studies in the Tāntras* (q.v.), pp. 87–92.

———. "On Foreign Element in the Tāntras," *IHQ*, VII, 1 (1931), 1–16. (Reprinted in his *Studies in the Tāntras*, pp. 45–55.)

———. "On Some Tāntrik Texts Studied in Ancient Kambuja," *IHQ*, V, 4 (1928), 754–69. (Reprinted in his *Studies in the Tāntras*, pp. 1–15.)

———, tr. *Pre-Āryan and Pre-Dravidian in India.* Essays by Sylvain Lévi, Jean Przyluski, and Jules Bloch. Calcutta, 1929.

———. "Primitive Elements of Jainism," *JDL*, V (1921), 349–64.

———. "The Sandhābhāṣā and Sandhāvacana," *IHQ*, VI, 2 (1930), 389–96. (Repr. in *Studies in the Tāntras*, pp. 27–33.)

———. *Studies in the Tāntras.* Calcutta, 1939.

BĀLA ŚĀSTRI, ed. *Bhāmatī, a Gloss on Śaṇkara Acharya's Commentary on the Brahmā Sūtras, by Vāchaspati Miśra.* Benares, 1880. (BI LXXXIII.)

BALFOUR, HENRY. "The Life History of an Aghorī Fakir," *Journal of the Anthropological Institute* (London), XXVI (1897), 340–57.

BALLANTYNE, J. R., tr. *The Sānkhya Aphorisms of Kapila.* London, 1885.

BANERJEA, JITENDRA NATH. "Some Folk Goddesses of Ancient and Mediaeval India," *IHQ*, XIV, 1 (1938), 101–09.

BANERJEE, CHARUCHANDRA, ed. *Śūnya Purāṇa.* [Details unavailable.]

BANERJEE, MANINDRA NATH. "Iron and Steel in the Ṛgvedic Age," *IHQ*, V, 3 (1929), 432–40.

———. "On Metals and Metallurgy in Ancient India," *IHQ*, III, 1 (1927), 121–33; III, 4 (1927), 793–802.

BANERJI, ADRIS. "Origins of Jain Practices," *Journal of the Oriental Institute* (University of Baroda), I (1952), 308–16.

BAREAU, ANDRÉ. "L'Absolu en philosophie bouddhique. Évolution de la notion d'*asaṃskṛta*." Diss. Paris: Centre de documentation universitaire, 1951.

———. "La Date du Nirvāna, *JA*, CCXLI (1953), 27–62.

BARNES, WILLIAM H. "Possible References to Chinese Alchemy in the Fourth or Third Century B.C.," *The China Journal* (Shanghai), XXIII (1935), 75–79.

———. and YUEN, H. B. "T'ao, the Recluse (A.D. 452–536), Chinese Alchemist," *Ambix* (London), II (1946), 138–47.

BARNETT, LIONEL DAVID. Review of *Rasopaniṣat*, ed. K. S. Śāstri, *JRAS* (1930), 445–46.

BARROW, H. W. "On Aghorīs and Aghorapanthīs," *Proceedings of the Anthropological Society of Bombay*, III (1893), 197–251.

BARTH, AUGUSTE. *Quarante Ans d'indianisme: Œuvres.* Paris, 1914–27. 5 vols.

BARUA, BENINADHAB. "The Ājīvikas: a Short History of Their Religion and Philosophy," *JDL*, II (1920), 1–80.

———. *A History of Pre-Buddhistic Philosophy.* Calcutta, 1921.

BASHAM, A. L. *History and Doctrines of Ājīvikas: a Vanished Indian Religion.* London, 1951.

BASU, ANATH NATH. "Tattvasvabhāvadṛṣṭigītikā dohā," *IHQ*, III, 4 (1927), 676–82.

BASU, BAMAN DAS. "Hindu System of Medicine," *Guy's Hospital Gazette* (London), 1889. (Reprinted in part in VASU, R. B. ŚRĪŚA CHANDRA, *Śiva Saṃhitā*, [q.v.], introd.)

BELVALKAR, SHRIPAD KRISHNA, ed. *The Brahmā-Sūtras of Bādarāyaṇa.* Poona, 1923. (Poona Oriental Series XIII.)

———. "*Māṭhara-vṛtti*," *ABORI*, V (1923–24), 133–68.

———. "*Māṭharavṛtti* and the Date of Īśvarakṛṣṇa." In *Commemorative Essays Presented to Sir Ramkrishna Gopal Bhāndārkar*, pp. 171–84. Poona, 1917.

Belvalkar, Shripad Krishna. "The So-called Kashmir Recension of the *Bhagavad Gītā*," *NIA*, II (1939), 211–31.

———. *Vedānta Philosophy*. Poona, 1929.

Bendall, Cecil, ed. "The *Megha-sūtra*, Text and Translation," *JRAS*, n.s. XII (1880), 286–311.

———, ed. *Śikṣāsamuccaya of Śāntideva*. St. Petersburg, 1902. (BB I.)

———, ed. "*Subhāṣitasaṃgraha*," *Le Muséon* (Louvain), n.s. IV–V (1903–04).

Benfey, Theodor, ed. *Pantschatantra*. Leipzig, 1859. 2 vols.

Benjamin, Samuel Greene W. *Persia and the Persians*. London, 1883.

Benz, Ernst. "Indische Einflüsse auf die frühchristliche Theologie," *Abhandlungen der Akademie der Wissenschaften und der Literatur* (Wiesbaden), geistes- und sozialwissenschaftlichen Klasse (1951), No. 3, pp. 172–202.

Beotra, B. R. "Gods and Temples in the Suket State," *JRASB*, n.s. XXVII (1933), 165–76.

Bernard, Theos. *Haṭha Yoga: the Report of a Personal Experience*. New York, 1944.

Bernier, François. *Voyages de François Bernier, docteur en médecine de la faculté de Montpellier*. Amsterdam, 1723. 2 vols.

Bhāndārkar, D. R. "Ājīvikas," *IA*, XLI (1912), 286–90.

Bhāndārkar, R. G. *Report on the Search for Sanskrit Manuscripts in the Bombay Presidency for the Year 1883–1884*. Bombay, 1887.

———. *Vaiṣṇavism, Śaivism and Minor Religious Systems*. Strassburg, 1913.

Bhattacharya, Kalipada. "Some Problems of Sāṅkhya Philosophy and Sāṅkhya Literature," *IHQ*, VIII, 3 (1932), 509–20.

Bhattacharyya, Benoytosh. "The Buddhists in Bengal," *The Dacca Review*, II, 7 (1921), 91–104.

———. "The Cult of Bhūtaḍāmara." In *Proceedings and Transactions of the Sixth All-India Oriental Conference* (*1930*), pp. 349–70. Patna, 1933.

———. "The Date of the Bauddha Gān O Dohā," *JBORS*, XIV (1928), 341–57.

———. "Glimpses of Vajrayāna." In *Proceedings and Transactions of the Third Oriental Conference* (*1924*), pp. 129–41. Madras, 1925.

———, ed. *Guhyasamāja Tantra*. Baroda, 1931. (GOS LIII.)

———. "The Home of Tantric Buddhism." In *B. C. Law Volume*, I, 354–61. Poona, 1945–46. 2 vols.

Bhattacharyya, Benoytosh. *The Indian Buddhist Iconography*. Oxford, 1924.

———. *An Introduction to Buddhist Esoterism*. London, 1932.

———, ed. *Niṣpannayogāvalī of Mahāpaṇḍita Abhayākaragupta*. Baroda, 1949. (GOS CIX.)

———. "Origin and Development of Vajrayāna," *IHQ*, III, 4 (1927), 733–46.

———, ed. *Sādhanamālā*. Baroda, 1925, 1928. (GOS XXVI, XLI.) 2 vols.

———, ed. *Śaktisaṅgama Tantra*. Baroda, 1932, 1941, 1947. (GOS LXI, XCI, CIV.) 3 vols.

———, ed. *Two Vajrayāna Works*. Baroda, 1929. (GOS XLIV.)

Bhoja Rāja. *See* Jhā, Gangānātha, and Mitra, Rājendralāla.

Bibliographie bouddhique. Paris, 1930–37. 8 vols.

Bīrūnī, al-. *See* Sachau, Edward C.; *also*, Addenda (A).

Bleichsteiner, Robert. *L'Église jaune*. Paris, 1937. (French tr. of *Die gelbe Kirche*. Vienna, 1937.)

Bloch, Jules. *L'Indo-aryen du Véda aux temps modernes*. Paris, 1934.

———. "Sanskrit et dravidien," *BSL*, XXV (1924), 1–21.

———. "Some Problems of Indo-Āryan Philology," *BSOS*, V, 4 (1928–30), 719–56.

Blochmann, H., and Jarrett, H. S., trs. *Ā'īn-i-Akbarī*. Calcutta, 1873–94. 3 vols.

Blofeld, John, tr. *The Path of Sudden Attainment: a Treatise of the Ch'an (Zen) School of Chinese Buddhism by Hui Hai of the T'ang Dynasty*. London, 1948.

Bloom, A. "Contemplation et ascèse, contribution orthodoxe," *Études carmélitaines* ("Technique et contemplation," 1948), pp. 49 ff.

———. "L'Hésychasme, Yoga chrétien?" in Masui, Jacques (q.v.), ed., *Yoga*, pp. 177–95.

Bloomfield, Maurice. "On the Art of Entering Another's Body: a Hindu Fiction Motif," *Proceedings of the American Philosophical Society* (Philadelphia), LVI (1917), 1–43.

———. "On False Ascetics and Nuns in Hindu Fiction," *JAOS*, XLIV (1924), 202–42.

Bose, Manindra Mohan. "An Introduction to the Study of the Post-Chaitanya Sahajiā Cult," *JDL*, XVI (1927), 1–162.

———. *The Post-Caitanya Sahajiā Cult of Bengal*. Calcutta, 1930.

Brahmānanda Bhaba, tr. *Haṭhayogapradīpikā of Svātmārāma Svāmin.* Bombay, 1889.

Briggs, George W. *The Chamārs.* Calcutta, 1920.

———. *Gorakhnāth and the Kānphaṭā Yogīs.* Calcutta, 1938.

Brown, George William. "Prāṇa and Apāna," *JAOS*, XXXIX (1919), 104–12.

———. "The Sources of Indian Philosophical Ideas." In *Studies in Honor of Maurice Bloomfield*, pp. 75–88. New Haven, 1920.

Buddhaghoṣa. *See* Davids, C. A. F. Rhys.

Bühler, Georg. "Barābar and Nāgārjuni Hill-Cave Inscriptions of Aśoka and Daśaratha," *JRASB*, XX (1901), 362.

———, tr. *The Laws of Manu.* Oxford, 1886. (SBE XXV.)

———, tr. *The Sacred Laws of the Āryas.* Oxford, 1879, 1882. (SBE II, XIV.)

Buitenen, J. A. B. van. "Studies in Sāṃkhya," *JAOS*, LXXVI (1956), 153–57; LXXVII (1957), 15–25, 88–107.

Burgess, James. "Digambara Jaina Iconography," *IA*, XXXII (1903), 459–64.

Burnouf, Eugène. *Introduction à l'histoire du bouddhisme indien.* 2nd edn., Paris, 1876.

Burrow, Thomas. "Dravidian Studies, IV: The Body in Dravidian and Uralian," *BSOS*, XI, 2 (1944), 328–56.

Caland, Willem, ed. *Vaikhānasasmārtasūtram. The Domestic and Sacred Laws of the Vaikhānasa School Belonging to the Black Yoga.* Calcutta, 1929. (BI CCLI.)

Caldwell, Robert. *A Comparative Grammar of the Dravidian or South-Indian Family of Languages.* 3rd edn., rev. and ed. J. L. Wyatt and T. Ramakrishna Pillai. London, 1913.

Carelli, Mario E., ed. *Sekoddeśaṭīkā of Naḍapāda (Nāropā), Being a Commentary of the Sekoddeśa Section of the Kālacakra Tantra.* Baroda, 1941. (GOS XC.)

Carpenter, Joseph Estlin. *Theism in Medieval India.* London, 1921.

Chakravarti, Chintaharan. "Antiquity of Tāntricism," *IHQ*, VI, 1 (1930), 114–26.

———. "The Cult of Bāro Bhāiyā of Eastern Bengal," *JRASB*, XXVI (1930), 379–88.

———. "The Soma or Sauma Sect of the Śaivas," *IHQ*, VIII, 1 (1932), 221–23.

CHALMERS, ROBERT, tr. *Further Dialogues of the Buddha [Majjhima-nikāya]*. London, 1926, 1927. (SBB V, VI.) 2 vols.

CHANDA, RĀMAPRASĀD. *Archaeology and Vaishnava Tradition*. Calcutta, 1920. (Memoirs of the Archaeological Survey of India V.)

———. *Bhanja Dynasty of Mayurbhanj and Their Ancient Capital Khiching*. Mayurbhanj, 1929.

———. *The Indo-Āryan Races*. Rajshahi, 1916.

———. "Medieval Sculpture in Eastern India," *JDL*, III (1920), 225–46.

CHANDLER, J. S. "Names of God in the Tamil Language Which Denote His Oneness," *JAOS*, XLV (1925), 115–18.

CHANG, CHUNG-YUAN. "An Introduction to Taoist Yoga," *Review of Religion* (New York), XXI (1956), 131–48.

CHARPENTIER, JARL. "Ājīvika," *JRAS* (1913), 669–74.

———. *Brahman: eine sprachwissenschaftlich-exegetisch-religionsgeschichtliche Untersuchung*. Uppsala, 1932.

———. "The Meaning and Etymology of Pūjā," *IA*, LVI (1927), 93–98, 130–35. (German tr., in Kirfel, W., ed., *Beiträge zur Literaturwissenschaft und Geistesgeschichte Indiens. Festgabe Hermann Jacobi*, pp. 276–97. Bonn, 1926.)

———. "Some Remarks on the *Bhagavadgītā*," *IA*, LIX (1930), 46–50, 77–80, 101–05, 121–26.

CHATTERJI, SUNITI KUMAR. *The Origin and Development of the Bengali Language*. Calcutta, 1926. 2 vols.

———. "The Study of Kōl," *The Calcutta Review* (Sept., 1923), 451–73.

CHAUDHURI, HEMCHANDRA RAY. *See* RAY CHAUDHURI, HEMCHANDRA.

CHAUDHURI, NANIMADHAB. "A Pre-historic Tree Cult," *IHQ*, XIX, 4 (1943), 318–29.

———. "Rudra-Śiva—as an Agricultural Deity," *IHQ*, XV, 2 (1939), 183–96.

CHAU JU-KUA. *See* HIRTH, FRIEDRICH, and ROCKHILL, WILLIAM W.

CHAVANNES, ÉDOUARD, ed. and tr. *Mémoire sur les religieux éminents qui allèrent chercher la loi dans les pays d'Occident, par Yi-tsing*. Paris, 1894.

———, ed. and tr. *Les Mémoires historiques de Se-ma-Ts'ien [Ssŭ-ma Ch'ien]*. Paris, 1895–1905. 5 vols.

———. *See also* LÉVI, SYLVAIN.

CH'ÊN KUO-FU. *See* DAVIS, TENNEY L.

CHIKASHIGE, MASUMI. *Alchemy and Other Chemical Achievements of the Ancient Orient.* Tokyo, 1936.

CHILDE, VERE GORDON. *New Light on the Most Ancient East.* London, 1934.

CHOU YI-LIANG. "Tantrism in China," *HJAS*, VIII (1945), 241–332.

CHRISTENSEN, ARTHUR. *Les Types du premier homme et du premier roi dans l'histoire légendaire des iraniens.* Uppsala, 1918.

CLARK, WALTER EUGENE. "Śākadvīpa and Śvetadvīpa," *JAOS*, XXXIX (1919), 209–42.

———, ed. *Two Lamaistic Pantheons.* Cambridge (Mass.), 1937. 2 vols.

COLEBROOKE, HENRY THOMAS, tr. *Sāṅkhya Kārikā of Īśvarakṛṣṇa.* Oxford, 1837.

COMBAZ, GISBERT. "L'Évolution du stūpa en Asie," *MCB*, II (1933), 163–305.

———. *L'Inde et l'Orient classique.* Paris, 1937. 2 vols.

———. "Masques et dragons en Asie," *MCB*, VII (1939–45), 1–328.

CONZE, EDWARD. *Buddhism, Its Essence and Development.* New York, 1951.

COOMARASWAMY, ANANDA K. "The 'Conqueror's Life' in Jaina Painting," *JISOA*, III (1935), 127–44.

———. *The Darker Side of the Dawn.* Washington, 1935.

———. *Elements of Buddhist Iconography.* Cambridge (Mass.), 1935.

———. *Figures of Speech or Figures of Thought.* London, 1946.

———. *Hinduism and Buddhism.* New York, 1943.

———. "Indian Architectural Terms," *JAOS*, XLVIII (1928), 250–75.

———. "Mudrā, muddā," *JAOS*, XLVIII (1928), 279–81.

———. "Notes on the *Kāṭha Upaniṣad*," *NIA*, I (1938), 43–56, 83–108, 199–213.

———. "Parāvṛtti: Transformation, Regeneration, Anagogy." In *Festschrift Winternitz*, pp. 232–36. Leipzig, 1933.

———. "The Philosophy of Mediaeval and Oriental Art," *Zalmoxis* (Bucharest), I (1938), 20–49.

———. "Recollection, Indian and Platonic," *JAOS*, Suppl. III (Apr.–June, 1944), 1–18.

———. "Sir Gawain and the Green Knight: Indra and Namuci," *Speculum* (Cambridge, Mass.), XIX (1944), 104–25.

———. "Some Pāli Words," *HJAS*, IV (1939), 116–90.

COOMARASWAMY, ANANDA K. *Spiritual Authority and Temporal Power in the Indian Theory of Government*. New Haven, 1942.

———. "The Tantric Doctrine of Divine Biunity," *ABORI*, XIX (1938), 173–83.

———. *Yakṣas*. Washington, 1928, 1931. 2 vols.

——— and DUGGIRALA, GOPALA KRISTNAYYA, trs. *The Mirror of Gesture, Being the Abhinaya Darpana of Nandikeśvara*. Cambridge (Mass.), 1917.

CORBIN, HENRY. "Le Livre du Glorieux de Jâbir ibn Hayyân. Alchimie et archétypes," *EJ*, XVIII (1949), 47–114.

COWELL, E. B., and GOUGH, A. E., trs. *Mahādeva's Sarva-darśana-saṇgraha*. 2nd edn., London, 1894.

CROOKE, WILLIAM. "Aghorī," in HASTINGS, JAMES (q.v.), ed., *Encyclopaedia of Religion and Ethics*, I, 210–13.

———. *An Introduction to the Popular Religion and Folk-lore of Northern India*. Westminster, 1896. 2 vols.

———. "Secret Messages and Symbols Used in India," *JBORS*, V (1919), 451–62.

———. *The Tribes and Castes of the North-western Provinces and Oudh*. Calcutta, 1896. 4 vols.

CUTTS, ELMER H. "Chinese-Indian Contacts Prior to the Latter Half of the First Century," *IHQ*, XIV, 3 (1938), 486–502.

Dabistān. *See* SHEA, DAVID, and TROYER, ANTHONY.

DAHLMANN, JOSEPH. *Das Mahābhārata als Epos und Rechtsbuch*. Berlin, 1895.

———. *Die Sāṃkhya-Philosophie als Naturlehre und Erlösungslehre*. Berlin, 1902.

DANIÉLOU, ALAIN. *Yoga: the Method of Re-integration*. London, 1949.

DĀRĀ SHIKŪH, MUḤAMMAD. *See* MAHFUZ-UL-HAQ.

DAS-GUPTA, HEM CHANDRA. "A Few Types of Indian Sedentary Games," *JRASB*, n.s. XXII (1926), 211–13.

———. "On a Type of Sedentary Game Prevalent in Shahpur," *JRASB*, n.s. XXVI (1930), 411–12.

DASGUPTA, SHASHI BHUSAN. *An Introduction to Tāntric Buddhism*. Calcutta, 1950.

———. *Obscure Religious Cults as Background of Bengali Literature*. Calcutta, 1946.

DASGUPTA, SURENDRANATH. *A History of Indian Philosophy*. Cambridge, 1922–55. 5 vols. (Vol. I, 1922. Vol. II, 1932.)

———. *Indian Idealism*. Cambridge, 1933.

———. *A Study of Patañjali*. Calcutta, 1920.

———. *Yoga Philosophy in Relation to Other Systems of Indian Thought*. Calcutta, 1930.

———. *Yoga as Philosophy and Religion*. London, 1924.

DAUBRÉE, M. A. "La Génération des minéraux métalliques dans la pratique des mineurs du Moyen Âge, d'après le *Bergbüchlein*," *Journal des savants* (Paris, 1890), 379–92, 441–52.

DAVID-NEEL, ALEXANDRA. "L'Entraînement psychique chez les thibétains," *Bulletin de l'Institut Général Psychologique* (Paris), XXVII (1927), 179–204.

———. *With Mystics and Magicians in Tibet*. London, 1931. (*Mystiques et magiciens du Thibet*. Paris, 1929.)

DAVIDS, C. A. F. RHYS, tr. and ed. *A Buddhist Manual of Psychological Ethics of the Fourth Century* B.C., *Being a Translation . . . of the . . . Dhammasangaṇi*. London, 1900.

———. "Dhyāna in Early Buḍdhism," *IHQ*, III, 4 (1927), 689–715.

———. "Religiöse Übungen in Indien und der religiöse Mensch," *EJ*, I (1933), 95–134.

———. "Sāṇkhya and Original Buddhism," *IHQ*, IX, 2 (1933), 585–87.

———, ed. *The Visuddhimagga of Buddhaghoṣa*, tr. P. M. Tin (*The Way of Purity*). London, 1920–21. (PTS XI, XVII, XXI.)

——— and AUNG, S. Z., trs. and eds. *The Compendium of Philosophy, Being a Translation . . . of the Abidhammattha-saṇgaha*. London, 1910.

——— and WOODWARD, F. L., trs. and eds. *The Book of the Kindred Sayings* [*Samyutta-nikāya*]. London, 1917–30. (PTS VII, X, XIII, XIV, XVI.)

DAVIDS, T. W. RHYS. *Buddhist India*. London, 1903.

———. *The Yogāvacara's Manual of Indian Mysticism as Practised by Buddhists*. London, 1896.

——— and DAVIDS, C. A. F. RHYS. *Dialogues of the Buddha*. Oxford, 1899, 1910, 1921. (SBB II, III, IV.) 3 vols.

——— and OLDENBERG, HERMANN. *Vinaya Texts*. Oxford, 1881–85. (SBE XIII, XVII, XX.) 3 vols.

DAVIES, JOHN, tr. *The Sānkhya Kārikā of Īswara Krishṇa*. London, 1881.

DAVIS, TENNEY L. "The Dualistic Cosmogony of Huai-nan-tzŭ and Its Relations to the Background of Chinese and of European Alchemy," *Isis* (Bruges), XXV (1936), 325–40.

———. "Ko Hung (Pao P'u Tzŭ), Chinese Alchemist of the Fourth Century," *JCE*, XI (1934), 517–20.

——— and CH'ÊN KUO-FU. "The Inner Chapters of *Pao-p'u-tzŭ*," *PAAAS*, LXXIV (1940–42), 297–325.

——— and WU, LU-CH'IANG. "An Ancient Chinese Treatise on Alchemy, Entitled *Ts'an T'ung Ch'i*, Written by Wei Po-yang about 142 A.D.," *Isis* (Bruges), XVIII (1932), 210–89.

———. "Chinese Alchemy," *The Scientific Monthly* (New York), XXXI (1930), 225–35.

———. "Ko Hung on the Gold Medicine and on the Yellow and the White, the Fourth and Sixteenth Chapters of *Pao-p'u-tzŭ*," *PAAAS*, LXX (1935), 221–84.

———. "T'ao Hung-ching," *JCE*, IX (1932), 859–62.

DE, D. L. "Pāñcarātra and the Upaniṣads," *IHQ*, IX, 3 (1933), 645–62.

DE, SUSHĪL KUMĀR. "Bhāgavatism and Sun-worship," *BSOS*, VI, 3 (1931), 669–72.

———. "The Bhakti-Rasa-Śāstra of Bengal Vaiṣṇavism," *IHQ*, VIII, 4 (1932), 643–88.

———. "The Buddhist Tantric Literature (Sanskrit) of Bengal," *NIA*, I (1938), 1–23.

DEFRÉMERY, CHARLES FRANÇOIS, and SANGUINETTI, B. R., trs. *Voyages d'ibn Batoutah*. Paris, 1853–59. 4 vols.

DEMIÉVILLE, PAUL, ed. *Hôbôgirin; dictionnaire encyclopédique du bouddhisme d'après les sources chinoises et japonaises*, published under the direction of Sylvain Lévi and J. Takakusu. Fasc. I–III. Tokyo, 1929–37.

———. Review of *Le Traité de la Grande Vertu de sagesse de Nāgārjuna*, ed. and tr. É. Lamotte, *JA*, CCXXXVIII (1950), 375–95.

———. "Sur la mémoire des existences antérieures," *BEFEO*, XXVII (1927), 283–98.

DERMENGHEM, ÉMILE. "Techniques d'extase en Islam," in MASUI, JACQUES (q.v.), ed., *Yoga*, pp. 274–83.

DEUSSEN, PAUL. *Allgemeine Geschichte der Philosophie*. Leipzig, 1899–1920. 7 vols.

———. *Die nachvedische Philosophie der Inder*. 3rd edn., Leipzig, 1920.

DEUSSEN, PAUL. *Die Philosophie der Upanishads.* 4th edn., Leipzig, 1920. (*The Philosophy of the Upanishads,* tr. A. S. Geden. Edinburgh, 1906.)

———. *Sechzig Upanishad's des Vedas aus dem Sanskrit übersetzt.* Leipzig, 1897.

DHRUVA, A. B. "Trividham Anumānam, or a Study in *Nyāyasūtra* I.1.5." In *Proceedings and Transactions of the First Oriental Conference (1919)*, II, 251–80. Poona, 1920. 2 vols.

DIKSHITAR, V. R. RAMCHANDRA. "Origin and Early History of Caityas," *IHQ*, XIV, 3 (1938), 440–51.

DIVANJI, P. C., "The *Yogayājñavalkya*," *Journal of the Bombay Branch of the Royal Asiatic Society*, n.s. XXVIII (1953), 99–158, 215–68; XXIX (1954), 96–128.

DRACOTT, ALICE E. *Simla Village Tales.* London, 1906.

DUBOIS, JEAN ANTOINE. *Mœurs, institutions et cérémonies des peuples de l'Inde.* Paris, 1825. 2 vols.

DUBS, HOMER H. "The Beginnings of Alchemy," *Isis* (Bruges), XXXVIII (1947), 62–86.

DUGGIRALA, G. K. *See* COOMARASWAMY, ANANDA K.

DUMÉZIL, GEORGES. *Flamen-Brahman.* Paris, 1935. (Annales du Musée Guimet. Bibliothèque de vulgarisation LI.)

———. *Horace et les Curiaces.* Paris, 1942.

———. *Jupiter, Mars, Quirinus. IV.* Paris, 1948. (Bibliothèque de l'École des Hautes Études LXII.)

———. *Légendes sur les Nartes.* Paris, 1930.

———. *Naissance d'archanges.* Paris, 1945.

DUMONT, PAUL ÉMILE, ed. *L'Aśvamedha.* Paris, 1927.

———. "Sunaphā. Note sur un passage de l'*Īśvaragītā* du *Kūrmapurāṇa*," *BCLS*, ser. V, vol. XVII (1931), 444–50.

DURME, P. J. VAN. "Notes sur le Lamaïsme," *MCB*, I (1931–32), 263–321.

DUTT, NALINAKSHA. "Notes on the Nāgārjunikoṇḍa Inscriptions," *IHQ*, VII, 3 (1931), 633–53.

EDGERTON, FRANKLIN, tr. *The Bhagavad Gītā.* Cambridge (Mass.), 1944. (HOS XXXVIII, XXXIX.) 2 vols.

———. "The Meaning of Sānkhya and Yoga," *AJP*, XLV (1924), 1–46.

EHRENFELS, OMAR ROLF VON. "Traces of a Matriarchal Civilization Among the Kolli Mailayālis," *JRASB*, IX (1943), 29–82.

EISLER, ROBERT. "Das Quainzeichen und die Queniter," *MO*, XXIII (1929), 48–112.

ELIADE, MIRCEA. *Alchimia asiatica*. Bucharest, 1935.

* ———. *Le Chamanisme et les techniques archaïques de l'extase*. Paris, 1951.

———. "Cosmical Homology and Yoga," *JISOA*, V (1937), 188–203.

* ———. *Forgerons et alchimistes*. Paris, 1956.

* ———. *Images et symboles*. Paris, 1952.

———. *Metallurgy, Magic and Alchemy*. Paris and Bucharest, 1938.

* ———. *Le Mythe de l'éternel retour*. Paris, 1949. (*The Myth of the Eternal Return*, tr. Willard R. Trask. New York, 1954. [BS XLVI].)

* ———. "La Nostalgie du paradis dans les traditions primitives," *Diogène* (Paris), III (1953), 31–45.

———. "Notes de démonologie," *Zalmoxis* (Bucharest), I (1938), 197–203.

———. "Symbolisme religieux et angoisse." In *Angoisse du temps présent et les devoirs de l'esprit*, pp. 55–71. Geneva, 1953.

———. "La Terre-Mère et les hiérogamies cosmiques," *EJ*, XXII (1953), 57–95.

* ———. *Traité d'histoire des religions*. Paris, 1949.

ELIAS, NEY, ed. *A History of the Moghuls of Central Asia, the Tārīkh-i-Raschīdī of Muḥammad Haidar Dughlāt*, tr. E. D. Ross. London, 1895.

ELLIOT, SIR HENRY MIERS. *The History of India as Told by Its Own Historians*, ed. John Dowson. London, 1867–77. 8 vols.

ELMORE, WILBER THEODORE. *Dravidian Gods in Modern Hinduism*. Lincoln (Neb.), 1915.

ESNOUL, ANNE MARIE, tr. *Maitrī Upaniṣad*. Paris, 1952.

EVANS-WENTZ, W. Y., ed. *The Tibetan Book of the Dead* (*Bardo Thödol*), tr. Lama Kazi Dawa-Samdup. 2nd edn., London, 1949.

———, ed. *Tibetan Yoga and Secret Doctrines; or, Seven Books of Wisdom of the Great Path*, tr. Lama Kazi Dawa-Samdup. Oxford, 1935.

———, ed. *Tibet's Great Yogī Milarepa; Being the Jetsün-Kahbum*, tr. Lama Kazi Dawa-Samdup. Oxford, 1928.

EVOLA, GIULIO CESARE. *La Dottrina del risveglio*. Bari, 1943.

———. *La Tradizione ermetica*. Bari, 1931.

———. *Lo Yoga della potenza* (*saggio sui Tantra*). Milan, 1949.

Ewing, Arthur H. "The Hindu Conception of the Functions of Breath," *JAOS*, XXII (1901), 249–308.

———. "The *Śāradā-tilaka Tantra*," *JAOS*, XXIII (1902), 65–76.

Faddegon, Barend. *The Vaiśeṣika-System, Described with the Help of the Oldest Texts*. Amsterdam, 1918.

Falk, Maryla. "Il Mito psicologico nell' India antica," *MRANL*, ser. VI, vol. VIII, fasc. V (1939), 289–738.

Farquhar, John Nicol. "The Fighting Ascetics of India," *Bulletin of the John Rylands Library* (Manchester), IX (1925), 431–52.

———. "The Organization of the Sannyāsīs of the Vedānta," *JRAS*, 479–86.

———. *An Outline of the Religious Literature of India*. Oxford, 1920.

———. "Temple and Image Worship in Hinduism," *JRAS* (1928), 15–23.

Fausbøll, Viggo, tr. *The Sutta-Nipāta*. Oxford, 1881. (SBE X, pt. II).

Feifel, Eugen, ed. and tr. "*Pao-p'u Tzŭ*," *MS*, VI (1941), 113–211; IX (1944), 1–33.

Festugière, R. P. *La Révélation d'Hermès Trismégiste*. Paris, 1944.

Filliozat, Jean. "La Doctrine des brâhmanes d'après saint Hippolyte," *RHR*, CXXX (1945), 59–91.

———. *La Doctrine classique de la médecine indienne*. Paris, 1949.

———. "Les Échanges de l'Inde et de l'Empire romain aux premiers siècles de l'ère chrétienne," *Revue historique* (Paris), CCI (1949), 1–29.

———. *Étude de démonologie indienne; le Kumāratantra de Rāvaṇa et les textes parallèles indiens, tibétains, chinois, cambodgiens et arabes*. Paris, 1937.

———. "Les Limites des pouvoirs humains dans l'Inde." In *Limites de l'humain*, pp. 23–38. Paris, 1943. (Études carmélitaines.)

———. "Liste des manuscrits de la collection Palmyr Cordier conservés à la Bibliothèque Nationale," *JA*, CCXXIV (1934), 155–73.

———. *Magie et médecine*. Paris, 1943.

———. "Nāgārjuna et Agastya, médecins, chimistes et sorciers." In *Actes du XXe Congrès international des Orientalistes* (*1938*), pp. 228 ff. Brussels, 1940.

———. "Les Origines d'une technique mystique indienne," *Revue philosophique* (Paris), CXXXVI (1946), 208–20.

———. Review of *Daśopanishads with the Commentary of Śrī Upanishad-Brahma-Yogin*, ed. Kunhan Rāja, *JA*, CCXXVIII (1937), 522.

FILLIOZAT, JEAN. Review of *Rasa-jala-nidhi*, by Rasacharya Kaviraj Mookerjee, *JA*, CCXXIII (1933), 110–12.

———. "Sur la 'concentration oculaire' dans le Yoga," *Yoga* (Harburg-Wilhelmsburg), I (1931), 93–102.

———. "Taoïsme et Yoga," *Dân Viêt-nam*, III (Aug., 1949), 113–20.

———. *See also* RENOU, LOUIS.

FINOT, LOUIS. "Manuscrits sanskrits de Sādhana's retrouvés en Chine," *JA*, CCXXV (1934), 1–86.

FORKE, ALFRED. "Ko Hung, der Philosoph und Alchimist," *Archiv für Geschichte der Philosophie* (Berlin), XLI (1932), 115–26.

———. *The World-Conception of the Chinese*. London, 1925.

FOUCHER, ALFRED CHARLES AUGUSTE. *Étude sur l'iconographie bouddhique de l'Inde*. Paris, 1900–1905. 2 pts.

———. *La Vie du Bouddha, d'après les textes et les monuments de l'Inde*. Paris, 1949.

FRANCKE, R. OTTO. "Mudrā = Schrift (oder Lesekunst)?" *ZDMG*, XLVI (1892), 731–34.

FRAZER, SIR JAMES GEORGE. *The Dying God*. London, 1918.

———. *Spirits of the Corn and of the Wild*. London, 1912. 2 vols.

FRYER, JOHN. *A New Account of East India and Persia*, ed. William Crooke. London, 1909–15. 3 vols.

GAIT, SIR EDWARD ALBERT. *A History of Assam*. 2nd edn., Calcutta, 1926.

———. "Human Sacrifices in Ancient Assam," *JRASB*, LXVII (1903), 56–65.

GARBE, RICHARD, tr. *Aniruddha's Commentary and the Original Part of Vedāntin Mahādeva's Commentary on the Saṃkhya Sūtras*. Calcutta, 1891–92. (BI CXXXI.)

———, ed. *Aniruddha's Sāṃkhya-sūtra-vṛtti*. Calcutta, 1888–89. (BI CXXII.)

———. "Der Mondschein der Sāṃkhya-Wahrheit, Vācaspatimiśra's *Sāṃkhya-tattva-kaumudī*," *ABAW*, Phil.-phil. Klasse, XIX (1890–92), 517–628.

———. "Pañcaśikha Fragmente." In *Festgruss an Rudolph von Roth*, ed. E. W. A. Kuhn, pp. 77–80. Stuttgart, 1893.

———. *Die Sāṃkhya-Philosophie, eine Darstellung des indischen Rationalismus*. Leipzig, 1894.

———, ed. *The Sāṅkhya-pravacana-bhāṣya; or, Commentary on the Exposition of the Sāṅkhya Philosophy*. Cambridge (Mass.), 1895.

(HOS II.) (In German, *Sāṃkhya-pravacana-bhāṣya, Vijñānabhikṣu's Commentar zu den Sāṃkhya-sūtras*, in *Abhandlungen für die Kunde des Morgenlandes* [Leipzig], IX [1889].)

———. *Sāṃkhya and Yoga*. Strassburg, 1896.

———. "Über den willkürlichen Scheintod indischer Fakirs." In *Beiträge zur indischen Kulturgeschichte*, pp. 199 ff. Berlin, 1903.

GARDET, LOUIS. "La Mention du nom divin (dhikr) dans la mystique musulmane," *Revue Thomiste* (Paris), LII (1952), 642–79; LIII (1953), 197–216.

GAUḌAPĀDA. *See* WILSON, HORACE HAYMAN.

GELPKE, F. "Induskultur und Hinduismus. Vorarische Elemente der indischen Kultur," *OZ*, n.s. XVII (1941), 201–05.

GETTY, ALICE. *The Gods of Northern Buddhism*. Oxford, 1914.

GHOSH, JAMINI MOHAN. *Sannyāsī and Fakir Raiders in Bengal*. Calcutta, 1930.

GHOSHA, PRATĀPACHANDRA. *Durgā Pūjā*. Calcutta, 1841.

GLASENAPP, HELMUTH VON. *Buddhistische Mysterien*. Stuttgart, 1940. (French tr., *Mystères bouddhistes*. Paris, 1944.)

———. "Ein buddhistischer Initiationsritus der javanischen Mittelalters," *Tribus* (Stuttgart), n.s. II–III (1952–54), 259–74.

———. "Die Entstehung des Vajrayāna," *ZDMG*, XC (1936), 546–72.

———. *Der Jainismus, eine indische Erlösungsreligion*. Berlin, 1925.

———. "Die Lehre Vallabhācāryas," *ZII*, IX (1932–34), 268–330.

———. *Die Philosophie der Inder*. Stuttgart, 1949. (French tr., *La Philosophie indienne*. Paris, 1951.)

———. "Tantrismus und Śaktismus," *OZ*, n.s. XII (1936), 120–33.

GODEL, ROGER. *Essais sur l'expérience libératrice*. Paris, 1952.

GOLDZIHER, IGNAZ. *Vorlesungen über den Islam*. Heidelberg, 1910.

GOLUBEV, VIKTOR. "Essais sur l'art de l'Indus: I: L'Homme au châle de Mohenjo-Daro," *BEFEO*, XXXVIII (1938; pub. 1940), 255–80.

GONDA, JAN. *Notes on Brahman*. Utrecht, 1950.

———, ed. *The Ṛgvidhāna*. Utrecht, 1951.

GOPĪNĀTHA RAO, T. A. *Elements of Hindu Iconography*. Madras, 1914–16. 4 vols.

GORDON, ANTOINETTE K. *The Iconography of Tibetan Lamaism*. New York, 1939.

———. *Tibetan Religious Art*. New York, 1952.

GOUGH, A. E. *See* COWELL, E. B.

GOUILLARD, JEAN. *Petite Philocalie de la prière du cœur*. Paris, 1953.

GOVINDACARYA SVĀMIN, A. "The Pāñcarātras or *Bhāgavat-Śāstra*," *JRAS* (1911), 935–61.

GRANET, MARCEL. *Danses et légendes de la Chine ancienne*. Paris, 1926. 2 vols.

———. *La Pensée chinoise*. Paris, 1934.

GRASS, KARL KONRAD. *Die russischen Sekten*. Leipzig, 1905–14. 3 vols.

GRIERSON, SIR GEORGE A., ed. *Linguistic Survey of India*. Calcutta, 1903–28. 11 vols. in 19.

———. "The Nārāyanīya and the Bhāgavatas," *IA*, XXXVII (1908), 251–62, 373–86.

GROOT, JAN J. M. DE. *The Religious System of China*. Leiden, 1892–1910. 6 vols.

GROWSE, FREDERIC SALMON. *Mathurā: a District Memoir*. 3rd edn., Allahabad, 1885.

GRÜNWEDEL, ALBERT. *Alt-Kutscha. Archäologische und Religionsgeschichtliche Forschungen an Tempera-Gemälden aus buddhistischen Höhlen der ersten acht Jahrhunderte nach Christi Geburt*. Berlin, 1920. (Veröffentlichung der Preussischen Turfan-Expeditionen.) 2 vols.

———. "Die Geschichten der vierundachtzig Zauberer (Mahāsiddhas) aus dem tibetischen übersetzt," *Baessler-Archiv* (Leipzig), V (1916), 137–228.

———. *Die Legenden des Nā-ro-pa, des Hauptvertreters des Nekromanten- und Hexentums*. Leipzig, 1933.

———. *Tāranātha's Edelsteinminne*. Petrograd, 1914. (BB VIII.)

———. "Der Weg nach Śambhala," *ABAW*, Phil.-phil. und hist. Klasse, XXIX, Abh. 3 (1915), 1–118.

GUÉRINOT, ARMAND ALBERT. *La Religion djaïna*. Paris, 1926.

GUHA, ABHAYAKUMAR. "Rasa-Cult in the *Chaitanya Charitāmṛta*." In *Sir Asutosh Mookerjee Silver Jubilee Volumes*, vol. III, pt. 3, pp. 368–88. Calcutta, 1921–27. 3 vols. in 5.

GULIK, ROBERT HANS VAN. *Erotic Colour Prints of the Ming Period, with an Essay on Chinese Sex Life from the Han to the Ch'ing Dynasty, 206 B.C.–A.D. 1644*. Tokyo, 1951 (pub. privately).

———. *Hayagrīva, the Mantrayānic Aspect of Horse-Cult in China and Japan*. Leiden, 1935.

GÜNTERT, HERMANN. *Der arische Weltkönig und Heiland*. Halle, 1923.

GURDON, PHILIP RICHARD THORNHAGH. *The Khāsīs*. London, 1907.

HALL, FITZ-EDWARD. *A Contribution Towards an Index to the Bibliography of the Indian Philosophical Systems*. Calcutta, 1859.

HARIYANNA, M. "*Ṣaṣṭi-tantra* and Vārsaganya," *JOR*, III (1929), 107–12.

HARTMAN, SVEN S. *Gayomart*. Uppsala, 1953.

HASTINGS, JAMES, ed. *Encyclopaedia of Religion and Ethics*. New York, 1928. 13 vols.

HAUER, J. W. *Die Anfänge der Yogapraxis*. Stuttgart, 1922.

———. *Die Dhāraṇī im nördlichen Buddhismus und ihre Parallelen in der sogenannten Mithrasliturgie*. Stuttgart, 1927.

———. "Das IV. Buch des *Yogasūtra*. Ein Beitrag zu seiner Erklärung und Zeitbestimmung." In Wüst, Walther, ed., *Studia Indo-Iranica, Ehrengabe für Wilhelm Geiger*, pp. 122–33. Leipzig, 1931.

———. *Glaubensgeschichte der Indogermanen*. Stuttgart, 1937. 2 vols.

———. *Das Laṇkāvatāra-Sūtra und das Sāṃkhya*. Stuttgart, 1927.

———. "Die *Śvetāśvatara-Upaniṣad*, ein monotheistischer Traktat einer Rudra-Śiva-Gemeinde," *ZDMG*, LXXXIV (1930), 37 ff.

———. "Eine Übersetzung der Yoga-Merksprüche des Patañjali mit dem Kommentar des Vyāsa," *Yoga* (Harburg-Wilhelmsburg), I (1931), 25–43.

———. *Der Vrātya. Untersuchungen über die nichtbrahmanische Religion Altindiens. I: Die Vrātya als nichtbrahmanische Kultgenossenschaften arischer Herkunft*. Stuttgart, 1927.

———. *Der Yoga als Heilweg*. Stuttgart, 1932.

HAUSCHILD, RICHARD. *Die Śvetāśvatara-Upaniṣad: eine kritische Ausgabe mit einer Übersetzung und einer Übersicht über ihre Lehren*. Leipzig, 1927.

HAUSHERR, IRENÉE. "L'Hésychasme: étude de spiritualité," *Orientalia Christiana Periodica* (Rome), XXII (1956), 5–40, 247–85.

———. *La Méthode d'oraison hésychaste*. Rome, 1927. (Orientalia Christiana, IX, 2.)

HAZRA, RAJENDRA CHANDRA. "Influence of Tantra on the Tattvas of Raghunandana," *IHQ*, IX, 3 (1933), 678–704.

HEIMANN, BETTY. *Studien zur Eigenart indischen Denkens*. Tübingen, 1930.

HEINE-GELDERN, ROBERT. "Ein Beitrag zur Chronologie des Neolithikums in Südostasien." In Koppers, W., ed., *Festschrift. Publication d'hommage offerte au P. W. Schmidt*, pp. 809–43. Vienna, 1928.

HEINE-GELDERN, ROBERT. "Kopfjagd und Menschenopfer in Assam und Birma und ihre Ausstrahlungen nach Vorderindien," *MAGW*, XLVII (1917), 1–65.

———. "Mutterrecht und Kopfjagd im westlichen Hinterindien," *MAGW*, LI (1921), 105–40.

———. "Die Osterinselschrift," *A*, XXXIII (1938), 815–909.

———. "Urheimat und früheste Wanderungen der Austronesier," *A*, XXVII (1932), 543–619.

HELD, G. J. *The Mahābhārata: an Ethnological Study*. London, 1935.

HEMBERG, BENGT. "Die Idaiischen Daktylen," *Eranos* (Uppsala), L (1952), 41–59.

———. *Die Kabiren*. Uppsala, 1950.

HENRY, VICTOR. "Physique védique," *JA*, ser. X, vol. VI (1905), 385–409.

HENTZE, CARL. "Zur ursprünglichen Bedeutung des chinesischen Zeichens *t'ou* = Kopf," *A*, XLV (1950), 801–20.

HERAS, HENRY. "More about Mohenjo Daro," *NIA*, I (1939), 637–41.

HERTEL, JOHANNES. *Indische Märchen*. Jena, 1921.

HERTZ, ROBERT. *Mélanges de sociologie religieuse et folklore*. Paris, 1928.

HEVESY, WILHELM VON. "The Easter Island and the Indus Valley Scripts," *A*, XXXIII (1938), 808–14.

HILL, WILLIAM DOUGLAS P., tr. *The Bhagavadgītā*. London, 1928.

HILLEBRANDT, ALFRED. *Vedische Mythologie*. 2nd edn., Breslau, 1927–29. 2 vols.

HIRTH, FRIEDRICH. *China and the Roman Orient*. Leipzig, 1885.

——— and ROCKHILL, WILLIAM WOODVILLE, trs. *Chau Ju-kua: His Work on the Chinese and the Arab Trade in the Twelfth and Thirteenth Centuries, Entitled Chu-fan-chï*. St. Petersburg, 1911.

History of the Sect of Mahārājas, or Vallabhāchāryas, in Western India. London, 1865.

HOCART, ARTHUR MAURICE. "Flying Through the Air," *IA*, LII (1923), 80–82.

HOENS, DIRK JAN. *Śānti: a Contribution to Ancient Indian Religious Terminology*. The Hague, 1951.

HOERNLE, A. F. R. "Ājīvikas," in HASTINGS, JAMES (q.v.), ed., *Encyclopaedia of Religion and Ethics*, I, 259–68.

———, ed. *The Bower Manuscript*. Calcutta, 1893–1912.

———, ed. and tr. *Uvāsagadasāo; or, The Religious Professions of an Uvāsaga*. Calcutta, 1885–90. (BI CV.) 2 vols. in 1.

Holl, Karl. *Enthusiasmus und Bussgewalt beim griechischen Mönchtum.* Leipzig, 1898.

Hommel, Fritz. "Pāli muddā = babylonisch musarū und die Herkunft der indischen Schrift." In Wüst, Walther, ed., *Studia Indo-Iranica. Ehrengabe für Wilhelm Geiger*, pp. 73–84. Leipzig, 1931.

Honigberger, John Martin. *Thirty-five Years in the East.* London, 1852. 2 vols. in 1.

Hopkins, Edward Washburn. "The Fountain of Youth," *JAOS*, XXVI (1905), 1–67, 411–15.

———. *The Great Epic of India.* New York, 1901. 2nd edn., New York, 1920.

———. "Yoga-Technique in the Great Epic," *JAOS*, XXII (1901), 333–79.

Hornell, James. "The Boats of the Ganges," *Memoirs of the Asiatic Society of Bengal* (Calcutta), VIII (1921), 173–98.

———. "The Origins and Ethnological Significance of Indian Boat Designs," *Memoirs of the Asiatic Society of Bengal*, VII (1920), 139–256.

Horner, I. B. "Gotama and the Other Sects," *JAOS*, LXVI (1946), 283–89.

Horten, Max. *Indische Strömmungen in der islamischen Mystik.* Heidelberg, 1927–28. 2 vols.

Hrozný, Bedřich. "Inschriften und Kultur der Proto-Inder von Mohenjo-Daro und Harappā," *Archiv orientální* (Prague), XII, 3–4 (1941), 192–259; XIII, 1–2 (1942), 1–102.

Hughes, Thomas Patrick. *A Dictionary of Islam.* London, 1885.

Hui Hai. *See* Blofeld, John.

Hultkrantz, Ake. *Conceptions of the Soul Among North American Indians.* Stockholm, 1953.

Hultzsch, Eugen. "Sāṃkhya und Yoga in Śiśupālayadha." In Negelein, Julius von, ed., *Aus Indiens Kultur: Festgabe, Richard von Garbe*, pp. 78–83. Erlangen, 1927.

Hume, Robert Ernest, tr. *The Thirteen Principal Upanishads.* London, 1921.

Hummel, Siegbert. "Die Lamaistischen Tempelfahnen und ihre Beziehung zu Yoga," *Tribus* (Stuttgart), I (1952–53), 239–52.

Ibn Baṭūṭah. *See* Defrémery, Charles François, and Sanguinetti, B. R.

ĪŚVARAKṚṢṆA. *See* COLEBROOKE, HENRY THOMAS; DAVIES, JOHN; GARBE, RICHARD; ŚĀSTRI, S. S. SURYANARAYANA; SINHA, NANDALAL, and WILSON, HORACE HAYMAN.

JACOBI, HERMANN. "The Dates of the Philosophical Sūtras of the Brāhmans," *JAOS*, XXXI (1910), 1–29.

———. *Gaina Sūtras*. Oxford, 1884, 1895. (SBE XXII, XLV.) 2 vols.

———. *Mahābhārata: Inhaltsangabe, Index und Konkordanz der Kalcuttaer und Bombayer Ausgaben*. Bonn, 1903.

———. "On Mahāvīra and His Predecessors," *IA*, IX (1880), 158–63.

———. Reviews of *Die Sāṃkhya-Philosophie*, by Richard Garbe, *Göttingische gelehrte Anzeigen*, CLVII (1895), 202–11; CLXXXI (1919), 1–30.

———. "Sind nach dem Sāṅkhya-Lehrer Pañcaśikha die *Puruṣas* von Atomgrösse?" *BSOS*, VI, 2 (1931), 385–88.

———. "Über das Alter der Yogaśāstra," *ZII*, VIII (1931), 80–88.

———. "Über das ursprüngliche Yogasystem," *Sitzungsberichte der preussischen Akademie der Wissenschaften* (Berlin), XXVI (1929), 581–624.

———. "Über das Verhältnis der buddhistischen Philosophie zu Sānkhya-Yoga und die Bedeutung des Nidānas," *ZDMG*, LII (1898), 1–15.

———. "Der Ursprung des Buddhismus aus dem Sānkhya-Yoga," *NGWG*, phil.-hist. Klasse (1896), 43–58.

JACOBY, ADOLF. "Zum Zerstückelungs- und Wiederbelebungswunder der indischen Fakire," *Archiv für Religionswissenschaft* (Leipzig), XVII (1914), 455–75.

JHĀ, GANGĀNĀTHA, ed. and tr. *Manu-Smṛti: the Laws of Manu with the Bhāṣya of Medhātithi*. Calcutta, 1920–26. 9 vols.

———, tr. *The Tattva-kaumudī* (*Vācaspati Miśra's Commentary on the Sāṃkhya-kārikā*). Bombay, 1896.

———, tr. *The Tattvasaṅgraha of Śāntarakṣita, with the Commentary of Kamalaśīla*. Baroda, 1937–39. (GOS LXXX, LXXXIII.) 2 vols.

———, ed. *The Yoga-Darśana. The Sūtras of Patañjali, with the Bhāṣya of Vyāsa, with Notes from Vācaspati Miśra's Tattvavaiśāradī, Vijñāna Bhikṣu's Yogavārtika and Bhoja's Rājamārtanda*. Bombay, 1907. 2nd edn., Madras, 1934.

———, tr. *Yogasāra-saṅgraha of Vijñānabhikṣu*. Bombay, 1894.

JOHNSON, OBED SIMON. *A Study of Chinese Alchemy*. Shanghai, 1928.

JOHNSTON, EDWARD HAMILTON. *The Buddhacarita; or, Acts of the Buddha.* Calcutta, 1935–36. (Panjab University Oriental Publications XXXI, XXXII.) 2 vols.
———. *Early Sāṁkhya.* London, 1937.
———. "Some Sāṁkhya and Yoga Conceptions of the *Śvetāśvatara Upaniṣad,*" *JRAS* (1930), 855–78.
JOLLY, JULIUS, tr. *The Institutes of Vishnu.* Oxford, 1880. (SBE VII.)
———. "Der Stein der Weisen." In *Festschrift Ernst Windisch,* pp. 98–106. Leipzig, 1914.
JUGIE, MARTIN. "Les Origines de la méthode d'oraison des hésychastes," *Echos d'Orient* (Paris), XXX, 162 (1931), 179–85.
JUNG, C. G. "Concerning Mandala Symbolism." In *Archetypes and the Collective Unconscious,* tr. R. F. C. Hull. New York and London, 1959 (Collected Works, 9, i.)
———. *Psychology and Alchemy,* tr. R. F. C. Hull. New York and London, 1953. (Collected Works, 12.)
———. "Psychology of the Transference," in *The Practice of Psychotherapy,* tr. R. F. C. Hull. New York and London, 1954. (Collected Works, 16.)
KALTENMARK, MAX, ed. and tr. *Le Lie-sien tchouan* (*Biographies légendaires des Immortels taoïstes de l'antiquité.*) Peking, 1953.
KAMALAŚĪLA. *See* JHĀ, GANGĀNĀTHA.
KAPILA. *See* BALLANTYNE, J. R.
KEITH, ARTHUR BERRIEDALE. *Buddhist Philosophy in India and Ceylon.* Oxford, 1923.
———. "The Doctrine of the Buddha," *BSOS,* VI, 2 (1931), 393–404.
———. *A History of Sanskrit Literature.* Oxford, 1928.
———. *Indian Logic and Atomism.* Oxford, 1921.
———. "The *Māṭhara-Vṛtti,*" *BSOS,* III, 3 (1924), 551–54.
———. "New Theories as to *Brahman.*" In *Jhā Commemoration Volume,* pp. 214 ff. Poona, 1937.
———. *The Religion and Philosophy of the Veda and Upanishads.* Cambridge (Mass.), 1925. (HOS XXXI, XXXII.) 2 vols.
———. *Rigveda Brāhmaṇas.* Cambridge (Mass.), 1920. (HOS XXV.)
———. *The Sāṃkhya System.* 2nd edn., Calcutta, 1924.
———. "Some Problems of Indian Philosophy," *IHQ,* VIII, 3 (1932), 425–41.
KENNEDY, MELVILLE T. *The Chaitanya Movement.* Calcutta, 1925.

KERN, JOHAN HENDRIK CASPAR. *Der Buddhismus und seine Geschichte in Indien*, tr. Hermann Jacobi. Leipzig, 1882–84. 2 vols.

———. *Manual of Indian Buddhism*. Strassburg, 1896.

KHAKHAR, DALPATRĀM PRĀNJIVAN. "History of the Kānphaṭās of Kachh," *IA*, VII (1878), 47–53.

KIMURA, R. "A Historical Study of the Terms Mahāyāna and Hinayāna and the Origin of Mahāyāna Buddhism," *JDL*, XI (1924), 1–43; XII (1925), 45–193.

KLEEN, TYRA DE. *Mudrās: the Ritual Hand-Poses of the Buddha Priests and the Shiva Priests of Bali*. London, 1924. 2nd edn., London, 1942.

KNOWLES, JAMES HINTON. *Folk-tales of Kashmir*. 2nd edn., London, 1893.

KONOW, STEN. "A European Parallel to the Durgāpūjā," *JRASB*, n.s. XXI (1925), 315–24.

———. *Das indische Drama*. Berlin and Leipzig, 1920.

———. *Mūṇḍā and Dravidian Languages*. Calcutta, 1906. (Sir George A. Grierson, ed., *Linguistic Survey of India*, vol. IV.)

KOPPERS, WILHELM. "Probleme der indischen Religionsgeschichte," *A*, XXXV–XXXVI (1940–41), 761–814.

KRAMRISCH, STELLA. *The Hindu Temple*. Calcutta, 1946. 2 vols.

KRISHNAMACHARYA, EMBAR, tr. and ed. *Tattva-saṅgraha of Śāntarakṣīta*. Baroda, 1926. (GOS XXX, XXXI.) 2 vols.

KRISHNAMURTI SARMA, B. N. "New Light on the *Gauḍapāda-Kārikās*," *Review of Philosophy and Religion* (Academy of Philosophy and Religion, Poona), II (1931), 35–56.

KROEBER, ALFRED LOUIS. *Anthropology*. New York, 1923. Rev. edn., New York, 1948.

KUIPER, F. B. J. "An Austro-Asiatic Myth in the *Rig-Veda*," *Mededelingen der koninklijke Nederlandse Akademie van Wetenschappen* (Amsterdam), n.s. XIII, 7 (1950), 163–82.

———. "Mūṇḍā and Indonesian," *Orientalia neerlandica* (Leiden, 1948), 372–401.

———. "Proto-Mūṇḍā Words in Sanskrit," *Verhandeling der koninklijke Nederlandse Akademie van Wetenschappen* (Amsterdam), LI, 3 (1948).

LACOMBE, OLIVIER. "Note sur Plotin et la pensée indienne," *Annuaire de l'École Pratique des Hautes Études*, Sciences religieuses (Paris), (1950–51), 3–17.

———. "Sur le Yoga indien," *Études carmélitaines* (Paris), XXVII (Oct., 1937), 107 ff.

LALOU, MARCELLE. *Iconographie des étoffes peintes (paṭa) dans le Mañjuśrīmūlakalpa.* Paris, 1930. (Buddhica Series I: Mémoires VI.)

———. *Répertoire du Tanjur d'après le catalogue de P. Cordier.* Paris, 1933.

———. *See also* PRZYLUSKI, JEAN.

LAMOTTE, ÉTIENNE. "La Légende du Buddha," *RHR*, CXXXIV (1947–48), 37–71.

———. *Notes sur la Bhagavadgītā.* Paris, 1929.

———. "Les Premières Relations entre l'Inde et l'Occident," *La Nouvelle Clio* (Brussels), V (1953), 83–118.

———. *Le Traité de la Grande Vertu de sagesse de Nāgārjuna (Mahāprajñāpāramitāśāstra).* Louvain, 1944, 1949. 2 vols.

———. *See also* PRZYLUSKI, JEAN.

LANGDON, STEPHEN HERBERT. "Gesture in Sumerian and Babylonian Prayer," *JRAS* (1919), 531–56.

LAUBRY, CHARLES, and BROSSE, THÉRÈSE. "Documents recueillis aux Indes sur les 'yogins' par l' enregistrement simultané du pouls, de la respiration et de l'électrocardiogramme," *Presse médicale* (Paris), LXXXIII (Oct. 14, 1936).

LAUFER, BERTHOLD. *Jade: a Study in Chinese Archaeology and Religion.* Chicago, 1912. (FMNH Anthropological Series X.)

———. *The Prehistory of Aviation.* Chicago, 1928. (FMNH Anthropological Series XVIII, No. 1.)

———. Review of *A Study of Chinese Alchemy*, by Obed S. Johnson, *Isis* (Bruges), XII (1929), 330–32.

———. *Sino-Iranica.* Chicago, 1919. (FMNH Anthropological Series XV, No. 3.)

———. *Use of Human Skulls and Bones in Tibet.* Chicago, 1923. (FMNH Department of Anthropology Publication X.)

LA VALLÉE POUSSIN, LOUIS DE, tr. and ed. *L'Abhidharmakośa de Vasubandhu.* Paris, 1923–26. 5 vols.

———. "À propos du *Cittaviśuddhiprakaraṇa* d'Āryadeva," *BSOS*, VI, 2 (1931), 411–15.

———. "Le Bouddha et les Abhijñās," *Le Muséon* (Louvain), XLIV (1931), 335–42.

———. *Bouddhisme: Études et matériaux.* London, 1898.

———. *Bouddhisme: Opinions sur l'histoire de la dogmatique.* 3rd edn., Paris, 1925.

La Vallée Poussin, Louis de. "Le Bouddhisme et le Yoga de Patañjali," *MCB*, V (1936–37), 223–42.

———. *Le Dogme et la philosophie du bouddhisme*. Paris, 1930.

———. *L'Inde aux temps des Mauryas et des barbares*. Paris, 1930.

———. *Indo-Européens et Indo-Iraniens. L'Inde jusque vers 300 av. J.-C.* New enlarged edn., Paris, 1936.

———. *La Morale bouddhique*. Paris, 1927.

———. "Musīla et Nārada," *MCB*, V (1936–37), 189–222.

———. *Nirvāṇa*. Paris, 1925.

———. "Notes de bibliographie bouddhique," *MCB*, III (1934–35), 355–407; V (1936–37), 243–304.

———. "Notes et bibliographie bouddhiques," *MCB*, I (1931–32), 377–424.

———. "Notes bouddhiques," *BCLS*, ser. V, vol. VIII (1922), 515–26.

———, tr. and ed. *Vijñaptimātratāsiddhi. La Siddhi de Hiuantsang*. Paris, 1928–48. 9 vols.

Law, Bimala Charan. "Gautama Buddha and the Paribrājakas," *JRASB*, n.s. XXI (1925), 123–36.

———. "Influence of the Five Heretical Teachers on Jainism and Buddhism," *JRASB*, n.s. XV (1919), 123–36.

———. "A Short Account of the Wandering Teachers at the Time of the Buddha," *JRASB*, n.s. XIV (1918), 399–406.

Law, Narendra Nath. "Mm. Dr. Haraprasād Śāstri," *IHQ*, IX, 1 (1933), 307–416.

Lehmann, Alfred. "Einige Bemerkungen zu indischen Gauklerkunststücken," *Jahrbuch des Museum für Völkerkunde zu Leipzig*, XI (1952), 46–63.

Leonard, G. S. "Notes on the Kānphaṭā Yogīs," *IA*, VII (1878), 298–300.

Leroy, Olivier. *Les Hommes salamandres*. Paris, 1931.

———. *La Lévitation*. Paris, 1928.

Lesimple, E., tr. *Māṇḍūkya Upaniṣad*. Paris, 1944.

Lévi, Sylvain. *La Doctrine du sacrifice dans les Brāhmaṇas*. Paris, 1898.

———. "Kaniṣka et Śātavāhana, deux figures symboliques de l'Inde au Ier siècle," *JA*, CCXXVIII (1936), 61–121.

———. *Le Népal: Étude historique d'un royaume hindou*. Paris, 1905–08. 3 vols.

———. "Notes chinoises sur l'Inde," *BEFEO*, V (1905), 253–305.

LÉVI, SYLVAIN. "Un Nouveau Document sur le bouddhisme de basse époque dans l'Inde," *BSOS*, VI, 2 (1931), 417–29.

———. "On a Tantrik Fragment from Kucha (Central Asia)," *IHQ, XII*, 2 (1936), 197–214.

———. "Pré-aryen et pré-dravidien dans l'Inde," *JA*, CCIII, (1923), 1–57.

———. *Le Théâtre indien*. Paris, 1890. 2 vols. in 1.

———. *Mémorial Sylvain Lévi*. Introd. Jacques Bacot. Paris, 1937.

——— and CHAVANNES, ÉDOUARD. "Les seizes Arhats protecteurs de la loi," *JA*, ser. XI, vol. VIII (1916), 5–50, 189–304.

LI AN-CHE. "Rñin-ma-pa: the Early Form of Lamaism," *JRAS* (1948), 142–63.

LIEBENTHAL, WALTER. *Satkārya in der Darstellung seiner buddhistischen Gegner*. Stuttgart and Berlin, 1934.

LIN LI-KOUANG. "Puṇyodaya (Na-T'i), un propagateur du tantrisme en Chine et au Cambodge à l'époque de Hiuan-tsang," *JA*, CCXXVII (1935), 83–100.

LINDQUIST, SIGURD. *Die Methoden des Yoga*. Lund, 1932.

———. *Siddhi und Abhiññā: eine Studie über die klassischen Wunder des Yoga*. Uppsala, 1935.

LINOSSIER, RAYMONDE. "Les Peintures tibétaines de la collection Loo." In *Mélanges Linossier*, I, 1–97. Paris, 1932. 2 vols.

LIPPMANN, EDMUND OSKAR VON. *Entstehung und Ausbreitung der Alchemie*. Berlin, 1919–54. 3 vols.

LIPSIUS, F. *Die Sāṃkhya Philosophie als Vorläuferin des Buddhismus*. Heidelberg, 1928.

LUBAC, HENRI DE. *La Rencontre du bouddhisme et de l'Occident*. Paris, 1952.

———. "Textes alexandrins et bouddhiques," *Recherches de science religieuse* (Paris), XXVII (1937), 336–51.

MACDONALD, A. W. "À propos de Prajāpati," *JA*, CCXL (1952), 323–38.

MACKAY, ERNEST. *The Indus Civilization*. London, 1935. 2nd edn., retitled *Early Indus Civilization*, rev. and enlarged by Dorothy Mackay. London, 1948.

MĀDHAVA. *Sarvadarśanasaṃgraha*. Poona, 1906. (Ānandāśrama Sanskrit Series LI.)

———. *See also* COWELL, E. B., and GOUGH, A. E., and SINHA, NANDALAL.

MAENCHEN-HELFEN, OTTO. "Svetadvīpa in Pre-Christian China," *NIA*, II (1939), 166–68.

MAHĀDEVA ŚĀSTRI, ALLĀDI, tr. and ed. *Yoga Upaniṣads with the Commentary of Srī Upaniṣad-Brahma-Yogin.* Adyar, 1920.

MAHFUZ-UL-HAQ, M., ed. and tr. *Majma 'ul-Baḥrain; or, The Mingling of the Two Oceans* [of Muḥammad Dārā Shikūh]. Calcutta, 1929. (BI CCXLVI.)

MAJUMDAR, ABHAY KUMAR. *The Sāṅkhya Conception of Personality.* Calcutta, 1930.

MAJUMDAR, DHIRENDRA NATH. "Notes on Kālī-Nautch in the District of Dacca in Eastern Bengal," *MI*, III (1923), 202–05.

MALLMANN, MARIE THÉRÈSE DE. *Introduction à l'étude d'Avalokiteçvara.* Paris, 1948.

MARSHALL, SIR JOHN (and others). *Mohenjo-daro and the Indus Culture.* London, 1931. 3 vols.

MARTIN, ROBERT MONTGOMERY. *History of the Antiquities of Eastern India.* London, 1838. 3 vols.

MARTIN, WILLIAM ALEXANDER PARSONS. *The Lore of Cathay; or, The Intellect of China.* New York, 1901.

MASPÉRO, HENRI. "Communautés et moines bouddhistes chinois aux IIe et IIIe siècles," *BEFEO*, X (1910), 222–32.

———. "Les Procédés de 'Nourrir le principe vital' dans la religion taoïste ancienne," *JA*, CCXXVIII (1937), 177–252, 353–430.

MASSIGNON, LOUIS. *Essai sur les origines du lexique technique de la mystique musulmane.* Paris, 1922.

———. *La Passion d'al-Hosayn-ibn-Mansour al-Hallâj, martyr mystique de l'Islam.* Paris, 1922. 2 vols.

———. "Le Souffle dans l'Islam," *JA*, CCXXXIV (1943–45), 436–38.

MASSON, JOSEPH. *La Religion populaire dans le canon bouddhique pāli.* Louvain, 1942. (Le Muséon Bibliothèque XV.)

MASUI, JACQUES, ed. *Yoga, science de l'homme intégral.* Paris, 1953.

MĀṬHARA. *See* SARMA, VISHNU PRASAD.

MAUSS, MARCEL. "Rapports historiques entre la mystique hindoue et la mystique occidentale," *Annales d'histoire du Christianisme* (Paris), III (1928).

MAX MÜLLER, F. *The Six Systems of Indian Philosophy.* London, 1899.

MEDHĀTITHI. *See* JHĀ, GANGĀNĀTHA.

MEERWARTH, A. M. "Les *Kathākalis* du Malabar," *JA*, CCIX (1926), 193–284.

MÉLY, FERNAND DE. "L'Alchimie chez les chinois et l'alchimie grecque," *JA*, ser. IX, vol. VI (1895), 314–40.

MERUTUNGA ĀCĀRYA. *See* TAWNEY, CHARLES HENRY.

MEYER, JOHN JACOB. *Trilogie altindischer Mächte und Feste der Vegetation.* Zurich and Leipzig, 1937. 3 vols. in 1.

MEYER, RUDOLF, ed. *Ṛgvidhāna.* Berlin, 1878.

MILAREPA. *See* EVANS-WENTZ, W. Y.

MITRA, KALIPADA. "Magic and Miracle in Jaina Literature," *IHQ*, XV, 2 (1939), 175–82.

MITRA, RĀJENDRALĀLA. *Buddha Gayā, the Hermitage of Śākya Muni.* Calcutta, 1878.

———. *The Sanskrit Buddhist Literature of Nepāl.* Calcutta, 1882.

———, ed. and tr. *The Yoga Aphorisms of Patañjali, with the Commentary of Bhoja Rāja.* Calcutta, 1881–83. (BI XCIII.)

MITRA, SARAT CHANDRA. "The Cult of the Lake-Goddess of Orissa," *JASB*, XII (1920–24), 190–97.

———. "The Cult of the Tortoise-shaped Deities of Midnapur and Bankura in Western Bengal," in "On Some Curious Cults of Southern and Western Bengal," *JASB*, XI (1917–20), 446–54.

———. "Notes on Tree-Cults in the District of Patna in South Bihār," *JBORS*, XIV (1928), 278–81.

———. "On the Conversion of Tribes into Castes in North Bihār," *JASB*, XII (1920–24), 735–43.

———. "On the Cult of Gorakshanātha in the District of Rangpur in Northern Bengal," *JASB*, XIV (1927/28–31), 1–5.

———. "On the Cult of Gorakshanātha in Eastern Bengal," *JDL*, XIV (1927), 1–41.

———. "On the Cult of the Jujube Tree," *MI*, V (1925), 115–31.

———. "On the Cult of the Tree-Goddess in Eastern Bengal," *MI*, II (1922), 230–41.

———. "On a Recent Instance of the Khāsī Custom of Offering Human Sacrifices to the Snake-Deity," *JASB*, XIII (1924–28), 192–98.

———. "On the Worship of Dakshina Rāya as a Rain-God," *JASB*, XIII (1924–28), 198–203.

———. "On the Worship of the Pipal Tree in North Bihār," *JBORS*, VI (1920), 572–74.

MITRA, UMESHA. "*Gauḍapādabhāṣya* and *Māṭharavṛtti*," *AUS*, VII (1931), 371–86.

———. "Physical Theory of Sound and Its Origin in Indian Thought," *AUS*, II (1926).

MODE, HEINZ. *Indische Frühkulturen und ihre Beziehungen zum Westen.* Basel, 1944.

MODI, JIVANJI JAMSHEDJI. *Asiatic Papers.* Bombay, 1905, 1917, 1929. 3 vols.

MONIER-WILLIAMS, SIR MONIER. "A Case of *Samādh* in India," *IA*, VII (1878), 264–66.

MONTADON, G. *La Race, les races.* Paris, 1933.

———. *Traité d'ethnologie culturelle.* Paris, 1934.

MOOKERJEE, RASACHARYA KAVIRAJ. *Rasa-jala-nidhi; or, Ocean of Indian Chemistry and Alchemy.* Calcutta, 1926–38. 5 vols.

MORENO, MARTINO MARIO. "Mistica musulmana e mistica indiana," *Annali Lateranensi* (Vatican City), X (1946), 103–212.

MUḤAMMAD HAIDAR DUGHLĀT. *See* ELIAS, NEY.

MUḤAMMAD MUḤSIN-I-FĀNI. *See* SHEA, DAVID, and TROYER, ANTHONY.

MUKHERJĪ, BRAJA LAL. "Tantra Shastra and Veda." In WOODROFFE, SIR John (q.v.), *Shakti and Shākta*, pp. 95–105.

MUS, PAUL. *Barabuḍur.* Hanoi, 1935 ff. 2 vols.

NĀGĀRJUNA. *See* LAMOTTE, ÉTIENNE.

NANDIKEŚVARA. *See* COOMARASWAMY, ANANDA K., and DUGGIRALA, G. K.

NANJIO, BUNYIU. *A Catalogue of the Buddhist Tripiṭaka.* Oxford, 1883.

NARAHARI, H. G. *Ātman in Pre-Upaniṣadic Vedic Literature.* Adyar, 1944.

NĀRĀYAṆASWAMI AIYAR, C. S. "Ancient Indian Chemistry and Alchemy of the Chemico-Philosophical Siddhānta System of the Indian Mystics." In *Proceedings and Transactions of the Third Oriental Conference* (1924), pp. 597–614. Madras, 1925.

NĀROPĀ. *See* CARELLI, MARIO E.

NEEDHAM, JOSEPH. *Science and Civilization in China.* Cambridge, 1954–56. 2 vols.

NEOG, MAHESWAR. "The Worship of Dharma in Assam," *Journal of the Asiatic Society of Bengal* (Letters), XVII (1951), 219–24.

NIGGEMEYER, HERMANN. "Totemismus in Vorderindien," *A*, XXVII (1932), 407–61; (1933), 579–619.

OBERMILLER, E. E. "Tson-kha-pa le Pandit," *MCB*, III (1934–35), 319–38.

O'GRADY, HAYES, ed. and tr. *Silva Gadelica: a Collection of Tales in Irish.* London, 1892.

OLDENBERG, HERMANN. *Buddha, sein Leben, seine Lehre und seine Gemeinde.* Berlin, 1881. 5th edn., Berlin, 1906. 9th edn., Berlin, 1921. (*Buddha, His Life, His Doctrine, His Order*, tr. W. Hoey. London, 1882.)

———. "Buddhistischen Studien," *ZDMG*, LII (1898), 613–94.

———. *Die Lehre der Upanishaden und die Anfänge des Buddhismus.* Göttingen, 1915.

———. *Das Mahābhārata; seine Entstehung, sein Inhalt, seine Form.* Göttingen, 1922.

———. *Die Religion des Veda.* 2nd edn., Berlin, 1917.

———. "Zur Geschichte der Sāṃkhya-Philosophie," *NGWG*, phil.-hist. Klasse (1917), 218–53.

———. *See also* DAVIDS, T. W. RHYS.

OLDFIELD, H. A. *Sketches from Nipal.* London, 1880. 2 vols.

OLDHAM, CHARLES FREDERICK. *The Sun and the Serpent.* London, 1905.

OLTRAMARE, PAUL. *L'Histoire des idées théosophiques dans l'Inde.* Paris, 1907. 2 vols.

———. *La Théosophie bouddhique.* Paris, 1923.

OMAN, JOHN CAMPBELL. *The Mystics, Ascetics, and Saints of India.* London, 1903.

OPPERT, GUSTAV. *On the Original Inhabitants of Bharatavarṣa or India.* Westminster, 1893.

OTTO, R. *Die Lehr-Traktate der Bhagavad-Gītā.* Stuttgart, 1935.

———. *Die Urgestalt der Bhagavad-Gītā.* Stuttgart, 1934. (*The Original Gītā*, tr. J. E. Turner. London, 1939.)

PARTINGTON, J. R. "Chinese Alchemy," *Nature* (London), CXIX (1927), 11; CXXVIII (1931), 1074–75.

———. "The Relationship Between Chinese and Arabic Alchemy," *Nature* (London), CXX (1927), 158.

PATAÑJALI. *Yoga-sūtras.* Poona, 1904; 2nd edn., 1919. (Ānandāśrama Sanskrit Series XLVII.)

———. *See also* JHĀ, GANGĀNĀTHA; MITRA, RĀJENDRALĀLA; RĀMA PRASĀDA; and WOODS, JAMES HAUGHTON.

PATEL, PRABBHUBHAI. "*Bodhicittavivaraṇa,*" *IHQ*, VIII, 4 (1932), 790–93.

———. "*Cittaviśuddhiprakaraṇam* of Āryadeva," *IHQ*, IX, 3 (1933), 705–21.

———. *Cittaviśuddhiprakaraṇa of Āryadeva.* Santiniketan, 1949.

PATHAK, K. B. "The Ājīvikas, a Sect of Buddhist Bhikshus," *IA*, XLI (1912), 88–90.

PATVARDHAN, R. V. "Rasavidyā or Alchemy in Ancient India." In *Proceedings and Transactions of the First Oriental Conference* (*1919*), I, clv. Poona, 1920. 2 vols.

PAYNE, ERNEST ALEXANDER. *The Śāktas: an Introductory and Comparative Study*. Calcutta, 1933. (The Religious Life of India.)

PELLIOT, PAUL. "Meou-tseu ou les doutes levés," *T'oung Pao* (Leiden), XIX (1919), 255–433.

PENZER, NORMAN MOSLEY, ed. *Somadeva's Kathā-sarit-sāgara, or Ocean of Streams of Story*, tr. C. H. Tawney. London, 1924–28. 10 vols.

PÉRI, NOËL. "Hārītī, la mère-de-démons," *BEFEO*, XVII (1917), 1–102.

PHELPS, MYRON H., ed. *Discourses on Radha-Swami Faith* (*Discourses Made by Babugi Sahib*). New York, n.d. (1914?).

PHILLIPS, GEORGE. "Mahuan's Account of Cochin, Calicut, and Aden," *JRAS* (1896), 341–51.

PIGGOTT, STUART. *Prehistoric India*. Harmondsworth and Baltimore, 1950. (A Pelican Book.)

PISCHEL, RICHARD. *Leben und Lehre des Buddha*. 2nd edn., Leipzig, 1910.

PODUVAL, R. VASUDEVA. *Kathākali and Diagram of Hand Poses*. Trivandrum, 1930.

POTT, P. H. *Yoga en Yantra*. Leiden, 1946.

POZDNEJEV, A. M. "Dhyāna und Samādhi im mongolischen Lamaismus," *ZB*, VII (1926), 378–421.

PRASAD, JVALA. "The Date of the *Yoga-sūtras*," *JRAS* (1930), 365–75.

PRZYLUSKI, JEAN. "Un Ancien Peuple du Penjab: les Udumbara," *JA*, CCVIII (1926), 1–59.

———. "Bengali Numeration and Non-Āryan Substratum," in BAGCHI, PRABODH CHANDRA (q.v.), tr., *Pre-Āryan and Pre-Dravidian in India*, pp. 25–32.

———. "Le Bouddhisme tantrique à Bali d'après une publication récente," *JA*, CCXVIII (1931), 159–67.

———. "De quelques noms anaryens en indo-aryen," *Mémoires de la Société de Linguistique* (Paris), XXII (1921), 205–10.

———. "Dragon chinois et Nāga indien," *MS*, III (1938), 602–10.

———. "Emprunts anaryens en indo-aryen," *BSL*, XXIV (1924), 118–23, 255–58; XXV (1925), 66–71; XXVI (1926), 98–103; XXX (1930), 196–201.

———. *La Légende de l'empereur Açoka*. Paris, 1923.

PRZYLUSKI, JEAN. "Mudrā," *Indian Culture* (Calcutta), II (1936), 715–19.

———. "La Numération vigésimale dans l'Inde," *Rocznik Orjentalistyczny* (Lwów), IV (1926; pub. 1928), 230–37.

———. "L'Or, son origine et ses pouvoirs magiques," *BEFEO*, XIV (1914), 1–17.

———. Le Parinirvāṇa et les funérailles du Buddha," *JA*, ser. XI, vol. XI (1918), 485–526; ser. XI, vol. XII (1918), 401–56.

———. "La Princesse à l'odeur de poisson et la nāgī dans les traditions de l'Asie orientale." In *Études asiatiques* II, 265–84. Paris, 1925. (Pub. on 25th anniversary of the École française d'Extrême-Orient.) 2 vols.

———. "Le Prologue-cadre des *Mille et une Nuits* et le thème du *svayaṃvara*," *JA*, CCV (1924), 101–37.

———. "La Théorie des *Guṇa*," *BSOS*, VI, 1 (1930), 25–35.

———. "Totémisme et végétalisme dans l'Inde," *RHR*, XCVI (1927), 347–64.

———. "Les Vidyārāja," *BEFEO*, XXIII (1923), 301–18.

——— and LALOU, MARCELLE. "Notes de mythologie bouddhique: 1. Yakṣa et Gandharva dans le *Mahāsamaya-suttanta*," *HJAS*, III (1938), 40–46.

——— and LAMOTTE, ÉTIENNE. "Bouddhisme et Upaniṣad," *BEFEO*, XXXII (1932), 141–69.

RADHAKRISHNAN, SARVEPALLI. *Indian Philosophy*. London, 1923, 1927. 2 vols.

RAFY, K. U. *Folktales of the Khāsīs*. London, 1920.

RĀHULA SĀNKṚTYĀYANA. "Recherches bouddhiques: I. Les Origines du Mahāyāna; II. L'Origine du Vajrayāna et les 84 Siddhas," *JA*, CCXXV (1934), 195–230.

RĀMĀNUJA. *See* THIBAUT, GEORGE.

RĀMA PRASĀDA, tr. *Patañjali's Yoga Sūtras, with the Commentary of Vyāsa and the Gloss of Vāchaspatimiśra*. Allahabad, 1910. 3rd edn., Allahabad, 1924. (SBH IV.)

RANADE, RAMCHANDRA DATTATRAYA. *A Constructive Survey of Upanishadic Philosophy*. Poona, 1926.

RAO, T. A. GOPĪNĀTHA. *See* GOPĪNĀTHA RAO, T. A.

RASMUSSEN, KNUD. *Intellectual Culture of the Iglulik Eskimos*, tr. William Worster. Copenhagen, 1929.

RAY, AMAR NATH. "The *Māṇḍūkya Upaniṣad* and the *Kārikās* of Gauḍapāda," *IHQ*, XIV, 3 (1938), 564–69.

RĀY, PRAFULLA CHANDRA. *A History of Hindu Chemistry.* 2nd edn., Calcutta, 1904–09. 2 vols.

RAY CHAUDHURI, HEMCHANDRA. *Materials for the Study of the Early History of the Vaishnava Sect.* Calcutta, 1920.

READ, B. F. "Chinese Alchemy," *Nature* (London), CXX (1927), 877–78.

RÉGAMEY, CONSTANTIN. "Bibliographie analytique des travaux relatifs aux éléments anaryens dans la civilisation et les langues de l'Inde," *BEFEO*, XXXIV (1934), 429–566.

REINAUD, JOSEPH TOUSSAINT. *Mémoire géographique, historique et scientifique sur l'Inde antérieurement au milieu du XIe siècle de l'ère chrétienne d'après les écrivains arabes, persans et chinois.* Paris, 1849. (Mémoires de l'Académie des Inscriptions XVIII.)

———. *Relations de voyages faits par les arabes et les persans dans l'Inde et à la Chine.* Paris, 1845. 2 vols.

RELE, VASANT GANGARAM. *The Mysterious Kuṇḍalinī.* Bombay, 1930.

RENOU, LOUIS. *Bibliographie védique.* Paris, 1931.

———, tr. *Kaṭha Upaniṣad.* Paris, 1943.

———. "Le Passage des Brāhmaṇa aux Upaniṣad," *JAOS*, LXXIII (1953), 138–44.

———. "Sur la notion du *brahman*," *JA*, CCXXXVII (1949), 7–46.

——— and FILLIOZAT, JEAN. *L'Inde classique, manuel des études indiennes.* Paris, 1947 [1949], 1953. 2 vols.

RISCH, HUBERT. "Le Haṭha Yoga. Exposé sommaire de la méthode, quelques expériences physiologiques et applications thérapeutiques." Diss. Paris: Faculté de Médecine, 1951.

RIVET, PAUL. "Les Océaniens," *JA*, CCXXII (1933), 235–56.

———. *Sumérien et Océanien.* Paris, 1929.

ROCKHILL, WILLIAM WOODVILLE. *Life of the Buddha.* London, 1884.

———. "Notes on the Relations and Trade of China with the Eastern Archipelago and the Coast of the Indian Ocean During the Fourteenth Century," pt. II, iv, *T'oung Pao* (Leiden), XVI (1915), 435–67.

———. "On the Use of Skulls in Lamaist Ceremonies," *Proceedings of the American Oriental Society* (New Haven, 1888), XL (1890), xxiv–xxxi.

———. *See also* HIRTH, FRIEDRICH.

ROERICH, GEORGE N., tr. *The Blue Annals.* Calcutta, 1949–53. 2 pts.

ROESEL, RICHARD. *Die psychologischen Grundlagen der Yogapraxis.* Stuttgart, 1928.

RÖNNOW, KASTEN. "Some Remarks on Śvetadvīpa," *BSOS*, V, 2 (1929), 253–84.

———. "Ved. *kratu-*, eine wortgeschichtliche Untersuchung," *MO*, XXVI (1932), 1–90.

ROY, SARAT CHANDRA. "Caste, Race, and Religion in India," *MI*, XIV (1934), 39–63, 75–220, 271–311.

———. *Orāon Religion and Customs.* Ranchi, 1928.

ROY, SATINDRA NARAYAN. "The Witches of Orissa," *JASB*, XIV (1927/28–31), 185–200.

RUBEN, WALTER. "Materialismus im Leben des alten Indien," *AO*, XIII (1934), 128–62.

———. *Die Philosophen der Upanishaden.* Bern, 1947.

———. "Schamanismus im alten Indien," *AO*, XVII (1939), 164–205.

———. "Über die Literatur der vorarischen Stämme Indiens," *Deutsche Akademie der Wissenschaften zu Berlin, Institut für Orientforschung, Veröffentlichung* XV (1952).

RUSSELL, ROBERT VANE (with RAI BAHADUR HĪRA LĀL). *The Tribes and Castes of the Central Provinces of India.* London, 1916. 4 vols.

SACHAU, EDWARD C., tr. *Alberuni's India.* London, 1910. 2 vols.

SANGUINETTI, B. R. *See* DEFRÉMERY, CHARLES FRANÇOIS.

ŚAṆKARA. *See* SARMA, HARADATTA, and THIBAUT, GEORGE.

ŚĀNTARAKṢITA. *See* JHĀ, GANGĀNĀTHA, and KRISHNAMACHARYA, EMBAR.

ŚĀNTIDEVA. *See* BENDALL, CECIL.

SARKAR, BENOY KUMAR. *The Folk-Element in Hindu Culture.* London, 1917.

SARMA, B. N. KRISHNAMURTI. *See* KRISHNAMURTI SARMA, B. N.

SARMA, HARADATTA, ed. *Jayamaṇgalā.* Introd. G. Kaviraj. Calcutta, 1926. (GOS XIX.)

———. "*Jayamaṇgalā* and the Other Commentaries on *Sāṅkhya-Saptati*," *IHQ*, V, 3 (1929), 417–31.

SARMA, VISHNU PRASAD, ed. *Māṭharavṛtti.* Benares, 1922. (Chowkhambā Sanskrit Series CCXCVI.)

ŚĀSTRI, ALLĀDI MAHĀDEVA. *See* MAHĀDEVA ŚĀSTRI, ALLĀDI.

ŚĀSTRI, JYOTIRBHUSAN V. V. RAMANA. "The Doctrinal Culture and Tradition of the Siddhas." In *The Cultural Heritage of India: Śrī*

Ramakrishna Centenary Memorial, II, 303–19. Calcutta [1937?]. 3 vols.

Śāstri, K. S., ed. *Rasopaniṣat*. Trivandrum, 1928. (Trivandrum Sanskrit Series XCII.)

Śāstri, Rāmakṛshṇa, and Śāstri, Keśava, eds. "*Yogavārttika* of Vijñānabhikṣu," *The Pandit* (Benares), n.s. V (1883), 39–48, 78–88, 123–33, 209–16, 263–75, 320–32, 379–92, 439–54, 477–95, 563–70, 583–94, 635–42; VI (1884), 24–32, 106–12, 129–43, 178–97, 249–58, 297–309, 337–52, 393–409, 449–68, 509–19, 561–76, 617–32.

Śāstri, S. S. Suryanarayana. "The Chinese *Suvarṇa-saptati* and the *Māṭhara-vṛtti*," *JOR*, IV (1930), 34–40.

———. "The *Maṇimēkalai* Account of the Sāṃkhya," *Journal of Indian History* (Madras), VIII (1929), 322–27.

———. "Māṭhara and Paramārtha," *JRAS* (1931), 623–39.

———, ed. and tr. *The Sāṃkhya Kārikā of Īśvara Kṛṣṇa*. Madras, 1930.

Saussure, Léopold de. *Les Origines de l'astronomie chinoise*. Paris, 1930.

Schebesta, Paul. *Les Pygmées*, tr. F. Berge. Paris, 1940.

Scherman, Lucian. "Siddha. Sanskrit Letters as Mystical Symbols in Later Buddhism Outside India." In K. Bharatha Iyer, ed., *Art and Thought, Issued in Honour of Dr. Ananda K. Coomaraswamy on the Occasion of His Seventieth Birthday*, pp. 55–62. London, 1947.

Schermerhorn, R. A. "When Did Indian Materialism Get Its Distinctive Titles?" *JAOS*, L (1930), 132–38.

Schmidt, P. Wilhelm. "Die Mon-Khmer Völker, ein Bindeglied zwischen Völkern Zentralasiens und Austronesiens," *Archiv für Anthropologie* (Brunswick), n.s. V (1906), 59–109. (Tr. into French by Mme J. Marouzeau, "Les Peuples Mon-Khmêr," *BEFEO*, VII [1907], 213–63; VIII [1908], 1–35.)

———. "Mutterrecht und Kopfjagd im westlichen Hinterindien," *A*, XIV–XV (1919–20), 1138–46.

Schmidt, Richard. *Fakire und Fakirtum im alten und modernen Indien*. Berlin, 1908. 2nd edn., Berlin, 1921.

Schrader, Friedrich Otto. "Dravidisch und Uralisch," *ZII*, III (1925), 81–112.

———. *Introduction to the Pāñcharātra and the Ahirbudhnya Saṃhitā*. Adyar, 1916. 2 vols.

———. *The Kashmir Recension of the Bhagavadgītā*. Stuttgart, 1930.

———. "Das *Ṣaṣṭitantra*," *ZDMG*, LXVIII (1914), 101–10.

SCHRÖDER, DOMINIK. "Zur Religion der Tujen des Sininggebietes (Kukunor)," *A*, XLVII (1952), 1–79; XLVIII (1953), 202–59.

SCHUBRING, WALTHER. *Die Lehre der Jainas, nach den alten Quellen dargestellt.* Berlin and Leipzig, 1935. (*Grundriss der indo-arischen Philologie und Altertumskunde*, ed. H. Lüders and J. Wackernagel, III, 7.)

SCHWAB, RAYMOND. *La Renaissance orientale.* Paris, 1948.

SEN, DINESH CHANDRA. *Chaitanya and His Age.* Calcutta, 1922.

———. *Chaitanya and His Companions.* Calcutta, 1917.

———. *History of Bengali Language and Literature.* Calcutta, 1911.

———. *The Vaiṣṇava Literature of Mediaeval Bengal.* Calcutta, 1917.

SENART, ÉMILE, tr. *La Bhagavadgītā.* Paris, 1922.

———. "Bouddhisme et Yoga," *RHR*, XLII (1900), 345–63.

———. *Essai sur la légende du Buddha, son caractère et ses origines.* Paris, 1875.

———. "*Rajas* et la théorie indienne des trois *guṇas*," *JA*, ser. XI, vol. VI (1915), 151–64.

———. "La Théorie des *guṇas* et la *Chāndogya Upaniṣad.*" In *Études asiatiques*, II, 285–92. Paris, 1925. (Pub. on 25th anniversary of the École française d'Extrême-Orient.) 2 vols.

SHAH, CHIMANLAL JAICHAND. *Jainism in North India, 800* B.C.–A.D. *526.* London, 1932.

SHAHIDULLAH, M., ed. and tr. *Les Chants mystiques de Kānha et de Saraha; les Dohā-koṣa et les Caryā*, Paris, 1928.

SHĀSTRI, DAKSHINARANJAN. *Chārvākashashti.* Calcutta, 1928.

———. "The Lokāyatikas and the Kāpālikas," *IHQ*, VII, 1 (1931), 125–37.

———. *A Short History of Indian Materialism, Sensationalism, Hedonism.* Calcutta, 1930.

SHĀSTRI, HARAPRASĀD, ed. *Advayavajrasaṃgraha.* Baroda, 1927. (GOS XL.)

———. *Bauddha Gān O Dohā.* Calcutta, 1916.

———. "Buddhism in Bengal since the Muhammadan Conquest," *JRASB*, X (1895), 55–61.

———. *Catalogue of Palm-Leaf and Selected Paper Mss. Belonging to the Darbar Library, Nepāl.* Calcutta, 1905, 1915. 2 vols.

———. "Chronology of Sāṃkhya Literature," *JBORS*, IX (1923), 151–62.

SHĀSTRI, HARAPRASĀD. *The Discovery of Living Buddhism in Bengal.* Calcutta, 1897.

———. "The Discovery of a Work by Āryadeva in Sanskrit," *JRASB,* XVII (1898), 175–84.

———. *Notices of Sanskrit Manuscripts.* 2nd ser. Calcutta, 1900.

SHĀSTRI, MUKUNDA RĀMA, ed. *The Tantrasāra of Abhinava Gupta.* Bombay, 1918. (Research Dept. Kashmir Series of Texts and Studies XVII.)

SHĀSTRI, UDAYA VIRA. "Antiquity of the *Sāṅkhya Sūtras.*" In *Proceedings and Transactions of the Fifth Indian Oriental Conference* (1928), II, 855–82. Lahore, 1930. 2 vols.

SHĀSTRI, VIDHUSHEKAR. "Sandhābhāṣā," *IHQ,* IV, 2 (1928), 287–96.

SHEA, DAVID, and TROYER, ANTHONY, trs. *The Dabistān; or, School of Manners.* Paris, 1843. 3 vols.

Si-do-in-dzou: Gestes de l'officiant dans les cérémonies mystiques des sectes Tendai et Singon. Tr. from the Japanese of Horyū Toki. Paris, 1899.

SILBURN, ALIETTE, tr. *Śvetāśvatara Upaniṣad.* Paris, 1948.

SIMPSON, WILLIAM. "Some Suggestions of Origin in Indian Architecture," *JRAS,* n.s. XX (1888), 49–71.

SINGH, MOHAN. *Gorakhnāth and Mediaeval Hindu Mysticism.* Lahore, 1937.

SINH, PAÑCHAM, tr. *Haṭhayogapradīpikā.* Allahabad, 1915. (SBH XV, 3.)

SINHA, NANDALAL, tr. *The Sāṃkhya Philosophy, Containing: (1) Sāṃkhya Pravachana Sūtram, with the Vritti of Aniruddha and the Bhāsya of Vijñāna Bhiksu and Extracts from the Vritti-sāra of Mahādeva Vedāntin; (2) Tattva Samāsa; (3) Sāṃkhya Kārikā; Pañchaśikhā Sūtram.* Allahabad, 1915 (SBH XI.)

SIRKAR, DINES CHANDRA. "The Śākta Piṭhas," *JRASB,* XIV (1948), 1–108.

SOMADEVA. *See* PENZER, NORMAN MOSLEY.

SOVANI, VENKATESA VAMANA. "A Critical Study of the Sāṅkhya System on the Line of Sāṅkhya-kārikā, Sāṅkhya-sūtra and Their Commentaries," *AUS,* VII (1931), 387–432. (Rep. separately, Poona, 1935. Poona Oriental Series XI.)

SSŬ-MA CH'IEN. *See* CHAVANNES, ÉDOUARD.

STCHERBATSKY, T. [FYODOR IPPOLITOVICH]. *Buddhist Logic.* Leningrad, 1930–32. (BB XXVI.) 2 vols.

———. *The Central Conception of Buddhism and the Meaning of the Word "Dharma."* London, 1923.

STCHERBATSKY, T. [FYODOR IPPOLITOVICH]. *The Conception of Buddhist Nirvāṇa.* Leningrad, 1927.

———. "The Doctrine of the Buddha," *BSOS*, VI, 4 (1932), 867–96.

———. *Erkenntnistheorie und Logik nach der Lehre der späteren Buddhisten.* Munich, 1924. (Tr. into French by Mme I. de Manziarly and Paul Masson-Oursel. Paris, 1926.)

STEIN, OTTO. "The Numeral 18," *Poona Orientalist*, I, 3 (1936), 1–37.

———. "References to Alchemy in Buddhist Scriptures," *BSOS*, VII, 1 (1933), 262–63.

STRAUSS, OTTO. "Eine alte Formel der Sāṃkhya-Yoga-Philosophie bei Vātsyāyana." In *Beiträge zur Literaturwissenschaft und Geistesgeschichte Indiens*, pp. 358–68. Bonn, 1926.

———. "Zur Geschichte des Sāṃkhya," *Wiener Zeitschrift für die Kunde des Morgenlandes*, XXVII (1913), 257–75.

SUALI, LUIGI. "Matériaux pour servir à l'histoire du matérialisme indien," *Le Muséon* (Louvain), IX (1908), 277–98.

ŚUBHADRA. *Jñānārṇava.* 2nd edn., Bombay, 1913.

SUBRAMANIAN, K. R. [SUBRAMANIA IYER]. *Buddhist Remains in Āndhra.* Madras, 1932.

SUGIURA, SADAJIRO. *Hindu Logic as Preserved in China and Japan*, ed. Edgar A. Singer, Jr. Philadelphia, 1900.

SUZUKI, BEATRICE LANE. "The School of Shingon Buddhism. Pt. II: The Mandara," *The Eastern Buddhist* (Kyoto), VII (1936), 1–38.

SUZUKI, DAISETZ TEITARO. *Essays in Zen Buddhism.* London, 1927, 1933, 1934. 3 vols. (so-called series).

———. *An Introduction to Zen Buddhism.* Kyoto, 1934.

———. *Manual of Zen Buddhism.* Kyoto, 1935.

SVĀTMĀRĀMA SVĀMIN. *Haṭhayogapradīpikā, with the Commentary of Brahmānanda and Glosses of Śrīdhara.* Bombay, 1889.

———. *See also* AYYAṆGĀR, T. R. ŚRĪNIVĀSA; BRAHMĀNANDA BHABA; SINH, PAÑCHAM, and WALTER, HERMANN.

TAJIMA, R. *Étude sur le Mahāvairocana-sūtra.* Paris, 1936.

TAKAKUSU, JUNJIRO. "*Sāṃkhyakārikā* étudiée à la lumière de sa version chinoise," *BEFEO*, IV (1904), 1–65, 978–1064.

TAKI, SHODO. *See* VIRA, RAGHU.

TĀRANĀTHA. *See* GRÜNWEDEL, ALBERT.

TARKATĪRTHA, PĀRVATĪ CHARANA, ed. *Kālīvilāsa Tantra.* London, 1917. (TT VI.)

TATIA, NATHMAL. *Studies in Jaina Philosophy*. Benares, 1951.

TATTABHUSAN, HEMCHANDRA GOSWAMI, ed. *Kāmaratna-tantra*. Sillong, 1928.

TAUBER, C. *Entwicklung der Menschheit von den Ur-Australiern bis Europa auf Grund der neuesten Forschungen über die Wanderungen der Ozeanier*. Zurich and Leipzig, 1932.

TAWNEY, CHARLES HENRY, tr. *The Prabandhacintāmaṇi; or, Wishing-stone of Narratives*. Calcutta, 1901. (BI CXLI.)

———. *See also* PENZER, NORMAN MOSLEY.

TAYLOR, F. SHERWOOD. *The Alchemists, Founders of Modern Chemistry*. New York, 1949.

———. "A Survey of Greek Alchemy," *The Journal of Hellenic Studies* (London), L (1930), 109–39.

TELANG, K. T., tr. *The Bhagavadgītā, with the Sanatsugātīya and the Anugītā*. Oxford, 1882. 2nd edn., Oxford, 1908. (SBE VIII.)

TESSITORI, L. P. "Yogīs (Kānphaṭā)," in HASTINGS, JAMES (q.v.), ed., *Encyclopaedia of Religion and Ethics*, XII, 833–35.

THIBAUT, GEORGE, tr. *The Vedānta Sūtra. With Rāmānuja's Commentary*. Oxford, 1904. (SBE XLVIII.)

———. *The Vedānta Sūtra. With Śaṇkara's Commentary*. Oxford, 1890, 1896. (SBE XXXIV, XXXVIII.) 2 vols.

THOMAS, EDWARD JOSEPH. *The Life of Buddha as Legend and History*. London, 1927.

TUCCI, GIUSEPPE. "Animadversiones Indicae," *JRASB*, n.s. XXVI (1930), 125–60.

———. "À Propos the Legend of Nāropā," *JRAS* (1935), 677–88.

———. *Il Buddhismo*. Foligno, 1926.

———. "Buddhist Notes," *MCB*, IX (1951), 173–220.

———. *Indo-Tibetica*. Rome, 1932–41. 4 vols. in 7.

———. "Linee di una storia del materialismo indiano," *MRANL*, ser. V, vol. XVII, fasc. VII (1924).

———. *"Mc'od rten" e "Ts'a-ts'a" nel Tibet indiano ed occidentale; contributo allo studio dell' arte religiosa tibetana e del suo significato*. Rome, 1932. (*Indo-Tibetica*, vol. I, pt. 1.)

———. *Pre-Diṅnāga; Buddhist Texts on Logic from Chinese Sources*. Baroda, 1929. (GOS XLIX.)

———. "Some Glosses upon the *Guhyasamāja*," *MCB*, III (1934–35), 339–53.

TUCCI, GIUSEPPE. *I Templi del Tibet occidentale e il loro simbolismo artistico.* Rome, 1935–36. 2 vols. (*Indo-Tibetica*, vol. III, pts. 1 and 2.)

———. *Teoria e pratica del maṇḍala.* Rome, 1949.

———. *Tibetan Painted Scrolls.* Rome, 1949.

———. "Tracce di culto lunare in India," in "Note indologichi," *Rivista degli studi orientali* (Oriental School, University of Rome), XII (1929–30), 419–27.

UI, HAKUJU. *The Vaiśeṣika Philosophy According to the Daśapadārthaśāstra*, ed. F. W. Thomas. London, 1917.

VĀCASPATIMIŚRA. *See* GARBE, RICHARD; JHĀ, GANGĀNĀTHA, and RĀMA PRASĀDA.

VARĀHAMIHIRA. *Bṛihajjātaka, with Utpala's Commentary. See* BHĀNDĀRKAR, D. R.

VASAKA, BHUVANANA CHANDRA, ed. *Gheraṇḍa Saṃhitā.* Calcutta, 1877.

VASU, NAGENDRA NATH. *Modern Buddhism and Its Followers in Orissa.* Calcutta, 1911.

———, ed. *Śūnya Purāṇa.* Calcutta, 1909.

VASU, RAI BAHADUR ŚRĪŚA CHANDRA, tr. *Gheraṇḍa Saṃhitā.* Bombay, 1895. Repr. Allahabad, 1914. (SBH XV, 2.) Repr. Adyar, 1933.

———. *An Introduction to the Yoga Philosophy.* 2nd edn., Allahabad, 1926. (SBH XV, 4.)

———, tr. *Śiva Saṃhitā.* Lahore, 1888. Repr. Allahabad, 1914. (SBH XV, 1.)

VASUBANDHU. *See* LA VALLÉE POUSSIN, LOUIS DE.

VATS, MADHO SARUP. *Excavations at Harappā.* Delhi, 1940. 2 vols.

VENKATA RAMANAYYA, N. *An Essay on the Origin of the South Indian Temple.* Madras, 1930.

VIDYĀBHŪṢAṆA, SATIS CHANDRA. *History of Indian Logic.* Calcutta, 1921.

———. "Sāṃkhya Philosophy in the Land of the Lamas," *JRASB*, n.s. III (1907), 571–78.

VIDYĀRATNA, TĀRĀNĀTHA, ed. *Kūlārṇava-tantra.* London, 1917. (TT V.)

———, ed. *Tantrābhidhāna, with Vījanighantu and Mudrānighaṇtu.* Calcutta, 1913. (TT I.)

VIDYĀRṆAVA, RAI BAHADUR ŚRĪŚA CHANDRA. *See* VASU, RAI BAHADUR ŚRĪŚA CHANDRA.

VIENNOT, ODETTE. *Le Culte de l'arbre dans l'Inde ancienne.* Paris, 1954.

VIJÑĀNABHIKṢU. *See* GARBE, RICHARD; JHĀ, GANGĀNĀTHA; ŚĀSTRI, RĀMAKṚSHṆA, and SINHA, NANDALAL.

VIRA, RAGHU, and TAKI, SHODO, eds. *Dakṣiṇāmūrti, Uddhārakoṣa. A Dictionary of the Secret Tantric Syllabic Code*. Lahore, 1938.

VISSER, MARINUS WILLEM DE. *Ancient Buddhism in Japan*. Paris, 1928–35. 2 vols.

———. *The Arhats in China and Japan*. Berlin, 1923.

VOGEL, JEAN PHILIPPE. *Indian Serpent-Lore; or, The Nāgas in Hindu Legend and Art*. London, 1926.

———. "Serpent Worship in Ancient and Modern India," *AO*, II (1924), 279–312.

———. "The Woman and Tree or *śālabhañjikā* in Indian Literature and Art," *AO*, VII (1929), 201–31.

VYĀSA. *See* JHĀ, GANGĀNĀTHA, and RĀMA PRASĀDA.

WADDELL, LAURENCE AUSTINE. *The Buddhism of Tibet; or, Lamaism*. London, 1895.

———. "The Dhāraṇī Cult in Buddhism, Its Origin, Deified Literature and Images," *OZ*, I (1912), 155–95.

———. " 'Dhāraṇī,' or Indian Buddhist Protective Spells," *IA*, XLIII (1914), 37–42, 49–54, 92–93.

———. "The Indian Buddhist Cult of Avalokita and His Consort Tārā 'the Saviouress,' " *JRAS* (1894), 51–89.

———. "Lamaism in Sikhim." In *The Gazetteer of Sikhim*, pp. 241–392. Calcutta, 1894.

WALEY, ARTHUR. "New Light on Buddhism in Medieval India," *MCB*, I (1931–32), 355–76.

———. "Notes on Chinese Alchemy," *BSOS*, VI, 1 (1930), 1–24.

———. "References to Alchemy in Buddhist Scriptures," *BSOS*, VI, 4 (1932), 1102–03.

———. *The Travels of an Alchemist: the Journey of the Taoist Ch'ang-ch'un from China to the Hindukush at the Summons of Chingiz Khan*. London, 1931.

———. *The Way and Its Power: a Study of the Tao Tê Ching and Its Place in Chinese Thought*. Boston and New York, 1942.

WALLESER, MAX. "The Life of Nāgārjuna from Tibetan and Chinese Sources." In Schindler, B., ed., *Hirth Anniversary Volume*, pp. 421–55. London, 1923.

WALTER, HERMANN, tr. "Svātmārāma's *Haṭhayogapradīpikā* (*Die Leuchte des Haṭhayoga*) aus dem Sanskrit übersetzt." Diss. Munich, 1893.

WARREN, HENRY CLARKE. *Buddhism in Translations.* Cambridge (Mass.), 1896. (HOS III.)

WASSILIEFF, W. *Der Buddhismus, seine Dogmen, Geschichte und Literatur.* St. Petersburg, 1860. (*Le Bouddhisme, ses dogmes, son histoire et sa littérature.* Paris, 1863.)

WATTERS, THOMAS. *On Yuan Chwang's Travels in India* A.D. *629–645,* ed. T. W. Rhys Davids and S. W. Bushell. London, 1904–05. 2 vols.

WAYMAN, ALEX. "Notes on the Sanskrit Term *Jñāna,*" *JAOS,* LXXV (1955), 253–68.

WELDEN, ELLWOOD AUSTIN. "I Metri delle *Sāṁkhya-Kārikās,*" *Studi italiani di filologia indo-iranica* (Florence), VIII, fasc. 3 (1912), Appendix.

———. "The Sāṁkhya Teachings in the *Maitrī Upaniṣad,*" *AJP,* XXXV (1914), 32–51.

WESTERMARCK, EDVARD ALEXANDER. *The History of Human Marriage.* London, 1891.

WHITEHEAD, HENRY. *The Village Gods of South India.* 2nd edn., rev. and enlarg. London, 1921. (The Religious Life of India.)

WIEGER, LÉON. *A History of the Religious Beliefs and Philosophical Opinions in China from the Beginning to the Present Time.* Ho-kien-fou, 1917. (*Histoire des croyances religieuses et des opinions philosophiques en Chine depuis l'origine, jusqu'à nos jours,* tr. E. C. Werner. 2nd edn., Hsien-hsien, 1927.)

WIKANDER, STIG. *Der arischer Männerbund.* Lund, 1938.

———. "La Légende des Pāṇḍava et la substructure mythique du *Mahābhārata,*" tr. and annotated in DUMÉZIL, GEORGES (q.v.), *Jupiter, Mars, Quirinus. IV,* pp. 37–53.

———. "Sur le fonds commun indo-iranien des épopées de la Perse et de l'Inde," *La Nouvelle Clio* (Brussels), I–II (1949–50), 310–29.

———. *Vāyu; Texte und Untersuchungen zur indo-iranischen Religionsgeschichte.* Uppsala, 1941.

WILHELM, HELLMUT. "Eine Chou-Inschrift über Atemtechnik," *MS,* XIII (1948), 385–88.

WILLS, CHARLES JAMES. *In the Land of the Lion and Sun, or Modern Persia.* London, 1891.

WILSON, HORACE HAYMAN, ed. and tr. *Sāṅkhya Kārikā . . . also the Bhāshya or Commentary of Gaurapāda* [*Gauḍapāda*]. Oxford, 1837.

WILSON, HORACE HAYMAN. *Sketch of the Religious Sects of the Hindus.* Calcutta, 1846. 2nd edn., London, 1861.

WINTERNITZ, MORIZ. *Geschichte der indischen Literatur.* Leipzig, 1905–22. 3 vols.

———. "Notes on the *Guhyasamāja-Tantra* and the Age of the Tantras," *IHQ*, IX, 1 (1933), 1–10.

———. "Der Sarpabali, ein altindischer Schlangencult," *MAGW*, XVIII (1888), 25–52.

———. *Some Problems of Indian Literature.* Calcutta, 1925.

———. "Die Vrātyas," *ZB*, VI (1924–25), 48–60, 311–12.

WOGIHARA, UNRAI, ed. *Asaṅga's Bodhisattva-bhūmi.* Leipzig, 1908.

WOODROFFE, SIR JOHN ("ARTHUR AVALON"), ed. *The Garland of Letters* (*Varnamālā*). Madras, 1922.

———. "Kuṇḍalinī Śakti," *Yoga* (Harburg-Wilhelmsburg), I (1931), 65–73.

———. *The Principles of Tantra.* London, 1914–16. 2 vols.

———. *The Serpent Power* (*Ṣaṭcakranirūpaṇa and Pādukāpañcaka*). 2nd edn., Madras, 1924. 3rd edn., Madras, 1931.

———. *Shakti and Shākta.* 3rd edn., Madras and London, 1929.

———. *Tantra of the Great Liberation* (*Mahānirvāṇa Tantra*). 2nd edn., Madras, 1927.

WOODS, JAMES HAUGHTON. "La Théorie de la connaissance dans le système du Yoga," *JA*, ser. XI, vol. IX (1917), 546 ff.; ser. XI, vol. XI (1918), 385–89.

———. "The *Yoga Sūtras* of Patañjali as Illustrated by the Comment Entitled 'The Jewel's Lustre,' or *Maṇiprabhā*," *JAOS*, XXXIV (1914), 1–114.

———. *The Yoga-System of Patañjali.* Cambridge (Mass.), 1914. (HOS XVII.)

WOODWARD, FRANK LEE. *Manual of a Mystic*, ed. C. A. F. Rhys Davids. London, 1916. (PTS VI.)

———. *See also* DAVIDS, C. A. F. RHYS.

WRIGHT, ARTHUR FREDERICK. "Fo-T'u-Têng. A Biography," *HJAS*, XI (1948), 321–70.

WRIGHT, DANIEL. *History of Nepāl.* Cambridge, 1877.

WU, LU-CH'IANG. *See* DAVIS, TENNEY L.

WULFF, KURT, ed. *Sang hyang kamahāyānam mantrānaya.* Copenhagen, 1935.

YI-TSING. *See* CHAVANNES, ÉDOUARD.

YUEN, H. B. *See* BARNES, WILLIAM H.

YULE, SIR HENRY. *The Book of Ser Marco Polo*, ed. Henri Cordier. 3rd edn., London, 1903. 2 vols.

ZIMMER, HEINRICH. *Kunstform und Yoga im indischen Kultbild.* Berlin, 1926.

———. "Lehren des Haṭhayoga, Lehrtexte," *Yoga* (Harburg-Wilhelmsburg), I (1931), 45–62.

———. *Myths and Symbols in Indian Art and Civilization*, ed. Joseph Campbell. New York, 1946. (BS VI.)

———. *Philosophies of India*, ed. Joseph Campbell. New York, 1951. (BS XXVI.)

* ———. "Zur Bedeutung des indischen Tantra-Yoga," *EJ*, I (1933), 9–94.

NEW TRANSLATIONS

The following translations, available since the first edition, are cited in this edition.

ELIADE, MIRCEA. *Le Chamanisme . . . = Shamanism: Archaic Techniques of Ecstasy*, tr. Willard R. Trask. New York and London, 1964. (BS LXXVI.)

———. *Forgerons et alchimistes = The Forge and the Crucible*, tr. Stephen Corrin. London and New York, 1962.

———. *Images et symboles = Images and Symbols: Studies in Religious Symbolism*, tr. Philip Mairet. New York and London, 1961.

———. *Le Mythe . . . = The Myth of the Eternal Return*, tr. Willard R. Trask. New York and London, 1954; reprinted 1965. (BS XLVI.) Also published as *Cosmos and History: The Myth of the Eternal Return* (Torchbooks paperback), New York, 1960.

———. "La Nostalgie du paradis . ." = "Nostalgia for Paradise in the Primitive Traditions," in *Myths, Dreams and Mysteries*, tr. Philip Mairet. London, 1960, New York, 1961 (pp. 59–72.)

———. *Traité d'histoire . . . = Patterns in Comparative Religion*, tr. Rosemary Sheed. London and New York, 1958.

ZIMMER, HEINRICH. "Zur Bedeutung . . ." = "On the Significance of the Indian Tantric Yoga," tr. Ralph Manheim, in *Spiritual Disciplines.* (Papers from the Eranos Yearbooks, 4.) New York and London, 1960. (BS XXX 4.)

INDEX

INDEX

C

F

G

H

J

M

N

O

W

Y

Index by Bart Winer

ADDENDA TO THE SECOND EDITION

ADDENDA

[The following bibliographical additions are keyed to the text and the Additional Notes at the points where asterisks occur. An index of authors is provided at the end. See also p. 480.]

(A) p. 9 and Note I, 2: J. W. Hauer, *Der Yoga. Ein indischer Weg zum Selbst* (Stuttgart, 1958) (see also review of Hauer's work by Paul Hacker, in *Orientalistische Literaturzeitung* No. 9–10 (1960), cols. 521–28); Jean Filliozat, "La Nature du Yoga dans sa tradition," in Thérèse Brosse, *Études Instrumentales des techniques du Yoga* (Publications de l'École Française d'Extrême-Orient, LII; Paris, 1963), pp. i–xxviii; Hellmut Ritter, "al-Bīrūnī's Übersetzung des Yoga-Sūtra des Patañjali," *Oriens* (Leiden), IX, 2 (1956), 165–200; Shlomo Pines and Tuvia Gelblum, "al-Bīrūnī's Arabic Version of Patañjali's *Yogasūtra:* a Translation of His First Chapter and a Comparison with Related Sanskrit Texts," *BSOS*, XXIX (1966), 302–325.

(B) pp. 47 ff.: A. Janáček, "The 'Voluntaristic' Type of Yoga in Patañjali's *Yoga-Sūtras*," *Archiv Orientální*, XXII (1954), 69–87.

(C) pp. 62–63 and 216 and Note VI, 6: G. C. Anawati and Louis Gardet, *Mystique musulmane* (Paris, 1961), pp. 187–89, 193–233, 238–55.

(D) pp. 63–65: W. Nölle, "Hesychasmus und Yoga," *Byzantinische Zeitschrift* (Leipzig), XLVII (1954), 95–103; E. von Ivanka, "Byzantinische Yogis?," *ZDMG*, LII, pp. 234–39. Jean-Marie Déchanet, *Yoga chrétien en dix leçons* (Paris, 1964).

(E) pp. 66 ff.: Gerhard Oberhammer, "Meditation und Mystik im Yoga des Patañjali," *Wiener Zeitschrift für die Kunde Süd- und Ostasiens*, IX (1965), 98–118.

(F) pp. 106 ff.: Chauncey Justus Blair, *Heat in the Rig Veda and Atharva Veda* (American Oriental Series, XLV; New Haven, 1961).

(G) pp. 107 ff.: Jan Gonda, *Change and Continuity in Indian Religion* (The Hague, 1965), pp. 315–462.

(H) pp. 124 ff.: Anton Zigmund-Cerbu, "The Ṣaḍaṅgayoga," *History of Religions* (Chicago), III, 2 (Summer, 1963), 128–34.

(I) pp. 200 ff. and Note VI, 1: Agehananda Bharati, *The Tantric Tradition* (London, 1965), with extensive bibliography, pp. 303–36; Chintaharan

Chakravarti, *Tantras; Studies on Their Religion and Literature* (Calcutta, 1963); Jan Gonda, *Die Religionen Indiens*, II: *Der jungëre Hinduismus* (Stuttgart, 1963), pp. 26–52; Kees W. Bolle, *The Persistence of Religion* (Leiden, 1965), especially pp. 1–78; Hakuyn Hadanu, "A Historical Study in the Problems Concerning the Diffusion of Tantric Buddhism in India," in *Religious Studies in Japan* (Tokyo, 1959), pp. 287–99; Herbert V. Guenther, *The Jewel Ornament of Liberation* (London, 1959); id., *Yuganaddha—The Tantric View of Life* (Chowkhamba Sanskrit Series, 2nd edn.; Varanasi, 1964); id., *The Life and Teachings of Naropa*, translated from the original Tibetan with a philosophical commentary based on the oral transmission (Oxford, 1963); D. L. Snellgrove, *Buddhist Himālaya* (Oxford, 1957), especially pp. 51–90, 202–11; id., *The Hevajra Tantra* (2 vols., London, 1959); Alex Wayman, "The Five-fold Ritual Symbolism of Passion," in *Studies of Esoteric Buddhism and Tantrism* (Koyasan, 1965), pp. 117–44; S. K. Chatterji, "Tantra and Brahmanical Hinduism," ibid., 145–66; E. Dale Saunders, "Some Tantric Techniques," ibid., 167–77; K. W. Bolle, "Devotion and Tantra," ibid., 217–28; André Padoux, *Recherches sur la symbolique et l'énergie de la parole dans certains textes tantriques* (Paris, 1963); *Le Vijñānabhairava*, text translated and edited by Lilian Silburn (Paris, 1961); *Le Paramārthasāra d'Abhinavagupta*, translated by L. Silburn (Paris, 1957); *Abhinavagupta, Essenza dei Tantra* (*Tantrasāra*), translated by Raniero Gnoli (Turin, 1960); L. Silburn, "Techniques de la transmission mystique dans le Shivaisme du Cachemire," *Hermes* (Paris), IV (1966–67), 158–75.

(J) pp. 212 ff.: J. Gonda, "The Indian Mantra," *Oriens* (Leiden), XVI (1963), 244–97.

(K) pp. 219 ff. and Note VI, 7: Erik Haarh, "Contributions to the Study of Maṇḍala and Mudrā," *AO*, XXIII (1958), 57–91; Johannes Schubert, "Das Reis-Maṇḍala," *Asiatica, Festschrift F. Weller* (Leipzig, 1954), 584 ff.; Ariane Macdonald, *Le Maṇḍala du Mañjuśrimūlakalpa* (Paris, 1962).

(L) pp. 221 ff. and Note VI, 7: Helmut Hoffmann, "Literarhistorische Bemerkungen zur *Sekoddeśaṭīka des Nādapāda*," *Beitrage zur Indischen Philologie und Altertumskunde* (Hamburg), VII (1951), 140–47.

(M) pp. 221 ff.: Gonda, op. cit. in (G), pp. 435–47; Agehananda Bharati, op. cit. in (I), pp. 185–98.

(N) pp. 245 ff.: E. D. Saunders, "A Note on Śakti and Dhyānibuddha," *History of Religions*, I, 2 (Winter, 1962), 300–306; Gerbrand Dekker, "Der Kuṇḍalinî-Yoga," *Asiatische Studien* (Bern), IX (1955), 45 ff. Bharati, op. cit., pp. 261 ff.

(O) pp. 249 ff. and Note VI, 10: Bharati, op. cit. in (I), pp. 164–84.

(P) pp. 254 ff. and Note VI, 11 and 12: Bharati, op. cit., pp. 244 ff.; A. Wayman, "Female Energy and Symbolism in the Buddhist Tantras," *History of Religions*, II, 1 (Summer, 1962), 73–111; Bharati, "Śakta and Vajrayana, Their Place in Indian Thought," in *Studies of Esoteric Buddhism and Tantrism* (Koyasan, 1965), 73–99.

(Q) pp. 264 ff.: Edward C. Dimock, *The Place of the Hidden Moon, Erotic Mysticism in the Vaiṣṇavasahajiya Cult of Bengal* (Chicago, 1966), especially pp. 166 ff., 222 ff., 241 ff.

(R) pp. 301 ff. and Note VIII, 3: Toni Schmidt, *The Eighty-Five Siddhas* (Stockholm, 1958).

(S) pp. 353 ff. and Note VIII, 11: Herbert P. Sullivan, "A Re-examination of the Religion of the Indus Civilization," *History of Religions*, IV, 1 (Summer, 1964), 115–25; Mario Cappieri, "Ist die Indus-Kultur und ihre Bevölkerung wirklich verschwunden?" *Anthropos* (Salzburg), LX (1965), 719–62; J. Gonda, op. cit. in (G), pp. 7–37.

(T) Note IV, 5: J.A.B. van Buitenen, "The Name 'Pañcarātra,' " *History of Religions*, I, 2 (Winter, 1962), 291–99.

(U) Note VI, 1 and 7: P. H. Pott, *Yoga en Yantra*: Rodney Needham, tr., *Yoga and Yantra: Their Interrelation and Their Significance for Indian Archaeology* (The Hague, 1966).

(V) Note VI, 3: Robert H. B. Williams, *Jaina Yoga: A Survey of the Mediaeval Śravakācāra* (London, 1963).

(W) Note VI, 4: E. Dale Saunders, *Mudrā: A Study of Symbolic Gestures in Japanese Buddhist Sculpture* (New York, 1960). (BS LVIII).

(X) Note VI, 8: Thérèse Brosse, op. cit. in (A); Jean Bruno, "Yoga et training autogène," *Critique* (Paris), No. 159–60 (August-September, 1960), 781–807.

(Y) Note VI, 12: R. H. van Gulik, *Sexual Life in Ancient China* (Leiden, 1961).

(Z) Note IX, 1: Li An-Che, "The Bkah-Brgyud Sect of Lamaism," *JAOS*, LXIX (April–June, 1949), 51–59; Ch'êng-chi Chang, *Teachings of Tibetan Yoga* (New York, 1963).

INDEX TO THE ADDENDA